To

Versra Atkuss, M.D.

with warmest regards,

[signature]

8. 1. 10

Oxygen and Aging

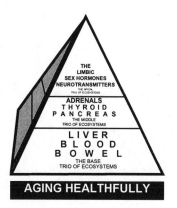

THE
LIMBIC
SEX HORMONES
NEUROTRANSMITTERS
THE APICAL
TRIO OF ECOSYSTEMS

ADRENALS
THYROID
PANCREAS
THE MIDDLE
TRIO OF ECOSYSTEMS

LIVER
BLOOD
BOWEL
THE BASE
TRIO OF ECOSYSTEMS

AGING HEALTHFULLY

Oxygen and Aging
©Majid Ali, 2000
All Rights Reserved

Library of Congress Catalog Card Number
On file
ISBN 1-879131-21-8

Ali, Majid
Oxygen and Aging
Majid Ali.--1st ed.

Includes bibliographical references and index
     1. Oxygen
     2. Aging
     3. Dysfunctional oxygen metabolism
     4. Dysoxygenosis
     5. Darwin and dysoxygenosis
     6. Oxidosis
     7. Oxygen: the molecular Dr. Jekyll/Mr. Hyde
     8. Primordial life forms
     9. Microbial pleomorphism
     10. Spiritual surrender for restoring oxygen metabolism

10 9 8 7 6 5 4 3 2 1

Oxygen and Aging
by
Majid Ali, M.D.

- President and Professor of Medicine, Capital University of Integrative Medicine, Washington, D.C.
- Former, Associate Professor of Pathology, College of Physicians and Surgeons of Columbia University, New York
- Editor, *The Journal of Integrative Medicine*
- President, Institute of Integrative Medicine, New York, New York, and Denville, New Jersey
- Former, President of Staff and Chief Pathologist, Holy Name Hospital, Teaneck, New Jersey
- Fellow, Royal College of Surgeons of England
- Diplomate, American Boards of Anatomic and Clinical Pathology
- Diplomate, American Board of Environmental Medicine

Aging Healthfully, Inc., New York
www.aginghealthfully.com

The trilogy of
dysfunctional oxygen metabolism:

1. Oxygen and Aging
2. Oxygen and the Hurt Children of a Hurt Earth
3. Oxygen and Fibromyalgia

From the author of:

- The Canary and Chronic Fatigue
- The Cortical Monkey and Healing
- The Ghoraa and Limbic Exercise
- The Butterfly and Life Span Nutrition
- RDA: Rats, Drugs and Assumptions
- What Do Lions Know About Stress
- Healing, Miracles and The Bite of the Gray Dog
- Integrative Allergy
- Pathology of Maintenance Dialysis (With Alfred Fayemi, M.D.)
- Surgical Pathology (With Alfred Fayemi, M.D. and Evalynne Braun, M.D.)
- Pathology Review Books 1974, 1975, 1976, 1977, 1978, 1979, 1980, 1981, 1982, 1983, and 1984 (with Alfred Fayemi, M.D., and others.)
- Curriculum of Department of Integrative Medicine, Capital University of Integrative Medicine

Acknowledgements

I am much indebted to the medical, nursing and administrative staffs of the Institute of Integrative Medicine for creating and sustaining an environment in which I can freely pursue my clinical work.

I am grateful to Jerrold and Dolores Finnie and Amy Lang for reviewing the manuscript and making valuable suggestions. I thank Barry Weiner for his sketches of the title pages for the book chapters as well as for helping me with the organization of this book.

Talat, my wife, continues to be my most treasured resource.

This book is about a simple idea:

Oxygen is the organizing influence of human biology and governs the aging process.

Deoxygenation of our air, water, and tissues of living beings is a growing global threat.

In the context of aging, the profound irony of our time is this: Intoxicated by the promises of Star Wars medicine, we blindly celebrate the possibilities of the future while ignoring the fact that our children are prematurely sickening and aging before our very eyes due to sugar overload, antibiotic abuse, poisoning by synthetic chemicals and hormones, and the anger that inevitably results when one discovers he has been the victim of the folly of others.

Rudolph Virchow, the German Pathologist and author of *Cellular Pathology* (1858), is rightfully considered the father of pathology. He wrote, "No matter how we twist and turn, we shall eventually come back to the cell." Fully in awe of Virchow's contribution to medicine, I take the liberty to paraphrase him thusly:

No matter how we twist and turn, we shall eventually come back to oxygen.

HUMAN CANARIES

Persons living with chronic fatigue, fibromyalgia, hyperactivity, chemical sensitivity syndrome, and other related "mystery" maladies are human canaries. They are sensitive and vulnerable. Their cells and tissues are injured by too much oxidation and too little oxygen. Their basic problem is *dysfunctional* oxygen metabolism.

In olden days, miners carried caged canaries deep into their mine shafts. The birds served as an early-warning intelligence system. When there were poisonous gases in the shaft, the birds collapsed or died, thus warning the miners to escape death by rushing out.

Human canaries are more prone to sugar overload, antibiotic abuse, metabolic poisons, pesticides, environmental toxins, and synthetic hormones. Their food sensitivities and allergic reactions go unrecognized.

They suffer many indignities at the hands of their ill-informed doctors. Their pain turns into anger, and so often their anger turns into depression. Each of the preceding factors threatens their oxygen metabolism.

Human canaries tell all of us something about the shape of things to come. No one is immune to what poisons them. It is merely a matter of time. As poisons accumulate to paralyze oxygen metabolism, everyone can be expected to become a canary. This is not a doomsday prophecy. In my travels from Beijing to Bangkok, from Moscow to Nairobi, from Oslo to the Honduras, I have seen human canaries of all colors, of all shapes, and of all ages. Everywhere I went, I saw human canaries in increasing numbers. *This book is a wake-up call about the pandemic of dysfunctional oxygen metabolism.*

A Scientist Has No Paradigm.

He has but one allegiance—to the truth in his observations. We begin to grow when we learn to observe. A theory may be proposed only to explain observations. *One must observe first.* I write this book to present my clinical and experimental observations about the oxygen order of human biology and how violation of that order leads to dysfunctional oxygen metabolism and premature aging.

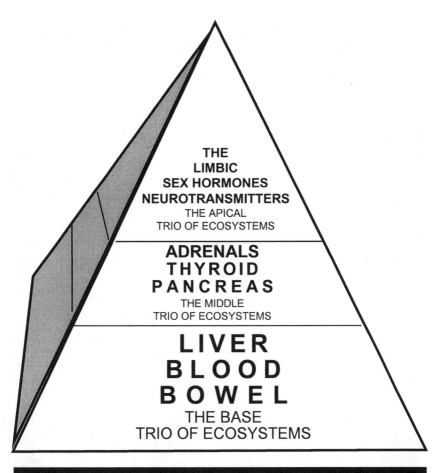

THE
LIMBIC
SEX HORMONES
NEUROTRANSMITTERS
THE APICAL
TRIO OF ECOSYSTEMS

ADRENALS
THYROID
PANCREAS
THE MIDDLE
TRIO OF ECOSYSTEMS

LIVER
BLOOD
BOWEL
THE BASE
TRIO OF ECOSYSTEMS

AGING HEALTHFULLY

The Pyramid
of the Trio of Trios of Human Ecosystems

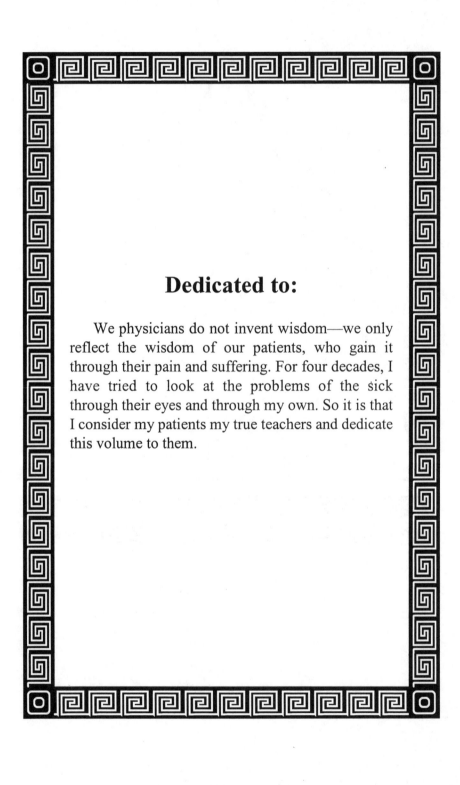

Dedicated to:

We physicians do not invent wisdom—we only reflect the wisdom of our patients, who gain it through their pain and suffering. For four decades, I have tried to look at the problems of the sick through their eyes and through my own. So it is that I consider my patients my true teachers and dedicate this volume to them.

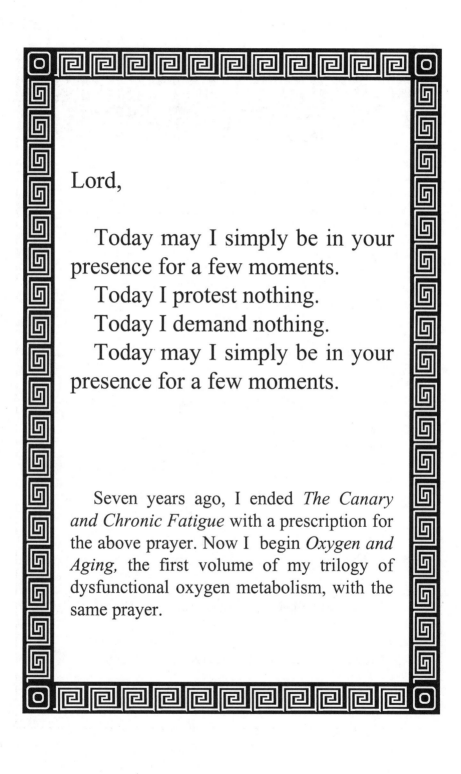

Lord,

Today may I simply be in your presence for a few moments.
Today I protest nothing.
Today I demand nothing.
Today may I simply be in your presence for a few moments.

Seven years ago, I ended *The Canary and Chronic Fatigue* with a prescription for the above prayer. Now I begin *Oxygen and Aging,* the first volume of my trilogy of dysfunctional oxygen metabolism, with the same prayer.

Table of Contents

Table of Contents

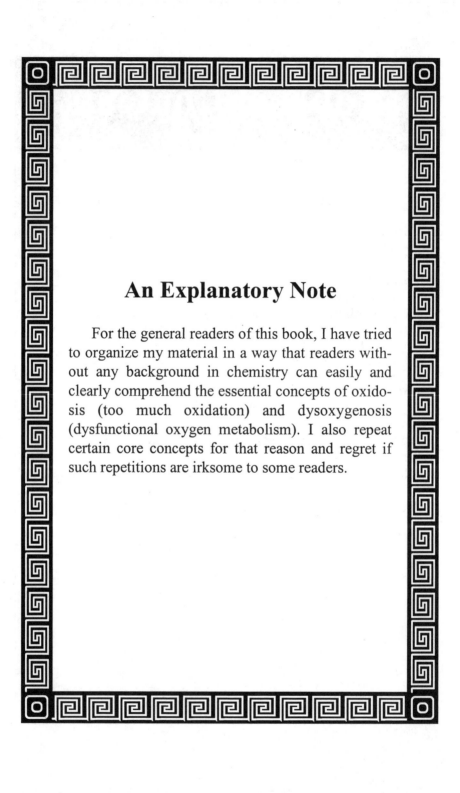

An Explanatory Note

For the general readers of this book, I have tried to organize my material in a way that readers without any background in chemistry can easily and clearly comprehend the essential concepts of oxidosis (too much oxidation) and dysoxygenosis (dysfunctional oxygen metabolism). I also repeat certain core concepts for that reason and regret if such repetitions are irksome to some readers.

Preface

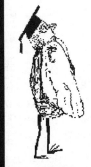

PREFACE

This book is about a simple idea: Oxygen is *the* organizing influence of human biology and governs the aging process.

From that idea I develop two other dominant themes of this book. First, *dysfunctional oxygen metabolism* (dysoxygenosis) is the *primary* mechanism of cellular aging and will be the single most important threat to the human life span in the coming decades. Second, a growing understanding of relationships among man's internal and external environments will govern *all* our plans for preserving health and reversing disease.

Those simple ideas form the core of my oxygen theory of aging.[1-4] But why shouldn't the aging-genes be on the center stage?, some readers might ask. Why not focus on antioxidants?, some others might ask. Should not those factors form the core of any theory of aging? My view is that neither genes nor antioxidants can work well in the presence of dysfunctional oxygen metabolism. I marshal several lines of evidence to support my view.

This book is not about low-fat diets for living longer. The Japanese eat a very low-fat diet and live longer than people in any other country of the world. The Swiss have a very high-fat diet and longer lifespan than any other people except the Japanese. So much for the low-fat and high-fat enthusiasts.

Neither is this book about taking cholesterol-lowering drugs to extend life. Cholesterol is an antioxidant. Coronary heart disease is caused by oxidative injury. Blaming healthy (unrancid, unoxidized) cholesterol for heart disease is as silly as blaming water for illness. Yes, excess rancid cholesterol threatens health just as drinking polluted water does, but the problem is rancidity of cholesterol as it is pollution in water. Nearly all trials of cholesterol-lowering drugs show a reduction in the *rate* of heart attacks of less than one percent. That means more than 990 of every 1,000 persons who take such drugs get no benefits at all. It is important to point out that *all* cholesterol-lowering drugs carry a risk of causing cancer, liver disease, chronic fatigue, and other problems. In 1997, for professional readers, my colleague, Omar Ali, and I discussed this subject at length in *The Journal of Integrative Medicine.*[1]

The true story of drug therapies for high blood pressure to prolong life is the same. A large number of recent studies clearly show that most people who were administered drugs for high blood pressure for years did not benefit from those therapies. There is broad consensus now that what was considered "mild" hypertension does not increase the risk of heart attacks, stroke, and kidney disease. Even the staunchest supporters of the use of drugs for mild hypertension now agree that millions of persons have been needlessly given drugs for decades. Indeed, over 95% of persons who are diagnosed with the so-called mild hypertension respond well to water therapy, meditation, optimal choices in the kitchen, and gentle, non-goal-oriented exercise.

This book is not about gene therapies for increasing longevity. I predict that gene therapies *will not* extend human life span. For several years now, the gene researchers have been intoxicated with the promise of extending life span and of miraculous cures with gene therapies of diseases by the bundle. I have believed for an equally long number of years that gene therapy will have limited benefits for a very small number of people with rare genetic disorders, but *only* if the oxygen metabolism of those persons can be preserved by natural supportive therapies. The principal reason for my belief is that the *language of genes* is far more complex than, say, the English language with its mere 26 letter-alphabet. There are an estimated

100,000 genes in the human genome and, in my view, this is likely to prove to be a gross underestimate. Beyond the simple matter of a 26-letter alphabet versus 100,000 genes is the far more important issue of genes reading and responding to their microenvironment, something that letters in words cannot do. Genes not only change their behavior in response to environment, but also alter the behavior of other genes. Of course, the environment also changes the structure of genes. In this volume I present my view that the *oxygen order of human biology profoundly affects the function of genes, and we will succeed with gene therapies only to the degree that we can preserve oxygen metabolism of the recipient of such therapies.* The claim of living longer by taking out the faulty genes and replacing them with new ones is pure Alice-in-Wonderland.

The use of drug therapies, though necessary for acute illness, is essentially blockade medicine. *All* commonly used drugs block essential cellular channels, receptors, enzymes, pumps, and mediators of the healing response. It is frivolous to think that the human lifespan can be prolonged by blocking essential cell functions. It is possible that some drugs may offer limited benefits to some people, but *only* as long as the fundamental oxygen order of human biology can be preserved. One simple but telling argument for my view is this: In the United States, more money is spent on health care than in any other country in the world and yet the life expectancy rate here is among the lowest in developed countries.

This is not an "anti-aging" book. I am much amused by the enthusiasm of the gurus of the anti-aging industry. Some of them have declared aging to be a *disease*, treatable with their favored products they sell. When I listen to them or read what they write, I wonder if *they* understand their stuff. I do not. I have never seen a spoiled peach become unspoiled, a rotten egg turn unrotten, or decomposed grass become undecomposed. Nor have I seen any anti-aging guru to "un-age" himself. I eagerly await the time that some 60-year-old expert will become 45 years old. I continue to search for any *reasonable* basis for their excitement. So far, what I have seen is nothing but misleading claims similar to those of merchants of cholesterol-lowering drugs.

This book is not about anti-aging hormones either. Many anti-aging gurus are full of ideas for prescriptions of anti-aging hormones. It is evidently true that natural hormones are essential for *healthful aging*. But there is a big difference between studying changes in the hormone levels as we advance in age and claims of the ability of hormones to anti-age people. Anti-aging gurus do not conduct any of their own studies. They fondly cite studies conducted by others with mice or medical students *for weeks or months*. Their game is to sell their products by promises of extended lifespan for decades, no matter how irrelevant the studies they cite are to their merchandise.

A scientist has no paradigm. He has but one allegiance —to the truth in his observations. We begin to grow when we learn to observe. A theory may be proposed only to explain observations. *One must observe first*. I write this book to present my clinical and experimental observations about the oxygen order of human biology and how violation of that order leads to dysfunctional oxygen metabolism. For the advanced and professional readers, I published my observations in a series of articles.[2-14] My guidelines for healthful aging are based on those observations made during the last four decades. The oxygen theory of aging I propose in this book is my attempt to shed some light on the mechanisms that underlie my observations.

Majid Ali, M.D.
New York
April 24, 2000

References

1.   Ali M. Spontaneity of Oxidation in Nature And Aging. Monograph. 1983. Teaneck, New Jersey.

2.   Ali M. Spontaneity of Oxidation in Nature Is the true cause of Aging in Humans and Root Cause of All Disease. page 199-304, RDA: Rats, Drugs and Assumption. 1995. Life Span Press, Denville, New Jersey.

3.   Ali M. Lifespan Molecules. The Cortical Monkey and Healing. page 18, 1990. Institute of Preventive Medicine, Bloomfield, New Jersey.

4.   Ali M, Ali O. AA oxidopathy: the core pathogenetic mechanism of ischemic heart disease. J Integrative Medicine 1997;1:1-112.

5.   Ali M. Oxidative coagulopathy in fibromyalgia and chronic fatigue syndrome. Am J Clin Pathol 1999; 112:566-7.

6.   Ali M. The basic equation of life. The Butterfly and Life Span Nutrition. 1992. The Institute of Preventive Medicine Press, Denville, New Jersey, pp 225-236.

7.   Ali M. Oxidative theory of cell membrane and plasma damage. RDA: Rats, Drugs and Assumptions. pp 281-302, 1995. Life Span, Denville, New Jersey.

8.   Ali M. Adrenergic hypervigilence. What Do Lions Know About Stress? pp 137-172, 1996. Life Span Press, Denville, New Jersey, .

9.   Ali M. Oxidative regression to primordial cellular ecology (ORPEC): evidence for the hypothesis and its clinical significance. J Integrative Medicine 1988;2:4-55.

10.   Ali M. Amenorrhea, oligomenorrhea, and polymenorrhea in CFS and fibromyalgia are caused by oxidative menstrual dysfunction. J Integrative Medicine 1998;3:101-124.

11.   Ali, M. Oxidative menopausal dysfunction (OMD-II): hormone replacement therapy (HRT) or receptor restoration therapy (RRT)? J Integrative Medicine 1998;3:125-139.

12.   Ali M. Ali O. Fibromyalgia: an oxidative-dysoxygenative disorder (ODD) J Integrative Medicine 1999;1:17-37.

13   Ali M. Darwin, oxidosis, dysoxygenosis, and integration. J Integrative Medicine 1999;1:11-16.

14.   Ali M. The oxidative-dysoxygenative perspective of allergic disorders. J Integrative Medicine 2000;4:15-24.

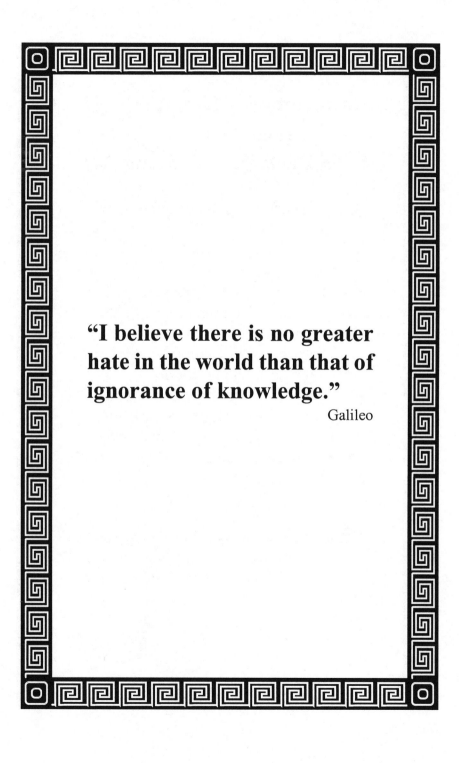

"I believe there is no greater hate in the world than that of ignorance of knowledge."

Galileo

Restoration of Dysfunctional Oxygen Metabolism Is an Ecologic Balancing Act

It's not about eradication of this virus nor
    that virus;
Nor about this mycoplasma nor
    that mycoplasma;
Nor about this yeast nor that yeast;
Nor about this bacterium nor
    that bacterium;
Nor about this parasite nor that parasite;
Nor about this drug nor that drug;
Nor about this vitamin nor that vitamin;
Nor about this mineral nor that mineral;
Nor about this enzyme nor that enzyme;
Nor about this toxic metal nor
    that toxic metal.

Human canaries need to look at their bodies, not as houses of disease to be filled with drugs, but as divine gardens to be nurtured holistically and spiritually.

Chapter 1

The
False
Promise

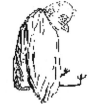

Today is the first day of the new year. My wife, Talat, and I returned from Greece yesterday afternoon and stayed up late last night watching CNN cover the New Year celebrations from New Zealand to New York. Oh, what a global party! What a view of the good life! Humankind wore a face I had never seen before. The excitement was immense and infectious—both for the stunning achievements of the past as well as for the predictions for the future that stretched credibility. What a feeling to be human on a day like that!

As I write this chapter, I hear two celebrated futurists on CNN share their great visions of the future. One of them holds an adopted Chinese baby in her arms and her face glows with joy. "She will live to be 115. All her needs will be met," she beams, then goes on to salute medical science and the projected miracles of gene therapy. The second futurist chimes in, "She will retire at age 29." Next, he goes on to wonder wistfully what else she might want to do with her life. It is easy to overlook the enthusiasm of the CNN futurists. They are not biologists. I recalled the words of a physicist-friend, "Medicine advances by trial and error. So far, gene therapies have only killed people. But I see a brilliant future. Don't you?" he asked. I shrugged but did not explain why I do not share his enthusiasm about gene therapy extending human life span to 115.

OF LIVING MARBLE AND DYING FROGS

The day before yesterday in Athens, Talat and I stood before the massive gleaming marble columns of the Parthenon, mesmerized by the temple's majesty. The remaining columns of Athena's temple are as alive today as when built over 2,500 years ago by the Greek goddess' cult. Some days earlier, in Istanbul I had read a short piece about red-legged frogs that have not been seen in Calveras County, California, for several decades. It had struck me odd then that *Turkish Daily News* was curious about why Mark Twain's frogs had disappeared without leaving any clues to their demise. My thoughts drifted from how much the ancients knew about the life span of marble to how little we know about the life span of frogs.

Of course, we humans are not the only victims of dysfunctional oxygen metabolism. We can learn much about oxygen metabolism by examining how excessive oxidation and dysfunctional oxygen metabolism cause disease and death in the animal kingdom. To underscore that point and to further illustrate my theme, I also explore disturbances in oxygen dynamics in the large bodies of waters and consequences of oxidosis suffered by many forms of life in fresh waters as well as in coastal waters, bays, and open seas. Below, I include some text from one of my articles published in *The Journal of Integrative Medicine*[1] to show that we can learn much about dysfunctional oxygen metabolism from disappearing frogs, shrimp, oysters, and other living beings.

> What do alpine meadows of Yosemite National Park, piney woods of South Carolina, and plains of Laramie, Wyoming, have in common? Answer: The warm summers there are unusually hushed. The reason for this is that the frog population in those areas—and many others in the world—has been decimated. By some estimates, up to a third of the nation's amphibians—frogs, toads, and salamanders—have disappeared. In 1988, in Costa Rica on a Monteverde ridge, half of the 40 amphibian species simply vanished. Some wags have speculated that

those amphibians were stolen by aliens—a global whodunit!

In Chesapeake Bay, during some summers, nearly *all* Eastern oysters are parasitized by dermo. Up to one-half of the total population succumbs. Similarly, grass shrimp suffer from heavy parasitic infestation. In Alaska, ten years after one of the largest oil spills in history, the Valdez accident, species which have failed to recover include the common loon, cormorant, harbor seal, harlequin duck, and pigeon guillemot.

Marine biologists report "mass mortalities" among plants and aquatic life forms. Consider the following quote from a recent issue of *Science*[2]:

In the past few decades, there has been a worldwide increase in reports of diseases affecting marine organisms. In the Caribbean, mass mortalities among plants, invertebrates, and vertebrates have resulted in dramatic shifts in community structure. Recent outbreaks of coralline algae lethal orange disease have affected Indo-Pacific communities on unprecedented scale.

The CNN futurists did not seem to know any of that. None of them so far this morning have broached the subject of dying frogs and vanishing marine life forms. Who wants to be a skunk in a garden party?

Did the CNN futurist who predicted a 115-year life span for her adopted daughter ever bother to *study* human genetics? Did the second futurist who foretold her retirement at age 29 ever bother to talk to millions of children all over the world whose lives have been severely diminished by chronic fatigue syndrome, fibromyalgia, and chemical sensitivity syndrome? I have seen hundreds of young people who were *disabled* by age 29, not retired by that age! Their active lives are truncated by excessive oxidation—a process of loss of energy through loss of electrons.

FROM GENOMICS TO PROTEOMICS

Gene researchers have spent billions of dollars of tax money and are coming close to mapping out the full human genome (gene structure). They have little, if anything, to show for all that money. Gene therapies simply have not helped the sick to date. Their claims to the contrary are superficial, deceptive, or both. Now they are changing the party line. Now the buzz word is *proteomics*. They want many more billions of dollars for mapping out all the proteins of cells. In its December 16, 1999, issue, *Nature* ran two remarkable editorials. Both pieces are very relevant to my subject of oxygen and aging. Consider the two headings and two direct quotes from the texts:

Gene Therapy for the Public[3]

The case of Jesse Gelsinger, whose death during a gene-therapy trial led to last week's hearing, reveals how poorly understood are the body's responses to those vectors [viruses that carry genes] in particular. But the uncertainties and violations revealed by the hearing should not halt pursuit of the adenovirus approach.

The Promise of Proteomics[4]

Analyzing the entire set of proteins of an organism is a far bigger challenge than anything in genomics...The inside of a cell is a crowded and dynamic place, where proteins are perpetually being created and discarded...Indeed, there is no such thing as proteomics—it will differ significantly not only between individuals (much more than do their genome), but also within one individual before and after, say, a millennium party.

Later, it was reported that "hundreds of gene-therapy deaths had gone unreported." A doctor on TV tried to defend such deaths by claiming that the persons who had received such therapies had no options. Was that really true? Had any of those patients been given vigorous oxygenative and nutrient therapies before deciding that there were no other options? My problem here is not that geneticists are twisting our arms for hundreds of billions of additional dollars of our tax money. My frustration is that they do not allow integrative physicians to apply for minimal grants of several thousand dollars to study the oxygen order of human life and how inexpensive oxygenative therapies outlined in this book can help hundreds of millions of people with chronic disorders. In their ignorance, they dismiss all such research as "unscientific."

A PREDICTION:
Gene Therapies Will Not Increase the Human Lifespan

It is generally believed that the structure of human DNA (genome) will be completely mapped out by 2002, and that such knowledge will open the way for genetic repair of damaged brain cells, weakened heart muscle, injured liver tissue, and bad backs. I hear of gene cures for cancer. Indeed, I often hear some geneticists exult that soon they will begin to toss out nonfunctioning body parts and insert genetically engineered new ones, just as car mechanics do now. I am much amused by such predictions. Nature did not build the human frame quite the same way carmakers makers build their machines.

I do agree that genes set the limits on the life span for an individual. But I strongly disagree with those who think gene therapies will soon let everyone live to the ripe old age of 115 years or more. I will make a clear prediction here: Gene therapies for extending human life span, whenever such therapies become available, will contribute to longevity and healthful aging only if oxygen metabolism can be maintained within the healthy range. As long as we continue to violate the oxygen metabolism of our children and young, no gene therapies will be able to correct their dysfunctional oxygen metabolism.

In the context of the dysoxygenosis theory of aging, there are two essential points:

1.   Within the limits set by genes, the lifespan of an individual is governed by oxygen metabolism.

2.   Genes function well only when oxygen metabolism is normal.

MUTANT MICE AND LIFE SPAN GENES

This is a time of great expectations in the world of genetics. Every week in my copies of *Nature* and *Science*, I read about fascinating discoveries of new genes and new behaviors of old genes. A paper by Italian researchers in the November 18, 1999, issue of *Nature*[5] reported that mutant mice live longer than mice in the wild. A longer life in mutant worms, yeast, and fruit flies was reported earlier. What distinguished the Italian report is that it was the very first time that life extension by a gene ($p66^{shc}$) modification was demonstrated in a mammal, hitting close to home for us humans. Heady times for geneticists!

Are there other things we should know about gene research? Did the yeast, worm, and fruit fly pay a price for their longer lives? Of course, they did, in smaller size and loss of fertility. Did the mutant Italian mice pay a price? Of course, they did, in abnormal lung tissue. Would such mice have reduced fertility? Most likely, yes. Are there likely to be many more long-term adverse effects? Almost certainly, in my opinion. There are yet other problems.

GENES THAT DO NOT FOLLOW OUR SCRIPTS

Gene enthusiasts seldom, if ever, temper their wild claims with the issues of genes affecting the structure and function of other genes. When I hear talk of production of genes to "mass cure" human diseases, my mind often drifts to the subject of 'gene silencers.' An interesting experiment was reported about ten years ago. Some geneticists came up with the idea of improving the color of flowers by inserting additional copies of pigment genes to petunias. The results startled them: Rather than showing the expected darker purple color, the flowers showed complete bleaching of the color in the form of white stripes.[6] My purpose in citing the preceding study is not to propose that gene therapy will not be valuable in any situations. Rather, it is to point out the possibility of the same happening to people receiving gene therapies. What genes will be silenced in people? What will those silenced genes do to them? What genes will take over when others are silenced? What will be the consequences of such a happenstance? Time alone will provide the answers. For now, I see the clear possibility of gene therapies playing out as antibiotics did: many short-term important benefits and many, many more long-term serious problems. It also seems likely to me that the problems created by silenced or silencing genes may be far worse than those of overgrowth of dangerous microbes created by antibiotics.

Another subject of interest in this context is that of "genome instability," in which genetic alterations are seen in cancer cells far in excess of what would be expected from random mutations alone. It has long been known that genes respond to environmental changes. The concept of genome instability, however, puts that in a much more sinister perspective since it indicates a dangerous instability of a growing part of the genome. For example, in the case of colon cancer it is increasingly recognized that such gene instability is related more to acquired genetic defects and less to inherited abnormalities. [7]

Human genes simply do not work well except when cellular oxygen metabolism is normal. This is my primary reason for believing that progress in gene therapy will be achieved only after we have learned how to maintain a healthful oxygen metabolism.

GENES AND DIABETES
Loser-Gainer Games and Diabetes-Cancer Trade-Off

Another good example to illustrate my reservation about the views of the gene therapy enthusiasts is the case of type II diabetes.

Type II is a widespread and *growing* problem in the United States, which puts an individual's lifespan in serious jeopardy. It usually develops slowly in older persons with a family history of diabetes and who have normal or high blood insulin levels. The reason that persons with type II diabetes have high blood sugar levels even though they have normal or *high* blood insulin levels is insulin resistance. In health, insulin is the primary hormone that facilitates entry of glucose into cells and its utilization there. Insulin resistance develops when the insulin receptors on the cell membranes fail to respond to insulin and blood sugar level rises. The pancreas produces more insulin to overcome the resistant insulin receptors, but to no avail. The blood sugar level continues to rise and type II diabetes is diagnosed.

Insulin resistance, in essence, is a cell membrane dysfunction.

In 1987, I introduced the term oxidative cell membrane dysfunction for a state in which oxidative injury to the cell membrane results in leaky cell membrane.[8] The result: What is outside the cell floods the cell innards and what is inside the cell hemorrhages out. For example, calcium enters the cell in excess through the leaky cell membrane and potassium leaks out. Other substances present in excess in or outside the cell are also affected by the increased "leakiness" (permeability) of the cells. All such changes put the cellular function and structure in serious jeopardy. In later chapters of this book, I present evidence for my view that *all* acquired cell membrane dysfunctions are oxidative-dysoxygenative in nature.

Doctors prescribe various drugs to lower the blood sugar level by increasing its entry and utilization in cells. However, none of those drugs address the fundamental issue of what causes the cell membrane to malfunction in genetically susceptible persons.

Enter gene therapy enthusiasts. Their approach is conceptually simple and seems logical on the surface: Find the culprit gene and replace it. That, of course, is easier said than done. I cite an example. One type of cell membrane receptor that plays an important role in insulin activity is called PPARy.[9,10] This receptor controls both the entry of glucose in cells and its metabolism there. Recent research has identified three different groups of mutations involving that receptor in a small number of type II diabetics: (1) a group of *loss*-of-function mutations; (2) a group of *gain*-of-function mutations; and (3) a group of other mutations that are associated with *variable* effects on insulin sensitivity. It can be safely predicted that many more mutations in each of those and other categories will be found in the future. In gene therapies, how will we assure that when we need a *gainer* gene, we will not end up with a *loser* gene? How will we tell both groups from the variable loss-gain genes? How will we know what genes will silence which genes to play havoc on the person? To date mutations of only PPARy receptors have been identified in a *small* number of type II diabetics. How many other receptors are there which affect insulin activity? How many other groups of mutations involving those receptors lurk behind the visible tip of the iceberg? The enthusiasm about curing diabetes by replacing the faulty genes must be tempered with the sobering thoughts concerning those questions.

WILL THERE BE A DIABETES-CANCER TRADE OFF?

The loser-gainer gene games in diabetes do not end there. The PPARy receptors are also involved in production of substances for immune cells and cells lining the blood vessels. Mutations in those functions are thought to contribute to cancer and obesity. Will there be a diabetes-cancer trade-off? How will we assure that while we try to cure diabetes with gene therapies, we do not cause cancer?

A different approach to the problem of insulin-resistant cell membranes is to restore the cell membrane function by integrative nutritional, herbal, and oxygenative therapies. It is a little known fact that many experienced integrative physicians can successfully manage high-insulin diabetics without prescribing drugs by focusing on all issues of cell membrane health. My colleagues and I have several examples of such patients in our practices.

Again, the issue here is not whether we continue to pour billions of dollars into gene therapy research. My point simply is this: Genes therapies will not work unless oxygen metabolism is preserved in healthy subjects and is restored in sick persons. And that restoration of oxygen metabolism calls for an "ecologic-restorative" approach.

A MENAGERIE OF MYSTERY MALADIES FOR THE MILLENNIUM

In matters of health, our legacy to the new millennium is a growing menagerie of mysterious maladies. It includes chronic fatigue syndrome, fibromyalgia, multiple chemical sensitivity syndrome, Gulf War syndrome, chronic Epstein-Barr syndrome, "candidiasis" syndrome, attention disorders, learning disabilities, and others. According to *The Wall Street Journal*, fibromyalgia alone disabled eight million Americans by 1999, and neurosurgeons were drilling parts of the skull bones off to treat muscle pain caused by that condition.[11] In some reports, up to one-quarter of patients presenting to general clinics complained of chronic fatigue.[12] Over ten years ago, the *Journal of the American Medical Association* reported that up to six percent of children in Baltimore County were prescribed drugs for attention and hyperactivity disorders.[13] I know of school systems in which up to nine percent of children take Ritalin and related drugs. Holistic doctors diagnose candidiasis in *most* of their patients. I return to this subject later.

The essential point I make concerning such mystery maladies is that none of those conditions can be understood without understanding dysfunctional oxygen metabolism (DOM). Beyond that, the readers will note that the concept of DOM also answers many questions concerning such common diseases as coronary heart disease, Alzheimer's disease, and rheumatoid arthritis. I refer the readers interested in pursuing the subject of oxidosis further to the companion volume, *RDA: Rats, Drugs and Assumptions.*

OXYOLOGY

Oxyology (oxy-olo-gy) is the study of oxygen, just as gemology is the study of gems. I recently introduced this term in an editorial published in *The Journal of Integrative* Medicine[14] for the following two reasons:

1.   The study of oxygen deserves to be considered as *the* core medical discipline; and
2.   Oxygen therapies have been badly neglected in clinical medicine.

Most doctors think of oxygen only when someone is near death in an intensive care unit. This is most unfortunate, because oxygen *is* what breathes life into all human cells at *all* times, in healthful aging and in disease states.

Oxygen ushers life in. Oxygen terminates life. As I amply demonstrate in this book, oxygen is the *most* important healing substance, the most effective detox agent, the premium blood cleanser, the most potent antibiotic, a versatile hormone, a blood clotter *and* declotter, and the conductor of the orchestra of the immune system. Without oxygen, the lungs cannot breathe, the heart cannot beat, the brain cannot think, the bowel cannot digest or absorb food, and the muscles cannot move. That is all very basic and essential.

A cancer cell hates oxygen; an immune cell loves it. That, in simple words, is the foundation of all oxygenative therapies my colleagues at the Institute and I prescribe for patients with malignant tumors. Indeed, I do not believe anyone can effectively manage any of the *systemic metabolic* issues involved in cancer treatment without an unrelenting focus on issues of oxidosis and dysoxygenosis.

Like cancer cells, primordial life forms (PLFs) also hate oxygen. PLFs is my term for a very large group of microbial families that include yeast-like microbes, nanobacteria, mycoplasma, the so-called stealth microbes, and bowel anaerobes. That is the primary reason why my colleagues and I prescribe oxygenative therapies for patients with acute and chronic infections, chronic fatigue syndrome, fibromyalgia, chemical sensitivity syndrome, multiple sclerosis, asthma, and many other immune and degenerative disorders. Most doctors will raise their eyebrows when they read this sentence, but that is because they have seldom, if ever, explored the enormous potential of oxygenative therapies. At present, not many physicians seem interested in oxygen metabolism in health and disease. I can confidently predict that will change in the future as the basic facts of dysfunctional oxygen metabolism get widely recognized.

NEED FOR ECOLOGIC THINKING

For healthful aging, we need to think of oxygen and oxidation within a larger ecological perspective. We must recognize and address the fundamental and global threats to our oxygen supply and dysfunctional oxygen metabolism. Or, we must prepare to watch helplessly while hundreds of millions of chronically ill persons continue to suffer from "mystery" maladies, as our Star Wars medical technology utterly fails to restore their health. Without an enlightened ecologic thinking and a clear understanding of the oxygen order of human life, we are doomed to wallow in ignorance as we encounter a growing menagerie of mystery maladies for the millennium. From extensive experience I know that, by and large, those maladies are reversible with broad-based, *ecologic-restorative* management plans. It is from the lessons learned from such experience that we can formulate preventive plans to stem the tide of those maladies and help people to age healthfully. That is the essential message of this book.

References

1.   Ali M. Fibromyalgia: an oxidative-dysoxygenative disorder (ODD). J Integrative Medicine 1999;3:17-37.
2.   Harvell CD, Kim K, Burkholder JM, et al. Emerging marine diseases, climate links and anthropogenic factors. Science 1999;285:1505.
3.   Editorial. Gene therapy for the public. Nature 1999;402:703.
4.   Editorial. The promise of proteomics. Nature 1999;402:703.
5.   Migliaccio E, Giogio M, Mele S, et al. The p66 shc adapter protein controls oxidative stress response and life span in mammals. Nature. 1999;402:309-13.
6.   Candidate 'gene silencers' found. News of the Week. Science 1999;286:886.
7.   Offit K. Genetic prognostic markers for colorectal carcinoma. N Eng J Med 2000;342:124-5.
8.   Ali M. Leaky Cell Membrane Dysfunction. Monograph. 1987. Teaneck, New Jersey.
9.   Schwartz MW, Kahn SE. Insulin resistance and obesity. Nature 1999;402:860-1.
10.   PPARy (perioxisome proliferator-activated receptor gamma) is both a receptor and a transcription factor. It belongs to a family of nuclear-hormone receptors. When activated by ligands, such as thiazolidinedione,

it binds to specific DNA sequence in gene promoters. Next, complexed with RXR (retinoid X receptor, another transcription factor), it activates the transcription of specific genes.

11.   Surgery on the skull for chronic fatigue? Doctors are trying it. The Wall Street Journal, November 11, 1999. pp, A1 and A8.

12.   Buchwald D, Sullivan JL, Karmaroff A. Frequency of chronic active Epstein-barr virus infection in general medical practice. JAMA 1987;257:2303.

13   JAMA 1988;260:2256

14.   Ali M. Oxyology: the need for a new discipline in clinical medicine. J Integrative Medicine. 1999;3:1-2.

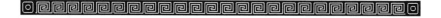

Genes are living beings. They talk and listen to each other. Their language is *living* and *creative*. They do not recognize simplistic mechanical models of replacing worn-out materials with spare parts. Genes read their environment and adapt. But human need a *living* environment to flourish, hence the core importance of optimal oxygen metabolism for their function.

Chapter 2

Seven Scientific Terms

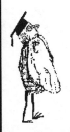
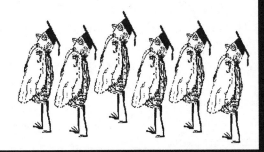

I have organize my material in this volume in a way that readers without any background in chemistry can easily and clearly comprehend the essential concepts of oxidosis (too much oxidation) and dysoxygenosis (dysfunctional oxygen metabolism). I also repeat certain core concepts for that reason and regret if such repetitions are irksome to some readers.

Seven scientific terms appear repeatedly in this book. It is essential to understand the meanings of those words. In this chapter, I give brief descriptions of those terms. Some readers without medical background may find the terms tedious in the beginning. I urge them to read the following pages slowly and take the time to grasp the full meanings of those terms. If necessary, the readers should re-read these pages to become familiar with the terms. Once that is done, I am confident the scientific knowledge presented in this book will become easily understandable. There are other rewards for that effort. I can promise the readers that with that knowledge they will be able to separate good from bad medical writings.

1. OXIDOSIS

Oxidosis (oxi-do-sis) is *excessive* loss of energy through rapid loss of electrons. In the context of aging, oxidosis causes disease and premature aging. Oxidation is loss of electrons. In chemical reactions, electrons are transferred from one atom or molecule to the other. The donor substance loses electrons and is so oxidized. The recipient gains electrons and so is reduced. The gainer becoming reduced seems strange but that is the awkwardness of the scientific terminology.

People *see* electrons every day. There is a spark when the plug on an electric appliance is pulled without first turning the unit off. That spark is a storm of electrons. In this example, a running appliance *gains* electrons from the source in the power company and uses it to produce energy for its function. That is exactly what happens in oxygen-driven oxidative reactions in the body. Oxygen first gains (steals) electrons from other substances and so begins the process of generation of energy. Those substances, in turn, are oxidized. Light is produced by a light bulb in a similar way. A high-energy beam of electrons loses some energy as light particles called photons and turns into a low energy beam of electrons.

Butter turns rancid, a flower wilts, meat decomposes—*that is oxidation.* A person develops a cataract and loses his eyesight. That happens when the proteins in the lens become oxidized. When a heart fails after a heart attack, that is because oxidosis in the heart muscle cells interferes with their function. In all tissues, excessive oxidation means a rapid breakdown in tissues. Thus, I see the hand of oxidosis at autopsy in *each and every* case, regardless of whether the death was caused by cancer or by chemotherapy, by coronary artery spasm or by a cardiologist's stent, by hepatitis or by pneumonia.[2]

Oxidosis leads to dysfunctional oxygen metabolism, which is the basis of all symptoms of fibromyalgia and chronic fatigue syndrome.[2] It is the molecular basis of pain, fatigue, and brain fog in those syndromes.

2. DYSOXYGENOSIS

Dysoxygenosis (dys-oxy-gen-o-sis) is my term for dysfunctional oxygen metabolism.[2] It is not merely lack of oxygen due to heart disease or asthma, nor poor transport of oxygen due to anemia. The scientific term for that is anoxia. Dysoxygenosis is the failure of *cellular* oxygen metabolism due to damage to the enzymes of oxygen metabolism. Thus, dysoxygenosis threatens the health of every cell, every tissue, every body organ.

Dysoxygenosis in muscle cells causes severe fatigue. In brain cells, it causes problems of mood, memory, and mentation. In the skin and eyes, it causes advanced dryness. In the cell membrane, it causes leaky membrane dysfunction, so that what is inside the cell hemorrhages out and what is outside floods the cell innards. Thus, the cell becomes dehydrated, shrunken, and loaded with toxins. Such a cell cannot function well.

3. ACIDOSIS

Acidosis (acid-o-sis) is excess acidity. Acidosis slows or blocks the enzyme systems of the body, including those involved with energy, digestion and absorption, detoxification, muscle function, and neurotransmitters. Enzymes are catalysts that facilitate life processes. Acidosis fans the flames of both oxidosis and dysoxygenosis which, in turn, cause more acidosis. As in the case of dysoxygenosis, acidosis in muscle cells causes severe fatigue.[3] In brain cells, it causes problems of mood, memory, and mentation. In the skin and eyes, it causes advanced dryness. And so on.

4. OXIDATIVE COAGULOPATHY

Oxidative coagulopathy (co-ag-u-lop-athy) is the process by which clean blood turns into "dirty" blood.

In health, the red blood cells are rounded, smooth in outline, and do not stick to each other. The hunter immune cells have irregular but sharp boundaries and move around like amoebae, searching for microbes to kill and digest. The antibody-forming immune cells are also smooth, rounded, and free of debris stuck to their surfaces. The plasma (fluid part of the blood) is clear and without any areas of congealing. There is no microclot or microplaque formations.

In 1997, my colleague, Omar Ali, M.D., and I introduced the term oxidative coagulopathy to describe a range of abnormalities in the blood of patients with coronary heart disease.[4] We observed the following changes in blood slides: deformities and clustering of red blood cells, death of immune cells, zones of congealed plasma, and microclot and microplaque formation. The blood clots and unclots all the time. However, in oxidative coagulopathy, microclot formation occurs at a rapid rate and unclotting cannot keep pace with clotting. Thus, microclots and microplaques accumulate in the blood and get stuck to the inside of small arteries in the heart and brain, causing heart attacks and strokes.

Later I described similar changes in fibromyalgia and chronic fatigue syndrome.[5] Adding bacterial culture to milk turns it into yogurt. Lemon juice squeezed into milk curdles it. That happens because microbes and certain acids solidify the proteins in milk, the same way microbes and certain acids entering the circulating blood curdle it. In health, such curdles (microclots) are readily dissolved by clot-busting enzymes. In fibromyalgia, a large number of microbes and large quantities of toxic oxidants enter the blood from the bowel, causing excessive microclot formation.

5. OXIDATIVE LYMPHOPATHY

Oxidative lymphopathy (lym-phop-athy) is my term for a process by which lymph becomes oxidized, rancid, thick and *gluey*. Lymph is the pale fluid that drains toxins from tissues. Such fluid stagnates in muscles and other tissues, preventing the free flow of oxygen-rich blood, causing soreness in tissues, and producing trigger points in muscles. I introduced this term in 1998 to focus on issues of stagnant lymph in tissues[4] and described its clinical significance in fibromyalgia in 1999.[6]

Blood and lymph channels exist in all body organs. Thus, damage caused by oxidative coagulopathy and oxidative lymphopathy quickly spreads to all cells of the body. 3M oxidopathy is my term for oxidative damage to cell membranes, matrix, and mitochondria. Matrix is the cement that holds cells together. Membranes are coverings of cells and their inner structures. Mitochondria are tiny power batteries of the cells. Since all three are continuously exposed to oxidized (rancid) blood and lymph, it should not surprise us that the oxidative coals in the blood and lymph (microclots) will also sear the 3M (matrix, membranes, and mitochondria).[5]

6. OXIDATIVE-DYSOXYGENATIVE DYSFUNCTION (ODD)

ODD is a state in which: (1) oxidosis is caused by oxidants of *all* three types (metabolic, microbial, and man-made) that threaten health; (2) oxidosis leads to dysoxygenosis (abnormal oxygen metabolism), which slows or blocks *all* life processes; (3) oxidosis and dysoxygenosis together cause acidosis; (4) all three elements (oxidosis, dysoxygenosis, and acidosis) feed upon each other and together fan the flames of oxidative injury. In fibromyalgia, an oxidative-dysoxygenative (OD) state leads to injury to *every microecologic cellular and macroecologic tissue-organ ecosystem of the body.*[6]

7. OXYOLOGY

Oxyology (oxy-olo-gy) is the study of oxygen, just as pathology is the study of diseases.[7] A sound knowledge of oxygen metabolism in health and of dysfunctional oxygen metabolism in disease and premature aging is of fundamental importance. Indeed, I believe neither health nor the aging process can be understood without such knowledge. In this volume, I present many aspects of oxygen that seldom, if ever, are discussed in medical textbooks.

References

1.   Ali M. Spontaneity of Oxidation in Nature and Aging. Monograph. Teaneck, New Jersey, 1983.
2.   Ali M. Darwin, oxidosis, dysoxygenosis, and integration. J Integrative Medicine 1999;1:11-16.
3.   Ali M. Oxidative regression to primordial cellular ecology (ORPEC): evidence for the hypothesis and its clinical significance. J Integrative Medicine 1988;2:4-55.
4.   Ali M, Ali O. AA oxidopathy: the core pathogenetic mechanism of ischemic heart disease. J Integrative Medicine 1997;1:1-112.
5.   Ali M. Amenorrhea, oligomenorrhea, and polymenorrhea in CFS and fibromyalgia are caused by oxidative menstrual dysfunction. J Integrative Medicine 1998;3:101-124.
6.   Ali M. Fibromyalgia: an oxidative-dysoxygenative disorder (ODD). J Integrative Medicine 1999;3:17-37.
7.   Ali M. Oxyology: the need for a new discipline in clinical medicine. J Integrative Medicine 2000;4:1-2.

Chapter 3

The
Spontaneity
of Oxidation
Theory of
Aging

The oxygen theory of aging presented in this book is an extension of the spontaneity of oxidation theory of aging originally proposed in 1983 in a monograph entitled, *The Spontaneity of Oxidation in Nature and Aging*.[1] The basic idea of that theory is simple: The primary drive for the aging process is the same as for the living process. All living and aging processes are driven by the same natural phenomenon that drives all life processes, i.e., the spontaneous process of living beings losing energy through a loss of electrons.

The basic idea of the oxygen theory of aging presented in this book is equally simple: The primary aging process involves *dysfunctional* oxygen metabolism (dysoxygenosis) so that cells, tissues, and body organs age because they cannot maintain normal oxygen metabolism. According to the proposed oxygen theory of aging, progressive dysoxygenosis develops in the following three phases:

1.   Oxidosis (too much oxidation);
2.   Acidosis (too much acidity);
3.   Dysoxygenosis (dysfunctional oxygen metabolism).

It is important to point out that oxidosis causes acidosis as well as dysoxygenosis. Acidosis, in turn, increases the rate of oxidation and interferes with oxygen metabolism, further increasing the degree of abnormal oxygen metabolism. Dysoxygenosis, in turn, feeds upon itself as well as fans the flames of both oxidosis and acidosis. Thus, each of the three elements feeds upon itself as well as increases the degrees of the other two. The following text is reproduced from that monograph and some previous publications[2-5] to provide a framework for the present discussion.

I want to prove that the boundaries set by the gods are not unbreakable.

Gilgamesh 2000 BC

Each living thing must one day die. If it had not been so for one single life form, that life form would have lived forever and would have crowded out all other forms of life from the planet Earth.

If one species of fish had lived forever, it would have filled up all the oceans, seas, rivers and lakes on our planet. There would have been no room for any other species of fish, nor for any other form of life in the water, any mollusk, any crab, any algae. If one single species of plant or animal on earth were to be exempt from nature's immutable "oxidative law of death," that plant or animal would have packed every inch of the land. There would have been no room for a new twig, a new bloom, a new plant, a new insect or a new baby. I wonder if Gilgamesh knew this.

New life must be preceded by death. Life, it seems to me, can be understood only through death. How did nature design this death-life-death cycle? Nature is a master planner. It is an ingenious designer. It has its own economy. It rarely errs. It is self-correcting.

RECYCLING LIFE IS ONE OF NATURE'S MASTER STROKES

Oxidation is nature's grand design for assuring that no life form lives forever. Nature made oxidation a spontaneous process. It requires no expenditure of energy. It needs no external cues or outside programming. In scientific jargon, oxidation is defined as *loss* of electrons by atoms and molecules. A molecule is a group of atoms bonded together. Electrons are the tiniest packets of energy. When atoms and molecules lose electrons, they lose energy. In oxidation, high-energy atoms and molecules are changed into lower-energy atoms and molecules. *This is the essence of the phenomenon of aging.*

HOW DO WE AGE?

Human frames age when their body organs age.
Human body organs age when their tissues age.
Human tissues age when their cells age.
Human cells age when their molecules age.
Human molecules age when they lose their plasticity.

How do molecules lose their plasticity? By oxidative injury. Oxidative molecular damage, then, is the *basic* mechanism of ongoing molecular aging.[2]

MOLECULAR DUALITY OF OXYGEN

Oxygen carries the seeds of life—and also of death. It builds molecules. It lacerates, mutilates and destroys molecules. Oxygen sustains life. Oxygen threatens life.

How does a log of wood burn to give us fire for cooking our meals? It requires oxygen to burn. It burns with oxygen. In the process of burning, the log yields its energy and turns into ashes. Oxygen serves our body tissues in exactly the same way. Food materials yield their chemical bond energy as they are burned by oxygen. We use this energy both for the processes of life and for building up our body stores of energy for periods when foods may not be available to us.

How do our enzymes build the molecules for the structure and function of the various tissues in our body? With oxygen. Oxygen and enzymes do not seem to care about our notions of eating or dieting. I am convinced our metabolic enzymes still do not know about our refrigerators, our food stamp programs, and about our grain silos. The enzymes maintain a high level of preparedness for a famine even when we indulge in heavy eating. They do not know where our next meal might come from or whether or not there will be a next meal.

What is the language of molecular injury?
Oxidation.

***

What is the language of molecular recovery?
Reduction.

***

What is the language of molecular aging?
Oxidative molecular injury.

***

What drives the aging process?
Spontaneity of oxidation in nature.

THE AGING-OXIDANT MOLECULES (AOMs)

During the early period of the development of my spontaneity of oxidation theory of aging, I coined the term "aging-oxidant molecules (AOMs)" for all substances that promote any or all of the oxidative reactions in the body.[3] In particular I wanted to explain to my patients that substances in nature were not always locked into oxidant or antioxidant roles. Thus, the term AOM is not synonymous with antioxidants. For example, milk is a strongly aging-oxidant food for a person with milk allergy, but not necessarily so in a nonallergic individual.

The AOMs exist in nature to assure that no life form lives forever. These molecules are present in each flower, each plant, each animal and each person. These are powerful molecules, fully capable of instantaneously burning all tissues. The AOMs can be divided into two broad categories: the internal metabolic AOMs and the external synthetic and natural toxic AOMs. The examples of the first category include aging-oxidant metabolic enzymes, minerals, proteins, fats and stress molecules. The external AOMs include industrial pollutants, petrochemicals, synthetic household chemicals, antibiotics, pesticides and herbicides. Radioactivity, ultraviolet waves and other forms of radiation do not come under the strict definition of AOMs, but readily generate AOMs by acting upon various atoms and molecules.

THE LIFESPAN MOLECULES

At that time I also introduced the term, "lifespan molecules (LSMs)" for molecules that provide a counterbalance to aging-oxidant molecules. These molecules exist to assure that the aging-oxidant molecules do not cause instant combustion of all living forms. As each flower, each plant, each animal and each person is made up of AOMs, so too they are made up of LSMs. LSMs exist to provide a counterbalance to AOMs. These molecules "neutralize" AOMs and prevent unwanted tissue damage. It is their responsibility to assure that each life form gets the opportunity to live out its normal life span in health, and with vigor and vitality. Examples of such molecules are vitamins, essential fatty acids, essential amino acids, essential minerals, and other antioxidants.

As in the case of AOM, the term LSM is also not synonymous with antioxidant. For example, ozone is a powerful oxidant in the laboratory that can serve as a potent antioxidant in the body of persons with certain types of viral infections and cancers. (See the chapter entitled, "The Oxygen Order of Life and Aging" for an explanation of this apparent paradox.)

I started using the two terms of AOMs and LSMs in my seminars on nutrition for life span. I soon discovered that patients without any biology background at all could understand these terms and the essential ideas behind their use easily and effortlessly. Indeed, people found the simplified concept of molecular aging, disease and death described with these two terms a useful framework for understanding nutrition. Below is a brief explanation of these terms.

THE BASIC EQUATION OF LIFE

The balance between the AOMs and LSMs is the basic equation of life. In scientific jargon, it is called *redox reaction.* Redox equilibrium (or potential, as it is sometimes called) determines the health and life of foods as it determines the health and life of people, animals and plants.

Human biology is an ever-changing kaleidoscope of molecular mosaics. AOMs and LSMs are in dynamic equilibrium at all times. Health and disease — at energy, electron and molecular levels — can be defined as the states created by the impact of AOMs and LSMs on an individual's genetic makeup. Health, in this light, may be seen as a dynamic state in which the LSMs have the upper hand and preserve the structural and functional integrity of cells and tissues. Disease, by contrast, is a state in which AOMs overwhelm the LSMs and cause dis-ease and disease.

I call the clinical practice of medicine founded on this basic equation of life molecular medicine,[4] a medicine of the future that seeks to reverse the basic cause of disease rather than simply suppress the symptoms with drugs. In acute illness, we need drugs or surgical scalpels. In chronic disease, nondrug treatment protocols of nutritional medicine, environmental medicine, medicine of self-regulation and fitness offer clearly superior long-term results.

THE SPONTANEITY OF OXIDATION THEORY OF AGING AS AN EXTENSION OF OTHER THEORIES

By now, the readers should clearly understand the basic and simple facts concerning oxygen, spontaneity of oxidation in nature, molecular duality of oxygen, and the dual roles of aging-oxidant and life-span molecules. That allows me to state my 1983 spontaneity of oxidation theory in the following simple words: Aging involves loss of energy triggered, perpetuated, and completed by the *ongoing and spontaneous* loss of energy through loss of electrons in all human cells and body organs.

In 1983, at the time of my proposing my theory, there were four major prevailing theories of aging: (1) Johan Bjorksten's cross-linking theory of aging[5]; (2) Denham Harmon's free radical theory of aging[6]; and (3) Roy Walford's immune theory of aging.[7] It was evidently necessary to ask: How does my theory stack up against the three major aging theories proposed earlier? Before publishing my monograph, I carefully considered each of those and recognized that the theory I was about to propose was fully consistent with all three. Indeed, my theory represented a clear extension—and, in my view at that time, a completion—of those theories. Below, I include some brief comments about each of those three theories.

THE CROSS-LINKING THEORY OF AGING

In 1955, Johan Bjorksten proposed his cross-linking theory of aging.[5] According to this theory, the basic aging process involves accumulation of damaged and insoluble (cross-linked) proteins, DNA, fats, and other large-sized molecules, such as vitamin A. Such cross-linked molecules cause aging by impeding or blocking the actions of enzymes, vitamins, and other substances. The process of cross-linking may be illustrated as follows: The structure of many healthy proteins resembles long threads of different sizes. Under heat or chemical stresses, individual molecules are bent, turned and twisted into many different shapes. Such misshapen molecules quickly regain their original shapes when the stresses clear up. The term cross-linking means that such turned and twisted molecules get permanently disfigured because of excessive stress. Thus, such molecules are torn apart and, when the ends unite, they get tangled with each other and form crooked protein molecules. Cross-linked molecules are two molecules wrapped around each other in such a way that neither can function normally. Since Bjorksten first proposed it, the cross-linking theory of aging has been fully validated.

In the context of the spontaneity of oxidation theory of

aging, the crucial question concerning the cross-linking theory is this: What is the molecular basis of cross-linking? Extensive review of the literature over a period of two decades has convinced me that all cross-linking that occurs during the aging process is oxidative in nature. I have not found any exceptions to that. And the primary drive for oxidation in human metabolism, as I indicate earlier, is spontaneity of oxidation in nature. Thus, the spontaneity of oxidation theory begins where the cross-linking theory leaves off.

THE FREE RADICAL THEORY OF AGING

In 1956, Denham Harmon proposed his free radical theory of aging.[6] According to this theory, the aging process involves molecular and cellular injury caused by free radicals. Free radicals are highly unstable, extremely reactive atoms or molecules that form during normal metabolism as well as during cellular injury caused by chemicals, microbes, radiation, and other types of injury. Since its introduction, this theory has also been validated by a huge body of longevity studies. Indeed, to my knowledge no evidence to the contrary has ever been put forth.

Again, in the context of the spontaneity of oxidation theory of aging, the crucial question concerning the free radical theory of aging is this: Where do free radicals come from? How do such radicals cause molecular and cellular aging? And again, a broad survey of the literature over a period of three decades has convinced me that all free radical generation is fueled by oxidative triggers. Furthermore, all molecular and cellular injury caused by free radicals is oxidative in nature. There are no studies to the contrary.

And again, the primary drive for free radical production as well as injury caused by such radicals is spontaneity of oxidation in nature. Thus, the spontaneity of oxidation theory extends the free radical theory of aging.

THE IMMUNE THEORY OF AGING

In 1962, Roy Walford proposed his immune theory of aging.[7] According to that theory, the aging process involves injury to the immune system of the body so that the injured system becomes confused and turns on the individual. Specifically, immune injury results in the production of abnormal antibodies that injure the body's own tissues rather than fighting microbes. Such antibodies are called autoantibodies. Like the cross-linking and free radical theories before it, the basic claim of this theory has also been validated. For example, increased production of autoantibodies directed against various body organs occurs with advancing age. Furthermore, there is much direct evidence for cellular injury (and aging) caused by such antibodies.

The core question concerning the immune theory of aging is the same as for the two preceding theories: What causes the immune injury? What is the molecular mechanism that triggers autoantibody production? Once again, the examination of the available clinical and experimental evidence leads us to the same conclusion: the immune injury is caused by oxidizing chemicals, microbes, and other agents. And once again, the primary drive for oxidative immune injury is spontaneity of oxidation in nature. Thus, the spontaneity of oxidation theory also extends the immune theory of aging.

There are some other less known theories of aging, including the following: (1) wear-and-tear theory; (2) preprogrammed senescence theory; (3) rate of metabolism theory; and (4) limited cell division theory.[8] A close examination of each of those theories also shows that it is equally compatible with the spontaneity of oxidation theory. It is clear from the basic facts of oxygen and oxidation presented here that the primary aging mechanism in the wear-and-tear, preprogrammed senescence, and rate of metabolism theories is oxidative injury. As for the genetically determined limited cell division theory, growing evidence seems to indicate that genes require optimal oxygen metabolism for proper functioning (discussed further in the following chapter). It seems safe to predict that future research will provide additional and conclusive evidence for that view.

OXIDATIVE RATES AND LIFE SPAN

Frozen meat left on a kitchen table thaws within hours and begins to decompose in several hours. Such decomposition is the result of spontaneous oxidation and is called auto-oxidation. The same process occurs when tissues of animals are removed and allowed to undergo spontaneous oxidation and decomposition. The rate at which such oxidation occurs is called the rate of auto-oxidation and is an indicator of the *rate of metabolism* of the animal species. In other words, those rates of oxidation represent the natural (innate) capacity of tissues for self-destruction. If the spontaneity of oxidation theory is valid, the rates of auto-oxidation of various animal species would be expected to correlate well with their lifespans. That possibility has been researched and the rates of oxidation in tissues of various animal species have been correlated with their lifespan.

Researchers at the National Institutes of Health measured the rates at which tissues undergo spontaneous oxidation in over 70 mammals. They observed that the animal species which showed the highest rates of auto-oxidation had the shortest life spans, and those with the lowest rates of auto-oxidation had the longest life spans. There was almost a perfect inverse correlation between the rates of oxidation and the species life spans. Selected data for rates of auto-oxidation in selected animal species and humans are shown in the table given below.

Rates of Auto-Oxidation and Life Spans of Mammalian Species [9]		
Species	**Oxidation Rate**	**Life Span (yrs)**
Man	24	90
Orangutan	25	50
Baboon	35	37
Green monkey	41	34
Squirrel monkey	74	18
Rat	104	4
Mouse	182	3.5

The above table illustrates clearly the inverse relationship between life spans and auto-oxidative rates: Animal species that oxidize their tissues rapidly live the shortest life spans, while those that oxidize their tissues slowly live the longest life spans. Man (with the lowest rate of tissue breakdown) has the highest longevity, while the mouse which has the highest rate among the species listed in the table has the lowest longevity.

References

1. Ali M. Spontaneity of Oxidation in Nature And Aging. Monograph. 1983. Teaneck, New Jersey.
2. Ali M. Spontaneity of Oxidation in Nature Is the true cause of Aging in Humans and Root Cause of All Disease. page 199-304, RDA: Rats, Drugs and Assumption. 1995. Life Span Press, Denville, New Jersey.
3. Ali M. Lifespan Molecules. The Cortical Monkey and Healing. page 18, 1990. Institute of Preventive Medicine, Bloomfield, New Jersey.
4. Ali M. Aging-Oxidant Molecules. The Cortical Monkey and Healing. page 17, 1990. Institute of Preventive Medicine, Bloomfield, New Jersey.
5. Bjorksten J. Crosslinking—key to aging. Chem and Engin News. 1955;33:1967.
6. Harmon D. Aging: a theory based on free radical and radiation chemistry. J Gerontol 1956;11:298.
7. Walford RI. Auto-immunity and aging. J Gerontol 1962;17:281.
8. Carrell A. Man, the Unknown. 1935. Harper Publishers, New York.
9. Tolmasoff JM, Ono T, Cutler RG. Superoxide dismutase: Correlation with life-span and specific metabolic rate in primate species. Proc Nat Acad Sci 1980;77:2777-81.
10. Cutler RG. Peroxide-producing potential of tissues: Inverse correlation with longevity of mammalian species. Proc Nat Acad Sci 1985;82:4798-4802.

"Spontaneity of oxidation is nature's grand scheme to assume that no life form lives forever. If a single life form was immune to the immutable law of oxidative death, the offspring of that species would have filled the planet earth long ago, and there would have been no space for any new insect, fish, or baby to be born."

Taken from *What Do Lions Know About Stress*

"All the days of Methuselah were nine hundred sixty and nine years, and he died."

Genesis 5:27

Chapter 4

Seven Insights and The Oxygen Theory of Aging

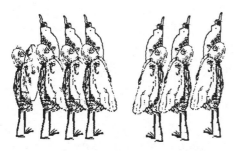

Seven insights form the basis of my clinical work with oxygen, the aging process, and healthful aging. My interest in aging arose as an extension of my search for the beginnings of diseases. Early in my pathology residency in the late 1960s, I recognized the principal limitation of my microscope: It showed me how cells and tissues looked *after* diseases had caused the damage. It could not show me events that happened *before* cellular and tissue injury occurred. I understood then that heat, cold, radiation, poisons, and microbes cause diseases. A handful of diseases were attributed to deficiency of nutrients. But there was no unifying concept of how such agents cause diseases. I learned how to diagnose many diseases by the examination of biopsy and autopsy material, but no one gave me a clear answer to how those disease processes *began.*

WITHERED FLOWERS DO NOT UN-WITHER

In 1983, a chance reflection on why stale buffers in the laboratory lose their buffering capacity led to the questions of why roses wither spontaneously but withered roses do not "un-wither" spontaneously and why cut grass decomposes spontaneously but decomposed grass does not "undecompose" spontaneously. Eggs rot but rotten eggs do not "unrot." People age but the aged do not "un-age." After months of struggling with those questions, I published my monograph, *Spontaneity of Oxidation in Nature and Aging,*[1] in which I linked the aging process to oxygen and spontaneity of oxidation. Since that first insight, I have had an abiding interest in oxygen, oxygenation (addition of oxygen), and oxidation (loss of electrons). Since writing that monograph and through two decades of my work as a hospital pathologist, I have rarely, if ever, thought about the cause of any disease except through my preoccupation with those three subjects.

Six other insights (listed and described in this chapter) followed during my research and clinical work, both as a hospital pathologist and as a clinical researcher.[2-7] That was followed by a series of publications in which I presented many of my observations concerning the subjects of excessive oxidative injury (oxidosis) and dysfunctional oxygen metabolism (DOM).

In this volume devoted to aging, I make several references to various chronic disorders of oxygen metabolism. My purpose is to illustrate several important aspects of oxidosis, acidosis, and dysoxygenosis. Indeed, my work with "mystery" maladies—such as chronic fatigue syndrome, fibromyalgia, chemical sensitivity syndrome, Gulf War syndrome, and the so-called candidiasis and Epstein-Barr syndromes—led me to the core idea of dysfunctional oxygen metabolism,[8] in which oxidosis (too much oxidation) leads to acidosis (too much acidity) and dysoxygenosis (too little oxygen). I introduced the term oxidative-dysoxygenative dysfunction (ODD) as a general model of oxygen disorders.[9] The ODD model has a strong explanatory power for symptom-complexes of not only the mystery maladies, but also for such common disorders as coronary heart disease, stroke, Alzheimer's disease, and others. Though this volume is devoted to presenting my oxygen theory of aging—dysoxygenosis theory, in technical language—most readers will find the material to be of direct relevance in understanding the beginnings of diseases mentioned in this paragraph and others included elsewhere in this book.

Beyond the issues of understanding the basic nature of the aging process and the underlying cause of oxygen disorders, the ODD model provides us with a rational and scientifically sound basis for formulating treatment plans for diverse disorders—such as coronary artery disease, asthma, Alzheimer's disease, multiple sclerosis, and others. It may surprise some that I attribute to dysfunctional oxygen metabolism all of the disorders listed above and many more mentioned later in this volume. Similarly, some may wonder how the same mechanism can explain brain fog in one person and heart palpitations in another. How can skin rashes in an eight-year-old allergic girl be attributed to the same process that causes Alzheimer's disease in an eighty-year-old woman? What could an acute asthma attack in a teenager and an acute attack of colitis in a middle-aged man have in common?

TENDER MEAT GETS COOKED FIRST

I give a simple analogy to explain my basic point. Suppose we put five different types of meat of varying degrees of tenderness in a pot full of water and turn on the heat. It is obvious that the most tender meat will get cooked first, then the less tender, next the tough meat, next the tougher meat, and finally the toughest type of meat in the pot. The heat beneath the pot provides the energy required for cooking the meat. *Dysfunctional oxygen metabolism in chronic disorders is the equivalent of heat in the meats-in-the-pot analogy.* Why some people are more troubled by persistent fatigue and others by brain fog or muscle pain depends on their genes—what body organ serves as the *spokesorgan* for their bodies. In other words, symptoms depend on how vulnerable to oxidative injury a given tissue or body organ is. That, of course, depends on an individual's genes. Thus, the genes determine which tissue is more tender and which tissue is tougher. If the oxidative fires burn uncontrolled, eventually every tissue will be affected.

The principal merit of dysfunctional oxygen metabolism (DOM) and oxidative-dysoxygenative dysfunction (ODD) models described in this book is that it keeps the focus on the central issue of *cellular oxygen metabolism* as the centerpiece of the aging process. Integrative nutritional and herbal therapies as well as tissue detoxification plans promote healthful aging. Below, I list those seven insights and include a thumbnail sketch of each. Later in this volume, I devote other chapters to an in-depth discussion of those subjects.

1.   Oxygen, spontaneity of oxidation in nature, and aging.
2.   Oxygen and its many Dr. Jekyll/Mr. Hyde roles.
3.   Oxygen, oxidative coagulopathy, and the absence of health.
4.   Oxygen, anger, guilt, and spirituality.
5.   Oxygen and microecologic cellular and macroecologic tissue-organ ecosystems.
6.   Oxidative regression to primordial cellular ecology (ORPEC).
7.   Oxidative-Dysoxygenative Dysfunction (ODD) [dysfunctional oxygen metabolism].

THE FIRST INSIGHT:
Oxygen, Spontaneity of Oxidation in Nature, and Aging

Fresh peaches left on my kitchen table spoil within days. That happens *spontaneously.* That means that those peaches are pre-programmed to spoil with time and do not need any external signals.

That natural process of decay is called oxidation. In scientific terminology, oxidation is a loss of electrons and energy.

I have not seen spoiled peaches become unspoiled. So spoiled peaches are not programmed to unspoil spontaneously. That means the process of spoiling of peaches (loss of electrons and energy) is unidirectional. Just as it is natural for water to flow downstream spontaneously, it is natural for fresh peaches to lose electrons and energy.

The human body is also preprogrammed to age spontaneously. Thus, aging is an oxidative process that does not require outside cues. People do not *un-age*. Notwithstanding the loud noises made by some in the "anti-aging industry," the notion of anti-aging is silly. A disease state, in essence, is a state of accelerated aging. The core health problem of human canaries is that they are trapped in the quicksand of dysfunctional oxygen metabolism that markedly speeds up the aging process.

What is the basis of oxidation being a spontaneous process? Here is a simple explanation: Electrons exist in atoms in spinning motion, and it is natural for electrons to spin off (fly away) unless something keeps them in place. That something is the weak pull on them by the nucleus of the atom. The electrons are forever looking to leave their nest as soon as they can break loose from that weak force.

An atom is in an eternal struggle to keep its electrons from running away. When electrons do finally break away, that is oxidation. That is the phenomenon of spontaneity of oxidation.

When an atom loses an electron, it loses energy. When a molecule loses electrons, it falls from a higher level of energy to a lower level. Every cell in every tissue in every organ is *forever* undergoing this loss of energy. Anything that "pushes" the electron will speed up that process of electrons running away. Many elements (such as anger, poisons, and microbial infections) increase the rate of oxidation.

We taste *life* in freshly squeezed vegetable juice. A stale juice is flat and lifeless. That happens because fresh vegetable juice loses electrons. That, in simple words, is the mechanism by which a flower wilts, cut grass decomposes, a fish rots, and iron rusts. That is also the mechanism by which lymph in the muscles of human canaries becomes stale and toxic. The result is muscle soreness and pain. This is a *core* concept, not only because it gives us the *essential and fundamental* theory of aging and disease, but also because it provides us a *sound and scientific* basis for developing our therapies.

The importance of the phenomenon of spontaneity of oxidation to issues of healthful aging and premature aging is this: Oxidation initiates itself and then feeds upon itself. Regardless of how oxidative injury begins, it fans its own fire. Thus, every moment of anger, every undiagnosed food reaction or mold allergy, every antibiotic abuse, every exposure to pesticides and industrial pollutants, and every addition to the toxic metal burden counts. All such oxidants speed up the aging process. In many cases, those oxidants turn simmering oxidative coals into leaping oxidative flames.

The opposite of oxidation is reduction, which does not happen spontaneously. That explains why an aging human does not spontaneously "un-age," why a wilted flower does not spontaneously become unwilted, why decomposed grass does not become un-decomposed, and why a rotten fish does not become unrotten. Nor can rusted iron unrust by itself. I devote the chapter, "The Oxygen Order of Life and Aging," to this subject. For additional reading, I suggest *RDA: Rats, Drugs and Assumptions.*

THE SECOND INSIGHT:
Oxygen and its Many Dr. Jekyll/Mr. Hyde Roles

I have been a student of medicine for forty-two years. In medical school, I learned to hold newborns upside down and gently slap their backs if they did not begin to breathe within moments after the delivery. Of course, breathing is about oxygen. I was taught that even a minute without oxygen can hurt the delicate brain of the baby. I also learned then about the other face of oxygen. Pure oxygen can make newborns blind. Thus, oxygen is essential for life, but it is also highly toxic. Ever since, the molecular duality of oxygen has fascinated me. The more I have studied it, the more I have discovered the Dr. Jekyll/Mr. Hyde roles of this element.

Oxygen is the master Dr. Jekyll/Mr. Hyde molecule of human existence. It is the ultimate spin master. It ushers life in. It terminates life. It drives the human metabolism. It is the currency of all human energy transactions. It is nature's most potent antibiotic, the most efficient scavenger, and the most competent detox molecule. Oxygen picks up an extra electron and becomes superoxide, a vile oxidant. It then spits out that electron and becomes an innocent bystander molecule. Then again, it picks up an electron and becomes a hormone.

Mothers pour hydrogen peroxide on the wounds of their children to clean them. The sight of the clear liquid hydrogen peroxide turning into bubbles symbolizes cleansing action. Of course, it kills microbes and that is why it is used for wounds. One way the hunter immune cells in the blood and tissues kill microbes is by producing hydrogen peroxide. But why does this clear liquid bubble when poured on wounds? How does it kill microbes? The simple answer: It liberates nascent (*active*) oxygen, which ruptures microbial walls by pulling out their electrons. When three atoms of oxygen dance as a threesome in a ring-around-the-rosie (ozone, as we call it in common language), they both protect us against cancer (by strengthening the immune system in the pure medical form) and increase risk of developing cancer (when in the polluted, highly toxic form). The mechanism for both effects is the same: Ozone breaks down to *safe* oxygen in the air as well as *unsafe* nascent oxygen. Whether ozone damages the DNA and sets the stage for the beginning of cancer or upregulates antioxidant defenses against the oxidative fires of cancer cells depends on many factors. I discuss this subject further in the chapter, "The Oxygen Order of Life and Aging."

We age healthfully when the body manages oxygen well. We age prematurely and often turn into human canaries when oxygen metabolism becomes dysfunctional.

This is a simple statement, but one that all students of the aging phenomenon as well as all human canaries must *truly* understand. The recovery of human canaries from disabling oxygen disorders literally depends on it.

THE THIRD INSIGHT:
Oxygen, Oxidative Coagulopathy, and the Absence of Health

It is one of the profound ironies of American medicine that mothers diagnose absence of health in their children long before pediatricians do. It is common for me to see children who suffered repeated ear infections and sore throats for years. Their mothers wondered why the children were always getting sick and finally concluded that something had to be wrong with the children's immune systems. And yet, their pediatricians repeatedly insist there was nothing wrong there. I have concluded following a careful review of thousands of case histories of persons with chronic fatigue syndrome, fibromyalgia, and multiple chemical sensitivity syndrome that *a state of absence of health preceded their chronic illnesses.* It took me many years of work as a surgeon and a pathologist to see that cells and tissues do not go to bed healthy one evening and wake up sick the next morning.

A clear zone of absence of health separates the domains of health and disease.

Below, I reproduce some text from the companion volume, *Canary Two: Oxygen and Fibromyalgia,* that describes one such case history in the words of the mother of a teenage fibro canary:

> I told Karen's first pediatrician that she sleeps all the time and her whole body aches. The pediatrician replied, "Take it from me. I'm a mother. Karen is eleven now. She will grow out of it. Give her

some Tylenol." Months later, she changed her mind and told us that Karen was making herself sick and that we should take her to a psychiatrist. Several months later, Karen's headaches became more frequent and we saw two more pediatricians. The same story. They had no clue to what made our daughter sick. Then Karen had episodes of dizziness and she passed out a few times. Her pediatrician referred us to a pediatric cardiologist. The cardiologist ordered a tilt-table test that turned out to be positive. He prescribed Florinef for six months. Initially we thought the steroid drug was helping, but that proved to be temporary. Karen's situation continued to get worse. She had abdominal cramps, cold hands and feet, and blurred vision. The eye symptoms really bothered her because she couldn't read for periods of time any more. We saw yet another pediatrician. The fourth pediatrician diagnosed chronic fatigue and said that it is something Karen had to live with and we had to cope with. And that there was no treatment for that, however she might get better on her own.

(Karen regained her health several months later after treatment at the Institute and went back to school. I saw her some years later. She was then a vigorous teenager.)

In my pathology work, I frequently diagnosed precancerous conditions. I recall clearly one particular conversation I had with an oncologist many years ago. The bone marrow biopsy I examined showed an excess of plasma cells, some with irregular features. I told him that the patient needed to be watched closely for a developing myeloma, a type of bone cancer. He replied, "Yes, I will watch him.

When he develops myeloma, I will hit him hard with chemotherapy."
Of course, I had heard similar comments many times before.
Somehow that time his words hit *me* hard. I simply could not shake
them off. We physicians love to pay lip service to preventive
medicine. But how does one prevent disease with blocker drugs such
as beta blockers, calcium channel blockers, enzyme inhibitors, and
other drugs that impair or block important molecular and cellular
mechanisms in the body? What drugs could he use to stop that
marrow from turning malignant?

It has been years since that conversation with that oncologist.
But the words often return to me. Every time I hear a fibro canary
describe how antibiotics and steroids were abusively prescribed for
him or her for years before fibromyalgia was diagnosed, I think of
that oncologist. How can we physicians not see something that
obvious? Between the state of health and a state of disease there must
be a state of dis-ease (a state of absence of health) that offers us an
opportunity to prevent disease. That requires that we think of
nutrition, food reactions, mold and other allergies, pesticides,
synthetic hormones, total body burden of toxic metals, industrial
pollutants, stress and anger. But all of that, of course, is considered
quackery in drug medicine. And so the opportunities for preventing
fibromyalgia, chronic fatigue, and other oxidative-dysoxygenative
disorders are missed.

Assessment of the State of Absence of Health

What is the molecular basis for the state of absence of health?
The answer: oxidosis, acidosis, and dysoxygenosis. How can it be
assessed? The most effective way for doing that is direct examination
of the slide of a drop of blood of the person with a special type of
microscope fitted with high-resolution (x15,000) and phase-contrast

optics. Indeed, my colleagues at the Institute and I regularly study the blood smears of our patients with oxygen disorders, such as Karen in the above case history, and readily observe direct microscopic evidence of oxidosis, acidosis, and dysoxygenosis. Many red blood cells in such slides are deformed, broken up, or clumped. Many hunter immune cells (white blood cells) are found dying or dead. Many zones of congealed plasma are encountered. In many cases, such areas of congealing advance into microclot and microplaque formation. In 1997, my colleague, Omar Ali, and I introduced the term *oxidative coagulopathy* to describe such abnormalities and published several dozen photographs fully illustrating the many abnormalities we observed.[10] We also published clear evidence that many changes of oxidative coagulopathy were reversible when antioxidants, such as vitamins C and E, taurine, and glutathione, were added to the drops of blood on microscopic slides.[11]

> **No body tissue is immune to oxidative damage caused by oxidative coagulopathy, hence no symptom-complexes are known not to develop in human canaries.**

The mischief of microclot formation, however, does not end with mere mechanical blockage of tiny blood vessels. The process of oxidative coagulopathy triggers many chemical reactions that cause spasms of blood vessels and further impede circulation. Microclots have sticky surfaces. They enlarge as blood cells stick to them. Bumping into the vessel wall, they are compacted to form what we termed microplaques. Such plaques cause even more blockages than the soft microclots and stick to the inner lining of the vessels, thus beginning the process of hardening of arteries (arteriosclerosis). More importantly, oxidative coagulopathy triggers many reactions that initiate, potentiate, and perpetuate yet other oxidative phenomena.

Thus, microclots and microplaques float in the circulating blood as simmering coals, lighting up brush fires in tissues wherever they reach. For an in-depth discussion of this subject, I refer the reader to *Canary Two: Oxygen and Fibromyalgia.*

THE FOURTH INSIGHT:
Oxygen, Anger, Guilt, and Spirituality

Healing is a spontaneous phenomena. This is the flip side of the coin of spontaneity of oxidation. Injury-healing-injury is the eternal drama of living beings. We have seen the central role of oxygen in oxidative injury. Amazingly, oxygen plays a similar central role in healing. It is my clinical observation that angry people do not heal well. A chronic sense of guilt has a similar effect on healing. I see the hand of oxygen in both.

How does oxygen fit into the world of anger and guilt? Simply stated, both anger and guilt are emotions solidly grounded in oxygen metabolism. The process of sensory perception in the sensory organs involves electron transfer events, and the hand of oxygen is visible everywhere. The physical signs of anger and guilt also involve electron transfer events, hence are also oxygen-related. Thus, oxygen mediates the physiological effects of anger and guilt that, in turn, stress oxygen metabolism by causing adrenaline rushes (adrenergic hypervigilence).

Nature seems to have designed adrenaline to alert us to danger. An adrenaline rush is nature's way of raising the oxygen metabolism to a higher gear for a maximal effort for coping with threats. In the natural order of things, adrenaline rushes end when the danger clears up. The problem with anger and guilt is that those feelings do not let up. Unless banished with spiritual work, both emotions continually feed the oxidative fires of adrenaline rushes.

Spirituality is a language without words.
Where there are words, there is a clutter.

In chronic illness, psychology keeps us trapped in old and obsolete models of pain and suffering. Spirituality sets us free. The common notion of stress being fight-or-flight response to a threatening situation is so inadequate as to be clinically irrelevant. The mind-over-body healing is a silly notion of those who never work with the sick. The mind does not even understand what healing is. How can it ordain healing in injured tissues? The thinking mind— cortical monkey, in my terminology—loves to recycle past misery. When that is not enough, it precycles feared future misery.

Pain causes anger. Anger interferes with healing. How does one cope with the demons of anger? Not by feeding them with the *Why me?* question. Not by unending and punishing analysis. That simply does not work.

Spirituality, Not Psychology,
Is the Answer to the Problem of Stress

How does one save oneself from oneself? By spiritual surrender. But, then, what is the spiritual? It is a language without words. To learn that language, first we need to unlearn the suffocating habits of the thinking mind. A tall order! Yes, it is. The demons of anger in chronic suffering cannot be banished with anything less. It is a linkage with the *Presence* that permeates and surrounds each of us at all times, without being troubled by the nature of that linkage. I devote *What Do Lions Know About Stress?* to an in-depth discussion of this subject.

THE FIFTH INSIGHT:
Oxygen and Microecologic Cellular and Macroecologic
Tissue-Organ Ecosystems

We physicians, by and large, are not ecologic thinkers. Gastroenterologists seldom, if ever, look at the stomach for answers to the problems of the colon. Cardiologists rarely, if ever, search for clues to heart palpitations in hormonal fluctuations (sugar-insulin roller coasters, in my terminology). Neurologists never seem to be interested in the bowel ecology. Pediatricians frequently refuse to listen when mothers describe how sugar affects the mood of their children. Dermatologists fail to see the obvious: Eruptions and rashes in chronic skin conditions worsen with prolonged antibiotic therapy. Rheumatologists do not study smears of their patients' blood with high-resolution microscopy to find out if the changes in the blood might yield some clues to muscle pain and fatigue in fibromyalgia and chronic fatigue syndrome. Why are we physicians not interested to see the obvious interrelatedness of everything in the body to everything else in it?

The possibilities of such relationships go unexplored in physicians' offices not because patients never bring those subject up, but because medical schools do not teach them and medical textbooks do not include them. Could it be because many doctors are so focused within the narrow confines of their respective specialties that they are blinded to even the most obvious realities surrounding them? Are we a nation of specialists that no longer can see the proverbial forest for the trees? Consider the following questions asked from me by some of my patients.

"Dr. Ali, it's very strange, but whenever I apply my frequency massage unit to my fissure my sinuses clear up. Can you believe that?" a young man with Crohn's colitis and a rectal fistula and fissure asked me.

"I believe that because you tell me, though I can't explain such a direct relationship between a rectal fissure and sinus congestion on the basis of known knowledge of human anatomy or physiology."

*****

"Whenever my chronic anal fissure hurts me after a bowel movement, my heels begin to hurt me. Weird! Isn't it? Has anyone else also told you something like that?" a man once asked me.

"That's a first for me," I replied.

"So you believe me," he went on with a grin. "My primary doctor didn't believe me. He told me that couldn't happen. It was just my imagination."

"I cannot explain how that might happen. But that doesn't mean I shouldn't believe you," I said.

***

"I swear to you, Dr. Ali, I get a severe headache every time I have sex with my wife unless I take three tablets of aspirin half an hour earlier. I have seen many, many doctors but none of them could explain that. Can you?"

"I can't with any degree of certainty," I replied, then added,

"But I have heard of such an association. It seems to me such reactions are allergic in nature," I replied.

"So, I'm allergic to my wife. Is that it?" he asked with a grin.

"Not to *all* of her, but perhaps to some of her fluids." I replied, half in jest.

We physicians often dismiss descriptions such as those given above as figments of patients' imaginations. Why do we do so? The obvious answer is because we cannot explain them. Something inexplicable happens to us during our medical training. We become uncomfortable when we think our knowledge or authority is challenged with questions that go beyond our models of diseases.

How often is the menstrual syndrome in young girls controlled with the right choices in the kitchen? How often do I see headaches clear up when the bowel issues are addressed? How often do their eczema rashes clear up when the bowel ecosystems are restored? How often do persons with chronic fatigue syndrome and fibromyalgia regain their health when all the issues of the bowel, blood, and liver ecosystems are effectively addressed with nutrient and herbal therapies? How often is the air hunger experienced by human canaries relieved when *all* of the tissue-organ ecosystems of their bodies are nurtured and restored with oxygenative and antioxidant protocols? Most mainstream physicians will find those questions irksome. Most holistic physicians will nod knowingly. None of those relationships can be understood except with ecologic thinking.

Whenever a fibromyalgia canary complains of severe brain fog, my mind turns to the state of dysfunctional oxygen metabolism in his circulating blood. When a young man reports disabling fatigue, I think of oxidized, toxic, and stagnant lymph in his tissues that interferes with cellular oxygen metabolism. When a teenager describes her cold hands and feet, in my mind's eye I see deformed and clumped red blood cells, microclots, and microplaques in her circulating blood that cause spasms in arteries and clog tiny capillaries. (Those are the changes I regularly see in the blood smears of such patients.) Patients with chronic fatigue, fibromyalgia, and severe immune disorders often have dry skin, dry mouths, and dry eyes. That is also caused by the same changes. All those symptoms are related to dysfunctional oxygen metabolism. When a young woman describes her abdominal pain and bloating, I see excessive fermentation in her colon caused by primordial microbes. That, of course, is also fundamentally an oxygen problem. In health, it is oxygen that keeps a lid on the overgrowth of primordial microbes in the bowel and blood. I discuss this critical issue in the chapter, "Oxygen and Primordial Life Forms."

In the chapter "Guidelines for Healthful Aging," I describe a simple ecologic model which I call The Pyramid of Trios of Human Ecosystems and which evolved in my mind several years ago. This simple model helps me think *ecologically* about the health/disease/disease continuum and to establish my clinical priorities for managing patients with cancer, immune disorders, and the so-called mystery maladies such as chronic fatigue syndrome and fibromyalgia. I also find this model helpful for explaining to my patients my ecologic concepts about their illnesses. With time, I realized that my pyramid of trios is just as relevant to my concept of aging healthfully as it is for reversing chronic disease.

A schema of that model is included here. The readers will note that I consider the base trio of the bowel, blood, and liver ecosystems as the foundation of health. I regard it imperative that I vigorously address all issues concerning that first trio for the sick, unwell, and those who enjoy good health and are eager to follow sound strategies for healthful aging.

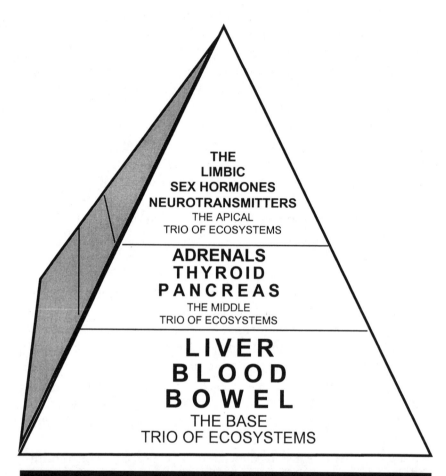

THE
LIMBIC
SEX HORMONES
NEUROTRANSMITTERS
THE APICAL
TRIO OF ECOSYSTEMS

ADRENALS
THYROID
PANCREAS
THE MIDDLE
TRIO OF ECOSYSTEMS

LIVER
BLOOD
BOWEL
THE BASE
TRIO OF ECOSYSTEMS

AGING HEALTHFULLY

THE SIXTH INSIGHT:
Oxidative Regression to Primordial Cellular Ecology
(ORPEC)

During my boyhood, I saw that some weeks our lawn was like a green velvet. During other weeks, weeds raised their ugly heads everywhere. I recognized then that our lawn contained seeds of both the grass and the weed. The condition of the soil determined whether the grass grew well or weeds overgrew the grass.

Many years later, in medical school I learned that the use of antibiotics in young women was sometimes followed by symptoms of vaginal irritation, discharge, and yeast infections. I knew that antibiotic pills do not carry yeast microbes. So where did the yeast microbes come from? Was that not the story of grass and weeds? Ecologic conditions must determine when the yeast microbes overgrew and when they didn't.

Many years later, my work with fatigue and fibromyalgia canaries led me to the study of their blood smears with a high-resolution microscope. I quickly confirmed what many holistic physicians were saying: The blood of such patients contained large numbers of white budding bodies which they designated as *Candida* organisms. Furthermore, such bodies diminished in number when patients were treated successfully with antifungal therapies. In 1994, Drs. Robert Bradford, Madhava Ramanarayanan, and Omar Ali, and I were able to stain some of those white bodies with anti-*Candida* antibodies and so established their identity with certainty.[12]

During my studies of the white bodies in the blood smears I discovered dark bodies that also occurred in large numbers, looked somewhat like blood platelets, and multiplied rapidly whenever acidity increased and oxygen levels fell under the coverslip on the slide.

I recognized then that those white and dark bodies represented many large families of microbes that hated oxygen, loved acid, and flourished on dead and dying organic matter.[6]

I introduced the term primordial life forms (PLFs) for such microbes because of their metabolic similarity to single-celled microbes that lived during the primordial era when there was no free oxygen on the planet Earth.

Next came the sixth insight. At about the time I struggled with the magnitude of the problem of PLF overgrowth in the blood of patients with serious chronic disorders, I chanced upon an important paper published in *Science*[13] that described the full genetic code of baker" yeast. It was reported that forty percent of yeast genes are identical to mammalian genes. For me, that was an eureka moment. *So, the seeds of yeast do not always have to come from without!* Those seeds are already there, as parts of the seeds of human cells. *The real issue is whether the prevailing ecologic conditions permit such seeds to grow.* That possibility flashed before me and led me to conduct an exhaustive search for evidence against such a possibility. Failing that, several months later I published my theory of oxidative regression to primordial cellular ecology (ORPEC).[6]

Essentially, the ORPEC theory was another version of the grass-weed story of my boyhood. Briefly, the ORPEC theory holds that uncontrolled oxidative injury (oxidosis) causes dysfunctional oxygen metabolism (dysoxygenosis) that leads to the creation of primordial cellular ecologic conditions in which oxygen-hating and acid-loving primordial microbes thrive on dead and dying organic matter. That represents a sharp departure from the healthful cellular conditions of normal oxygen metabolism in which PLFs cannot multiply and in which oxygen-loving, acid-hating hunter immune cells flourish and rapidly kill the primordial microbes. In other words, the human body works the same way. It also has seeds of healthy cells as well as those of disease-causing primordial life forms (PLFs). This simple fact is of enormous importance to fibro canaries as I demonstrate later in the chapter, "Oxygen and Primordial Life Forms." PLF is my term for early single-celled life forms that appeared during the primordial period in the history of the planet Earth. PLFs hate oxygen, love acids, and thrive on dead organic matter. By contrast, our healthy hunter immune cells love oxygen, hate organic acids, and are suffocated by dead and dying organic matter.

THE SEVENTH INSIGHT:
Oxidative-Dysoxygenative Dysfunction (ODD)

On hot days, my peaches spoil much more rapidly. Thus, heat *speeds up* the process of oxidation. Sometimes when an apple slips through my hands, I pick it up and look for bruises. I know the bruised skin will turn brown before the other parts of the apple's skin turn color. Bruising (the oxidative process triggered by the crushing injury) *speeds up* the process of rotting of that apple. The injury to the apple's skin quickens decay of its innards. The decaying innards quicken the rate of decomposition of the rest of the skin.

The human body also works the same way. Oxidosis triggers dysoxygenosis. Oxidosis also causes acidosis. Dysoxygenosis and acidosis, in turn, speed up the process of oxidosis. Oxidosis (accelerated oxidative molecular injury) is the primary cause of the failure of the digestive-absorptive, energy, detox, and neurotransmitter enzymes. The above simple statements permit me to state the basic concept of the ODD state in simple words: The three fibro furies (oxidosis, dysoxygenosis, and acidosis) create primordial conditions in the cells. Since human cells share many genes with primordial life forms, those genes can move in one direction under one set of conditions and in another direction under others. What separates cellular oxygen metabolism in health and in a primordial state, of course, is oxygen.

In the context of the ORPEC state, three simple facts are of great importance to all persons with serious chronic oxidative-dysoxygenative disorders, including cancer. First, primordial life forms multiply rapidly when excessive oxidative injury causes dysoxygenosis and creates primordial conditions. Second, PLFs cause microclot formation in the blood, just as adding culture to milk causes it to form curdles. Third, microclots cause dysfunctional oxygen metabolism in many ways. For the professional readers, I discuss this subject at length in *Integrative Medicine: The Principles and Practice*.

THE OXYGEN THEORY OF AGING

The basic idea of the oxygen theory of aging presented in this book is simple: The primary aging process involves *dysfunctional* oxygen metabolism (dysoxygenosis) so that cells, tissues, and body organs age because they cannot maintain normal oxygen metabolism. In this book, I introduce the terms *oxygen theory of aging* for the general readers and *dysoxygenosis theory of aging* for advanced and professional readers. The second term is more specific—and hence preferable—since it directly points to the fundamental abnormality of oxygen metabolism that is the centerpiece of my theory. However, the term oxygen theory is simpler for use by the general reader. The important point here is that the two terms are used interchangeably in this volume.

The concept of dysoxygenosis—defined as dysfunctional oxygen metabolism—evolved during my work with over 5,000 patients with chronic fatigue syndrome and fibromyalgia over a period of several years. Extensive clinical and research studies convinced me that the basic problem in those patients was *abnormal cellular* oxygen metabolism. I marshaled evidence for my view in a series of articles.[1,6-11] I introduced the term dysoxygenosis for what I believe is a serious dysfunction of *cellular* oxygen metabolism.[8,9] Those articles are reproduced in the companion volume, *Canary Two: Oxygen and Fibromyalgia.*

According to the proposed oxygen theory of aging, progressive dysoxygenosis develops in the following three phases:

1.   Oxidosis (too much oxidation);
2.   Acidosis (too much acidity);
3.   Dysoxygenosis (dysfunctional oxygen metabolism).

It is important to point out that oxidosis causes acidosis as well as dysoxygenosis. Acidosis, in turn, increases the rate of oxidation and interferes with oxygen metabolism, further increasing the degree of abnormal oxygen metabolism. Dysoxygenosis, in turn, feeds upon itself as well as fans the flames of both oxidosis and acidosis. Thus, each of the three elements feeds upon itself as well as increases the degrees of the other two.

Dysoxygenosis is not merely a lack of oxygen, the medical term for which is anoxia. The concept of dysfunctional oxygen metabolism is much broader and includes the following:

1.   Decreased availability of oxygen to cells due to impaired oxygen transport.
2.   Failure of cells to metabolize oxygen properly due to improper function of enzymes involved in oxygen metabolism.
3.   Abnormal oxygen metabolism due to accumulation of toxic organic acids due to factors included in the first two categories.

The number of individual factors included in each of the above three categories is very large. All such issues are discussed at length in various chapters of this book. In this context, I consider the chapter titled, "The History of Oxygen and Dysfunctional Oxygen Metabolism," especially valuable.

GENES AND OXYGEN THEORY

Why do I neglect the issue of genes in my oxygen theory of aging?, some readers are likely to ask. Is it not true that the human life span is genetically determined? Shouldn't that mean that we must focus on genetic research both for understanding the true nature of the aging process as well as for designing plans for reversing the aging process? Or, as is more chic these days, for anti-aging strategies? I addressed this subject in the first chapter, "The False Promise." I can reiterate my point here succinctly: All attempts to take out faulty genes (gene deletion), put in new ones to replace those that malfunction (gene insertion), or change their structure or function (gene modulation) *simply will not work for long in the presence of dysfunctional oxygen metabolism.*

ANTIOXIDANTS AND OXYGEN THEORY

Why do I neglect the issue of antioxidants in my oxygen theory of aging?, other readers might ask. If excess oxidation is the centerpiece of my theory of aging, why not focus on antioxidants? Is it not true that antioxidants can increase the human life span? Shouldn't antioxidant therapies be the mainstay of all anti-aging therapies? The answer to those questions is equally simple:

Antioxidants have limited efficacy in the presence of dysfunctional oxygen metabolism.

Indeed, if that were not true, everyone suffering from chronic fatigue syndrome and/or fibromyalgia would have been cured with antioxidants. As for the studies demonstrating longevity advantage obtained with vitamin C and other antioxidants, it is important to recognize that: (1) The observed benefits are very limited in the reported studies; and (2) The subjects included in such studies were generally healthy and without oxygen dysfunction.

The health/dis-ease/disease continuum is a spectrum of energetic-molecular events. The enormous healing potential of spiritual surrender and certain energetic phenomena is well known to all astute observers in medicine. That statement will be questioned by only those who limit their work to mechanistic aspects of illness and have little, if any, passion for the healing phenomena. However, technology sufficiently sensitive to measure subtle energy fields — and molecular and cellular resonance created in them — is not yet forthcoming. Thus, as far as observable and reproducible phenomena are concerned, in clinical medicine we are left with the molecular components of the energetic-molecular healing phenomena. In this volume, I argue that *all* molecular events that determine whether a person is healthy and ages healthfully or becomes ill and undergoes premature aging are related to oxidosis and dysoxygenosis. *Thus, the molecular basis of both the state of absence of health and premature aging is the same: dysfunctional oxygen metabolism or dysoxygenosis.* Health, by contrast, is optimal management of oxygen metabolism.

A NOTE ABOUT THE SECOND LAW OF THERMODYNAMICS

Some readers familiar with the Laws of Thermodynamics will readily see that my theory of spontaneity of oxidation and the oxygen theory of aging are direct applications of the Second Law of Thermodynamics to human health and aging. They might wonder why I do not refer to that law in presenting my theories. The answer is that I myself did not see that direct relevance when I wrote my initial monograph and some earlier papers. Perhaps I missed the lecture about the law when that was taught in college. Or, what seems more likely to me, I was in one of my frequent and serious ADD drifts when that subject was covered.

Years later, when I finally recognized that my theories were founded on the Second Law of Thermodynamics, I dug out some interesting aspects of that law. In 1824, Sadi Carnot, a French engineer, discovered the law which establishes that energy tends to turn into its degraded forms with time. His book and idea had a few takers. Not unlike most *significant* advances in science, his law was ignored for decades. In the 1850s, Rudolph Clausius, the German physicist, introduced the term entropy (derived from two Greek stems meaning "turning into") for heat dissipating (turning into) degraded forms. He famously put the first two laws of thermodynamics in two brief sentences: "The energy of the universe is constant. The entropy of the universe tends to a maximum."

The story of the First Law of Thermodynamics, which actually was discovered *after* the Second Law, is also of interest in this context. In 1842, Julius Mayer, a German surgeon, wrote: "A force once in existence cannot be annihilated." His paper was rejected by the physics journals. Disappointed but not defeated, he published his theory in a self-published pamphlet. Five years later, Hermann von Helmholtz, a German physicist and physician, propounded Mayer's law in greater detail. Apparently he was unaware of Mayer's pamphlet. His paper met the same fate as that of his predecessor. The physics journals would have none of that. He also self-published his paper as a pamphlet. (Was there a pattern?) Then followed a long period in which the credit for two of the *greatest* laws of physics went to others. In the 1860s, the record was finally set right by fair-minded John Tyndall, a history-conscious Irish physicist.[14]

References

1.   Ali M. Spontaneity of Oxidation in Nature and Aging. Monograph. 1983. Teaneck, New Jersey.
2.   Ali M. The Cortical Money and Healing, 1991, p. 18. Life Span, Denville, New Jersey.
3.   Ali M. Rats, Drugs and Assumptions, 1995, pp. 281-302. Life Span, Denville, New Jersey.
4.   Ali M. The Canary and Chronic Fatigue, Second Edition, 1994, Life Span, Denville, New Jersey.
5.   Ali M. The Altered States of Bowel Ecology and Health Preservation, Monograph, 1993, Life Span, Denville, New Jersey.
6.   Ali M. Oxidative regression to primordial cellular ecology (ORPEC): evidence for the hypothesis and its clinical significance. J Integrative Medicine 1988;2:4-55.
7.   Ali M. Spontaneity of Oxidation in Nature Is the True Cause of Aging in Humans and Root Cause of All Disease. RDA: Rats, Drugs and Assumptions. 1995, pages 199-304. Life Span Press, Denville, New Jersey.
8.   Ali M. Darwin, oxidosis, dysoxygenosis, and integration. J Integrative Medicine 1999;1:11-16.
9.   Ali M. Ali O. Fibromyalgia: an oxidative-dysoxygenative disorder (ODD) J Integrative Medicine 1999;1:17-37.
10.   Ali M, Ali O. AA oxidopathy: the core pathogenetic mechanism of

ischemic heart disease. J Integrative Medicine 1997;1:1-112.

11.   Ali M. Ascorbic acid reverses abnormal erythrocyte morphology in chronic fatigue syndrome. Am J Clin Pathol 1990;94:515.

12.   Ali M, Ali O, Bradford R. et al Immunostaining of candida organisms in peripheral smears. (Abstract). American Academy of Otolaryngic Allergy. Spring Meeting, Palm Desert, CA.

13.   Botstein D, Chervitz SA, Cherry JM. Yeast as a model organism. Science 1997;277:1259-1260.

14.   Loewenstein WR. The Touchstone of Life: Molecular Information, Cell Communication, and the Foundations of Life. 1998. Oxford University Press. Oxford. page 338.

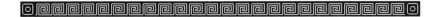

"I know that most scientific discoveries can be stated in a few words and that their demonstration requires only a small number of decisive experiments. But if one tries to find out how they came about, and if one carefully follows their development, one realizes how slowly these discoveries have come into being."

In Debre's *Louis Pasteur* (page 121)
The Johns Hopkins University Press, Baltimore, 1998.

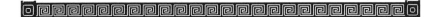

Chapter 5

The
Oxygen
Order of
Life and
Aging

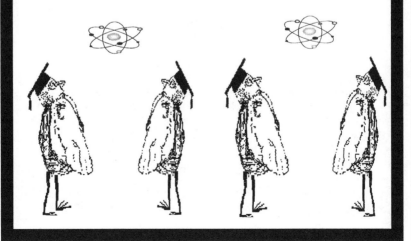

I have been a student of oxygen for over forty years. The more I study this element, the deeper its mystery becomes. I now believe that we can understand the aging process only to the degree we can understand oxygen.

Oxygen is the conductor of the orchestra of life. It is a life giver and a life exterminator. It is the ultimate spin doctor of biology. Oxygen causes cell death by its presence as well as by its absence. Oxygen is the ultimate molecular Dr. Jekyll and Mr. Hyde. It is the spark for the furnace of human metabolism. *It is the primary nutrient of life*. It is the primary detox molecule of the body. It turns poisons into harmless materials and innocent substances into poisons. Oxygen is nature's primary antibiotic. Oxygen referees the match between a hunter immune cell and a microbe. Then, it *determines* who wins that match. In the same way, it referees the match between a hunter immune cell and a cancer cell, then *determines* who wins. When needed, it becomes a hormone (by picking up an extra electron). In short, the oxygen metabolism of an individual determines the state of his health. The oxygen dysmetabolism (dysoxygenosis) leads to the continuum of the absence of health, dis-ease, disease, and death.[1-10]

The art of aging healthfully
is the art of managing oxygen metabolism.

THE SPOONMAKER'S DIAMOND

Some years ago, I saw the fabled Spoonmaker's Diamond in the museum of Topkapi Palace in Istanbul. It is a rare jewel and was one of the most coveted treasures in the Ottoman Empire. Legend has it that it was found in a dustbin by a streetsweeper. Unaware of what the dirty stone in his palm was, the streetsweeper took it to a spoonmaker, who agreed to give him a newly carved wooden spoon in return for the stone. The streetsweeper was ecstatic with the trade. Such spoons came in handy when some rich man offered free food to the poor. Also, a carved wooden spoon then was considered a prestigious possession. The spoonmaker washed the stone and was impressed by its glitter. He thought that it might be of some value and decided to visit a jeweler. The jeweler's apprentice examined the object for a few moments and knew that it was valuable. At first he pretended not to be interested, but then bought the stone for all the money he had on him. The spoonmaker left happily. When the new owner of the diamond showed his purchase to his master, the jeweler immediately recognized the rarity of the gem. He offered his apprentice a handsome profit and acquired the jewel.

When left alone, the jeweler began to polish the diamond. "Behold! It is a rare gem worthy of the Grand Vizier," he cried out as he saw its brilliance. After finishing his work of setting the big diamond in gold and arranging two rows of smaller diamonds around it, the jeweler made an appointment with the Grand Vizier of the Sultan. The Grand Vizier took one look at the rare diamond and immediately knew that a glorious diamond like that could only be part of the Sultan's private treasures. "What a great diamond for presenting to the Sultan!" he exulted. He then offered a large sum for the diamond. The jeweler was happy to receive a fortune for something that he had paid little for. Back in his palace, the Grand Vizier had the diamond wrapped in elegant red velvet and placed it on a gold plate. He then rushed to the Sultan's court in Topkapi Palace. Once in the Sultan's audience, he bowed repeatedly and then slowly unveiled the diamond. "God be praised!" the Sultan spoke in his regal tone as he lifted the diamond for a close examination. "God be praised," the throne hall resonated as the courtiers joined in unison. The Sultan stared at the diamond for several moments and then pronounced, "I have never seen a diamond this large and this unique. It will be forever a symbol of the Turkish Empire. It will always be treasured."

***

I often think of the Spoonmaker's Diamond in Topkapi Palace when I reflect on the nature of the aging process and the mysterious ways of oxygen. This Dr. Jekyll-Mr. Hyde element can be seen at many different levels just as the Spoonmaker's Diamond was. In this chapter, I describe my search for the meaning of oxygen in matters of health and healthful aging. I believe this chapter will give the readers not only a sense of how my "oxygen thinking" evolved, but will also give them a much deeper understanding of the many roles that oxygen plays in health as well as in dysfunctional oxygen metabolism that leads to premature aging.

OXYGEN: THE CONDUCTOR OF THE ORCHESTRA OF LIFE

In elementary school, I learned that I needed oxygen to live. I do not recall if I ever wondered then about what oxygen is or why it is necessary for life. In middle school, I was taught that oxygen is a colorless and odorless gas that makes up a little more than one fifth of the air I breathe. And that one atom of oxygen combines with two atoms of hydrogen to produce water. I realized oxygen is necessary both as a free gas and as a part of water. In high school, I read about experiments that showed that oxygen is necessary for things to burn. A matchstick cannot be lighted in a jar of nitrogen, and a lighted matchstick goes out as soon as it is put into such a jar. I also remember learning that when iron is exposed to oxygen it turns into iron oxide and rusts.

In college, oxygen seemed to find its way into most equations of chemistry. It was evident to me that oxygen is necessary for thousands of chemical reactions in my body as well as in nature. In medical school, I learned that my body exchanges oxygen with carbon dioxide in an amazingly complex fashion. My lungs do not merely expand to pull in air, but house a complex machinery for extracting oxygen from the air I breathe. Furthermore, my whole body participates in the gas exchange. Things seemed to become ever more complex in medical school, and certainly oxygen had its growing share of things to do in that complexity. A few more lessons in physiology and I recognized that oxygen was essential for *all* of my metabolic functions.

As a freshly minted doctor doing his emergency room rotation, I learned that the easiest way to avoid criticism in the care of accident victims was to begin oxygen therapy. Oxygen comes in handy for junior doctors. Accident victims are hard to evaluate when they first land in emergency rooms. The senior doctors who visit such patients after the initial care always seem wiser, simply because there has been more time for the injured to fully reveal their injuries. Thus, junior doctors are easy targets for the senior ones, especially when the older ones have no better way of claiming superiority. If things go well for the patient, young doctors who give oxygen to the accident victim are merely smiled at as simpletons overreacting to the situation. If things turn sour, the act of administering oxygen is seen as commendable vigilance and promptness in recognizing a serious situation. Thus, I learned to look at the oxygen cylinder as my guardian angel in the emergency department. And, of course, the accident victims receiving oxygen come out ahead either way.

As a young house surgeon in training in Pakistan, I learned about other ways oxygen gets young doctors-in-training into trouble with older surgeons. Many of my patients were nutritionally deficient. Others were anemic. Such patients do not heal surgical wounds well. Those conditions also stress the heart during surgery. Thus, episodes of rapid heart rate, skipped heartbeats, and rhythm disturbances were not uncommon in the operating room. Then there was the ominous threat of a cardiac arrest on the operating table. The management of all factors that lead to such complications was considered to be the responsibility of the house surgeon. Thus, junior surgeons were held responsible for all poor surgical outcomes. Years later, I recognized the hand of oxygen in *all* surgical complications, except when the operating surgeon cut the wrong tissues and couldn't hide that fact from anyone. Early on during my surgical training, I made two observations: (1) Older surgeons were *always* right; and (2) When surgical complications developed, it was always the fault of the younger surgeons-in-training. Years later, I made a third observation: Oxygen was the nemesis of the poor surgeon-in-training.

OXYGEN IS UNFORGIVING

As a pathologist, I had a rude awakening. While in surgery I saw the lack of oxygen as an ever-present threat to the patient, in pathology I began to see the other face of oxygen. I performed autopsies on patients who had been on respirators in our intensive care unit who had been given oxygen for days. There I saw unmistakable evidence of oxygen toxicity. Their lungs were dark, heavy, and hard to compress. It was not simply a matter of excess fluid or blood in the lungs. The lung tissue had lost its elasticity. My microscope revealed the cause: I observed thick layers of protein deposits on the inner lining of the air sacs, blocking air exchange. The patients had been literally choked to death. I knew that such deposits had formed when oxygen had oxidized and denatured proteins in the lung tissue. I think it was then that I first told myself that oxygen is a molecular Dr. Jekyll and Mr. Hyde (sometime in the late 1960s, nearly fifteen years before I published my first monograph about the molecular duality of oxygen in 1983).

Years earlier, I had read in my textbooks about newborns who had been blinded by oxygen. That type of blindness occurs when excess oxygen stimulates overproduction of collagen by a type of cell called a fibroblast and is termed retrolental fibroplasia. The newborns affected by such blindness had been given pure oxygen. That was before anybody had suspected that oxygen could be toxic to the delicate eye tissues of the newborn. Peering through my microscope at the lung tissue and recalling the descriptions of blinding oxygen toxicity in premature newborns, I recognized that *oxygen is unforgiving.*

ENVIRONMENTAL MEDICINE IS ALL ABOUT NUTRITION AND NUTRITIONAL MEDICINE IS ALL ABOUT OXYGEN

My view of oxygen changed once again when I began the practice of environmental medicine. There were two important issues:

First, patients with environmental illness react to minute amounts of chemicals that others tolerate without any symptoms. So it seemed obvious to me that I should look into their detox chemistry. How does the body detoxify itself? Of course, it utilizes nutrients to trap, degrade, or otherwise neutralize chemicals. So I recognized that the chemistry of detox is the chemistry of nutrition.

The second obvious thing was to ask my friends about therapies they employed for their patients with environmental illness. The answer was nutrients, especially those that play important detox roles, such as vitamin B complex and C, glutathione, coenzyme Q10, N-acetylcysteine, minerals (such as magnesium and zinc), taurine, and others. What is in common among those nutrients?, I asked. The answer was quite obvious: All those nutrients were directly or indirectly involved with fighting excess oxidative stress.

So I realized that environmental medicine is in reality nutritional medicine. Recognition and avoidance of environmental triggers were primarily things the patients had to do themselves.

Many of my patients with environmental sensitivity looked very well and had no known lung disease, and yet experienced persistent air hunger. They insisted they felt oxygen-starved even though their skin color looked healthy and their pulmonologists had reassured them that all lung function tests were normal. What's this mystery?, I wondered. There is no recognizable lung disease, anemia, heart disease, or cellular poisoning. Then why this oxygen starvation?, I asked myself, with growing frustration.

Next came my research with fatigue and fibro canaries. The more I listened to them describe their suffering, and the more I studied their blood samples with my microscope or with chemistry analyzers, the more clearly I saw their *two basic* problems: (1) Their enzyme and immune defenses were shattered by excess oxidative injury; and (2) Their symptoms could be explained only by understanding their dysfunctional oxygen metabolism.

Through their suffering, my fatigue and fibro canaries began to give me yet new insights into the many seemingly contradictory roles of oxygen. It was then that I began to see the essential oxygen order of human biology. The more I searched for the Dr. Jekyll-Mr. Hyde roles of oxygen, the more varied such roles became. I recognized that oxygen determines who wins the battle between man and the primordial microbe. A primordial microbe (an anaerobic bacteria is an example) hates oxygen and loves excess acidity. It also thrives on many organic acids that are highly toxic to human immune and other cells. A primordial microbe also feeds well on cellular debris. By contrast, an immune cell loves oxygen and hates excess acidity. Many organic acids damage immune cells. Finally, cellular debris suffocates healthy cells. This subject is of crucial importance for understanding fibromyalgia. I discuss this at length in the chapter, "Oxygen and Primordial Life Forms."

Many of my patients with cancer also suffer severe fatigue. I recognized that oxygen determines who wins the battle between a cancer cell and an immune cell. A cancer cell hates oxygen and loves excess acidity. It also thrives on many organic acids that are highly toxic to human immune and other cells. A cancer cell also feeds well on cellular debris. As I wrote earlier, an immune cell loves oxygen and hates excess acidity. Many organic acids damage immune cells. Finally, cellular debris suffocates healthy cells. So a cancer cell and a primordial microbe had similar metabolism, and the central figure in both is dysfunctional oxygen metabolism.

My work with patients with neurologic disorders, such as Alzheimer's disease, Parkinsonism, multiple sclerosis, and others led me to conclude that dysfunctional oxygenation and oxidation were the primary mechanisms of brain and nerve cell injury in those mechanisms. Those and my earlier clinical and experimental findings led me to propose my theory that *all disease processes are caused by excessive oxidative injury*. I devoted a large section of *RDA: Rats, Drugs and Assumptions* to this theory and cited a large number of studies to support my view.

Sometime during those years, I read an article entitled, "Did radicals strike Lou Gehrig?" published in *Nature*.[11] It cited a report firmly linking Lou Gehrig's disease with a defect in the SOD1 (superoxide dismutase 1) gene which is responsible for saving brain cells from toxicity of reactive oxygen (superoxide). (Another famous victim of that disease is the famous British physicist, Stephen Hawking.) It also explained how brain cell injury caused by *lack* of oxygen causes overstimulation of a neurotransmitter called glutamate. How amazing! I wondered out loud. In how many other diseases does oxygen injure tissues *both by its presence as well as its absence*?

Oxygen picks up an extra electron and turns into superoxide.
In that highly reactive form, oxygen can:

     A.   *Act as an oxidant.*
     B.   *Act as an antioxidant.*
     C.   *Beget many other oxidant molecules.*

Such is the mind-numbing mystery of oxygen!

That a superoxide can function as an antioxidant, I am certain, will surprise most people. Indeed, it may even stretch the credibility of many scientists with considerable knowledge of free radical chemistry. I ask them to consider the following quote from *Nature*:

Although O2- (superoxide) was previously known as a product of the radiolysis of oxygenated water, it is now understood to be a common product of both spontaneous and enzyme-catalyzed oxidations. It is chemically active both as a reductant and as anoxidant.[11]

Finally, I recognized that the *metabolism of oxygen is fundamentally abnormal* in fibro and fatigue canaries. To write about this subject, I introduced the term dysoxygenosis for the professional readers and dysfunctional oxygen metabolism for the general readers.

Though the three volumes of my oxygen trilogy are devoted to aspects of oxygen (as well as oxidosis), the lessons learned from my fibro and fatigue canaries are equally important for patients with cancer, immune disorders (such as lupus and multiple sclerosis), and degenerative diseases (such as heart disease, Alzheimer's disease, and kidney failure).

In the following pages, I include some passages from my original article about molecular duality of oxygen and spontaneity of oxidation published in 1983[1] as well as from my expanded discussion of those subjects in *RDA: Rats, Drugs and Assumptions.*[9] I ask the readers to accept some repetition in the interest of clarity. A full comprehension of the basic scientific facts concerning Dr. Jekyll-Mr. Hyde roles of oxygen in health and disease is essential for understanding my theory as well as the scientific basis of therapies I recommend. The same is true of the subject of spontaneity of oxidation as the primary mechanism of cell injury. For the advanced and professional readers, I suggest the second volume of this book, which contains seven articles originally published in *The Journal of Integrative Medicine.* For additional reading, I suggest some of my other publications cited at the end of this chapter.[1-10,12-15]

THE OXYGEN ORDER OF HUMAN LIFE

An oxygen order governs human life. In this order, oxygen provides the basic drive for human biology. The basis of life is energy, and the basis of energy in humans is oxygen. (Other forms of energy undoubtedly influence human health, but technology for measuring such energy dynamics is not yet available.) Oxygen is the currency of life. It provides the spark for all metabolic fires. It initiates and regulates all digestive-absorptive, energy, and detoxification enzyme pathways.

Oxygen drives human metabolism. It is essential for building substances in the body. It is also necessary for breaking them down. Oxygen drives digestion in the gut and detox enzymes in the liver. It allows brain cells to talk to each other. It is also a primary communication molecule in the rest of the body. It also serves as a hormone.

Oxygen is nature's primary antibiotic. Oxygen is the weapon used by the immune system to kill bacteria, viruses, yeasts, and parasites. The mechanisms used by the hunter immune cells to immobilize, capture, kill, and digest microbes (as their food) are *all* triggered and maintained by oxygen-related biochemical events. For example, when a hunter immune cell (phagocyte) comes in contact with a microbe, it releases reactive (nascent) oxygen, which directly oxidizes the components of the microbial surface and kills it.

Oxygen is a powerful oxidant. Butter left on the kitchen table turns rancid. That is because oxygen in the air oxidizes and denatures its fatty acids. Flowers on a window sill wilt—that is also oxidation. Cut grass decomposes—that involves the same chemical process. Many years ago, I looked down at the Grand Canyon and saw layers of red rock. I then realized that centuries earlier oxygen in the air had oxidized the iron in the rock into red-colored iron oxide.

A woman becomes blind with cataracts. That happens when the clear protein in the lens of the eye is oxidized into an opaque gray-white substance. Her skin wrinkles with age. That occurs due to damage to collagen proteins in the skin caused by oxygen. Many persons die of a sudden heart attack. This happens when coronary arteries go into spasm and choke the heart muscle, or plaques in the arteries rupture and cause sudden blockage. Both conditions occur due to damage caused by oxidative stress which, in turn, is triggered by oxygen, in some direct and many indirect ways. I can go on citing one such example after another, but my point is simply this: I see the hand of oxygen behind *all* cellular injury. This basic scheme of things in nature repeatedly appears in this book as I discuss in greater detail the various patterns of oxidative injury to the various ecosystems of the body, especially those of the bowel, blood, and liver ecologies. For additional information, I recommend to the readers *RDA: Rats, Drugs and Assumptions,* a large part of which is devoted to this subject.

OXYGEN: THE MOST VERSATILE
DR. JEKYLL AND MR. HYDE

Oxygen is the angel of life. Oxygen is the messenger of death. Health is a balance between the good and bad roles of oxygen. Dis-ease and disease are caused when the health-giving role of oxygen is dominated by its dis-ease-causing role. The more I have pursued the study of oxygen, the more oxygen has become like the Spoonmaker's Diamond.

It is common knowledge that we use oxygen to burn the calories in our food to release energy for our life processes. Rarely do we appreciate that *the process by which oxygen breaks down food is exactly the same by which oxygen breaks down our tissues and causes us to age and finally die.* Oxygen sustains life. Oxygen degrades life.

It is also common knowledge that we cannot live without breathing oxygen in the air. If denied air for more than five minutes (as in drowning), a person dies. So we recognize that oxygen is essential for life. We usually do not realize that oxygen is also a killer molecule. Pure oxygen is highly toxic. I cite earlier the cases of oxygen toxicity in ICU patients as well as in newborns blinded by pure oxygen.

There are many molecular Dr. Jekylls (that promote healing) and Mr. Hydes (that interfere with healing) in human biology. For example, iron is a molecular Dr. Jekyll. Oxygen in the blood is carried by a protein called hemoglobin. Anemia is a condition of hemoglobin deficiency, which causes the skin and eyes to look pale and is a cause of fatigue. Anemia in an extreme form is also a recognized cause of heart failure. Iron is essential for production of hemoglobin. Another important function of iron among its many Dr. Jekyll roles is its part in the liver detoxification as a component of several essential enzymes, including the all-important cytochrome oxidase system. Without iron, the adrenal glands cannot produce their hormones.

Iron is also a molecular Mr. Hyde. When present in excess, it causes serious cellular injury and leads to heart failure. Other problems caused by too much iron are diabetes (injury to pancreas), liver scarring, and adrenal gland failure. I might add here that nature has provided the human body with a shield for the iron dagger. It is a protein called transferrin, which keeps the iron dagger "covered" until it is needed for production of hemoglobin and essential enzymes. Thus, the body can keep adequate iron stores without being cut up by the iron dagger itself.

Copper is another Dr. Jekyll-Mr. Hyde mineral. It is also an essential component of several important enzymes. And as in the case of iron, excess copper causes cellular injury, including liver cirrhosis. Nitric oxide and the family of endothelins are substances that regulate blood flow. Both are good examples of molecular Dr. Jekylls and Mr. Hydes. Indeed, the more I reflect on the molecular duality of substances in the body, the more I am mystified by nature's sense of economy. Everywhere I look, I see the same basic design.

The essential point I want to make here is this: *Oxygen is the most versatile Dr. Jekyll and Mr. Hyde.* This must be clearly understood by all fibro and fatigue canaries for the following three reasons:

1. The basic oxidative-dysoxygenative nature of common chronic disorders can be understood only through a good working knowledge of the many Dr. Jekyll-Mr. Hyde roles of oxygen.
2. All symptoms of the human canaries are caused by dysfunctional oxygen metabolism, which can be understood only through an understanding of the many Dr. Jekyll-Mr. Hyde roles of oxygen.
3. Effective treatment plans for recovery from common chronic disorders must also be based on an understanding of the many Dr. Jekyll-Mr. Hyde roles of oxygen.

The last-mentioned reason becomes fully evident in the chapters devoted to treatment plans for reversal of fibromyalgia.

OXYGEN: AN ACCOMPLISHED MOLECULAR CHAMELEON

Dr. Jekyll-oxygen is a life-giver molecule. When two atoms of oxygen are linked together with a *full* number of electrons in their orbits, it is called molecular oxygen. This form of oxygen is the safe form of oxygen that we breathe. It makes up one fifth of the air and provides just the right spark to ignite the needed (healthful) fires of physiologic metabolism. For me it is one of the most profound mysteries in nature that oxygen seems to understand this role so well and plays it with such astounding efficiency. Except when studying oxygen in a classroom, no one ever seems to be conscious of its existence. It is different for fibro and fatigue canaries. They *know* what air hunger and oxygen starvation is all about.

Oxygen is also a killer molecule. Mr. Hyde-oxygen is toxic oxygen—a reactive (nascent), atomic, and dangerous toxic oxygen that kills life. The main health hazard we face today is this: Most of our technology is rapidly turning safe, life-sustaining oxygen into a toxic life-threatening form. It is ironic that to solve the health problems caused by toxic oxygen (and related toxic oxidants), we use drugs that further increase oxidative injury. Oxidant molecules are like little matches, ready to set things on fire when lit. A little match can burn the whole forest. How? It is ignited by oxygen, and the oxyradical formation triggered by this process perpetuates the process of burning.

Nature designed life-span antioxidant molecules to provide a counterbalance to the oxidant molecules. These molecules prevent ignition by oxygen and hold in check other types of oxidant molecules. Living things generate these molecules so they can save themselves from immediate destruction by oxidant molecules.

Life is self-sustaining. Life is lethal. This *is* the fundamental paradox of all considerations of health and disease. At the risk of annoying some readers, I approach this paradox from many angles because that simply must be done if anyone is to understand oxygen. Without *knowing* oxygen, no fibro canary can hope to understand dysfunctional oxygen metabolism. And without *knowing* dysfunctional oxygen metabolism, no canary can hope to understand the true nature of his/her suffering.

OXYGEN: THE ULTIMATE SPIN DOCTOR

Molecular oxygen has an interesting "love-hate" relationship with electrons. It avidly picks up free electrons in its vicinity, then just as avidly spins them out. During the production of ATP, the basic energy molecule of the body (in a process called oxidative phosphorylation), the safe molecular oxygen steals an electron and becomes an unsafe free radical called superoxide. *Note that safe Dr. Jekyll-oxygen turns into the unsafe Mr. Hyde-oxygen in the same process that sustains life, i.e., production of ATP.*

Next, an equally amazing event takes place. The unsafe superoxide spins out extra electrons spontaneously, turning back into the safe oxygen, and begins its eternal spin cycle again. However, this ultimate spin doctor does something else while it spins that electron: It triggers a domino effect called free radical chain reactions. In that wave of electron shuffle, electrons spun by oxygen tear into every molecule in their way. They oxidize sugars, proteins, and fats. At each oxidative step, those sources of energy are broken down to release energy contained in them, a process called digestion. Those are the Dr. Jekyll sides.

But we know Dr. Jekylls cannot exist except in the company of Mr. Hydes. So who are the Mr. Hydes unleashed along the way? They are the highly toxic aldehydes from sugars, reactive radicals from proteins, and fat peroxides. Other ever-present free radicals unleashed by the grand spin master include single oxygen and hydrogen peroxide. Nature also came up with first-line antioxidant defenses against the mischief mongers in the form of superoxide dismutase, catalase, and glutathione peroxidase. The second-line defenses include antioxidants such as vitamins C and E, taurine, coenzyme Q10, lipoic acid, and others. The ultimate spin doctor has tricks yet up its sleeve. Recall, it is a killer molecule whose ultimate purpose is to recycle life. *No one must be allowed to live forever*, that's the grand design of this spin doctor. So what does it do? It slowly robs the living being of its enzymes. Each time it does its spin thing, a part of some enzyme dies somewhere.

OXYGEN TRIGGERS CELL DEATH
ABSENCE OF OXYGEN TRIGGERS CELL DEATH

In dog experiments, clamping of the main artery to the lungs cuts off the blood and oxygen supply to the tissue. If the clamp is not released within minutes, serious cell injury and the death of tissues occur due to lack of oxygen, called anoxia in medical terminology. Anoxia causes tissue injury by unleashing a huge number of free radicals. What is not so well known is that if the clamp is removed before tissue death occurs, tests show a markedly increased free radical activity. In other words, oxygen increases free radical injury and tissue injury both by its lack as well as its presence.[16-19]

Oxygen is oxidizing, hence it is expected to be toxic when present in higher concentrations. Amazingly, oxygen is also oxidizing when present in lower than physiologic concentrations. Those two faces of oxygen make another fascinating duality of this spin master. This is not fully appreciated by most doctors, who think of anoxia only in acutely ill patients with advanced diseases of the heart and lung. They seldom, if ever, think in terms of the abnormal oxygen metabolism in chronically ill persons. This, in my view, is one of the reasons why dysfunctional oxygen metabolism is ignored by mainstream doctors in managing fibromyalgia, chronic fatigue, and other chronic disorders. (The main reason, of course, is that most of them do not learn anything about oxygen unless it is about patients in intensive care units.)

That the lack of oxygen in cells directly leads to oxidosis may seem counterintuitive to some. That should not be so. It is well known that cellular anoxia leads to excessive production of lactic acid and many related organic acids, some of which directly poison enzymes that regulate oxygen metabolism. Excess acidity (acidosis) caused by accumulation of lactic acid and its related organic acids further increases oxidative stress on cells. Anoxia also damages cell membrane channels, causing oxidative leaky cell membrane states in which excess calcium accumulates in the cells. Calcium in excess directly kills cells by triggering a process of death called apoptosis.

Lower than physiologic concentrations of oxygen activate many genes to produce strongly oxidizing substances which further fan the oxidative fires. There is also evidence that lack of oxygen also results in damage to DNA and is another way oxidative mechanisms may be triggered. I believe these issues of oxidative mutation of genes and oxidative dysfunctional genetics will be the subject of vigorous research in the near future, which will strongly support the oxidative-dysoxygenative dysfunction (ODD) hypothesis which I put forth last year[14] and which I describe at length in this book.

OXYGEN AND THE BIG YELLOW BALL

Sunlight supports all life on the planet Earth. What would happen if all the heat of sunlight were to reach the Earth's surface all at once? Every living being would be instantaneously scorched. Sunlight sprouts seeds. Sunlight, when not tempered by rain, also burns plants. So the energy of the big yellow ball up above sustains life in one way and exterminates it in another.

Gasoline fuels an automobile. What would happen if all the fuel in a car were to get ignited all at once? The car would go up in flames. That is why a carburetor is built into an automobile engine to regulate the entry of the mixture of gasoline and air into its combustion chamber. So gasoline, like the sun, moves a car one way and can burn it down in another.

The above observations about the energies of sunlight and gasoline raise another fundamental question about oxygen. Oxygen brings forth delicate life. Without oxygen we cannot digest and absorb foods, nor can we "burn" foods to produce energy for life functions. But oxygen is also a ruthless oxidative monster that has no respect for life. In a dry season, a fire started by lightning can burn down thousands of acres of a forest. That happens because oxygen in the air feeds the fire sparked by lightning, and the fire so begun feeds the frenzy of oxidation triggered by oxygen. So oxygen, like the big yellow ball in the sky and gasoline in a car tank, nurtures life one way and terminates it another. How does oxygen do that?

How does oxygen save us from its own fire as well as the fires it ignites to break down foods we eat? At a more basic level, how does oxygen regulate itself? This is a *core* question in our search for the cause of dysfunctional oxygen metabolism. I repeat that it is only through a clear understanding of dysfunctional oxygen metabolism that we can understand fibromyalgia and the suffering of fibro canaries. To unravel those secrets, we need to understand the energy systems of another kind of yellow ball, the citric acid "ball" of human metabolism. In scientific terminology, this ball is called Krebs' cycle (or citric acid cycle) of energy enzymes that break down sugars, proteins, and fats to release energy. It is this yellow citrus ball spun by oxygen that regulates the even release of energy for cell functions, not too fast to burn them, not too slow to cause energy depletion and fatigue.

**One important cause of dysfunctional oxygen
metabolism in fibromyalgia is the malfunctioning
of the yellow ball of the citric acid cycle spun by
oxygen. Disabling fatigue, unending pain, brain
fog, and other fibro symptoms develop when
tissues starve for oxygen.**

THE TAMING OF THE OXYGEN-SHREW

The many mischiefs of oxygen should be evident to the reader
by now. How do cells tame this shrew? It turns out that oxygen is one
shrew that can be tamed only by itself. In this taming is hidden
another important clue to understanding the debilitating fatigue of
fibro and fatigue canaries.

Two things should be obvious from my discussion of oxygen
so far. First, that oxygen is temperamental, often explosive, and plays
many different Dr. Jekyll-Mr. Hyde roles. Second, that it is the
currency of human biology. That creates an obvious problem. For a
healthy economy, a currency must be stable and dependable. How
can an unpredictable and explosive substance like oxygen serve as the
currency of life? The answer to that question reveals yet another
mystery of oxygen and gives us another window to understanding
dysfunctional oxygen metabolism in fibromyalgia. How does oxygen
do all that? That was another of many oxygen riddles that
preoccupied me for some time.

One day I stood before a statue of Zeus seducing Lydia at the Metropolitan Museum of Art in New York City. Mesmerized by the stunning beauty of the statute, it seemed to me that the ancient Greeks had an answer for everything. Could it be that they also had an answer for my oxygen riddle as well? It occurred to me those Greeks must have understood oxygen well. How else could they create Zeus, their supergod, so perfectly in its image?

Zeus suffered from attention deficit and hyperactivity syndrome. Like oxygen, Zeus was a Dr. Jekyll-Mr. Hyde without peer among the Olympian immortals. He was well known for throwing unprovoked temper tantrums, just like oxygen. He struck hapless mortals with his thunderbolt, often without knowing why he did so. He was promiscuous. He tried to make love to everything that moved, again just like oxygen. Who could have been the role model for Zeus?, I wondered. Oxygen alone, I recognized, could have been his inspiration. In the museum statue, Zeus climbed Lydia in the form of a swan. He often turned himself into animal forms to escape the notice of Hera, his wife, during his sexual escapades. (Looking at Zeus' swan, my mind drifted to two recent young American presidents who also had the same inclinations. Who was the role model of those lustful presidents, Zeus or oxygen?, I wondered.)

So, how does oxygen keep peace and incite riots of free radicals at the same time? The statue of the swan gave me the answer. Zeus begot Athena, the goddess of wisdom. Athena, we are told, gave the Greeks their sense of order and civility. Athena, we are also told, had a way with Zeus, just as many cool and collected daughters have with their volatile dads. She knew how to pacify her old man. So far, so good. But, how did the Greeks figure that out? In whose image did those clever Greeks create goddess Athena?, I wondered. Enter ATP.

The Greeks created their benevolent and impetuous supergod Zeus in oxygen's image. Then they created the wise Athena in ATP's image. "I am on to your clever little game," I chuckled aloud at my insight, standing before the swan Zeus. "Oxygen begot ATP, just as Zeus begot Athena. Then ATP tames oxygen, just as Athena tamed Zeus. Neat stuff! Your ATP's Athena was the answer to the shenanigans of your oxygen's Zeus. You hid the answer to the volatile unpredictability of the dad in the wisdom and dependability of the daughter. Makes sense, doesn't it?" I had my answer. The swan had unraveled that oxygen riddle. ATP is the answer. This prime energy molecule conducts all energy transactions in the cells, but does so without any of oxygen's volatility.

ATP AND CELLULAR ENERGETICS

ATP is a high-energy substance present in all cells. It releases a large quantity of free energy (12,000 calories per mole under physiologic conditions) to drive nearly all reactions in the cells, including the following:

1.   ATP energizes the production of the various substances in the cells. That is important to fibro canaries because they are so often deficient in: (a) enzymes, protective antibodies, and other proteins; (b) essential oils; (c) neurotransmitters; (d) antioxidants; (e) detox molecules; and (f) many other substances.

2.   ATP energizes muscles to contract so that the heart can beat and the muscles in the arms, legs, and the bowel can move those body parts. That is important to fibro canaries because

they so often have severe fatigue, muscle weakness, and heart rhythm problems.

3.   ATP energizes transport of digested food substances across the membranes of cells lining the gut. That is important to fibro canaries because they so often have severe digestive-absorptive problems.

4.   ATP energizes transport of substances across the membranes of cells in other parts of the body, including those in the liver and the kidney. That is important to fibro canaries because they so often have oxidative leaky cell membrane dysfunction. That leads to hemorrhage of nutrients from inside the cells, such as of magnesium, potassium, taurine, and other essential healthful substances. That also causes flooding of cell innards by undesirable substances, such as excess calcium that triggers cell death. That explains why the fibro canaries suffer from so many nutritional deficiencies and weakness.

5.   ATP energizes glands to produce their secretions. That is important to fibro canaries because they so often have severe dryness of eyes, mouth, and vaginal tract.

ATP is composed of a sugar (5-carbon ring ribose), a nitrogen base (adenine), and three phosphate groups. The phosphate groups (called radicals in chemistry) are attached to the rest of the molecule by *high-energy bonds*. Oxygen produces ATP through metabolism of starches and sugars, proteins, and fats. For example, thirty-eight molecules of ATP are produced when each molecule of glucose is broken down to carbon dioxide and water. The following is the breakdown of such ATP production:

1.   Two molecules are produced during glycolysis, a process by which oxygen turns one molecule of glucose into two

molecules of pyruvate. Many readers will recall that pyruvate has made quite a few headlines in recent years.

2.   Two molecules are produced in the Krebs cycle (the oxygen-driven yellow citric acid ball) as pyruvate is broken down to carbon dioxide and water.

3.   Thirty-four molecules are formed when hydrogen produced during the above two reactions is oxidized (a process called oxidative phosphorylation).

OXYGEN IN A RING-AROUND-THE ROSIE

Some amazing things happen when three atoms of oxygen dance together, like three little girls holding each other's hands in ring-around-the-rosie. Those familiar with Italian art may see that as the three muses in Botticelli's *Primavera*. Oxygen atoms dancing in threesomes (ozone in common language) have the potential of both seriously threatening human health as well as saving lives of the very sick. Such is the mystery of oxygen in a ring-around-the-rosie!

Ozone is a good player. Ozone is a bad player. I read articles published by public health officials warning readers about the dangers of rising levels of ozone in smog. They write about ozone toxicity and consider it as one of the important factors in the rising incidence of lung disorders, including asthma, in polluted cities. That makes ozone bad. Then I hear scientists on TV forecasting doom because there is not enough ozone up in the sky. They show maps of gaping holes in the ozone layer. They teach us that ozone in the sky protects us from cancer-causing ultraviolet rays in sunlight, and that we get skin cancer when holes in the ozone layer fail to block those rays. That makes ozone a good player. Many people do not seem to realize that ozone in pure form and ozone mixed with pollutants behave differently. (Furthermore, the ozone layer in the stratosphere has a different impact on humans than that on a beach.)

Ozone is an oxidant. Ozone is an antioxidant. "Of course, ozone is an oxidant. That's basic chemistry," the chemists chime, in supporting drug doctors. "Don't those quacks who inject ozone into the blood understand something that simple? Doesn't everyone know we need antioxidants such as vitamin C and E to protect our tissues from oxidative injury? Don't they know anything about science?" That shows ozone is an oxidant. "Yes, ozone is an oxidant in a test tube," the ozone therapists refuse to yield. "The point is that ozone works for the chronically ill, whether it is oxidant or antioxidant." So the proponents of ozone therapy are steadfast in their defense of the empirical value of their chosen therapy.

For several years, I sided with the chemists on the above issue. How could I reject established chemistry? So I stayed clear of ozone and hydrogen peroxide therapies. But then I conducted some other experiments and, to my great surprise, found that ozone and hydrogen peroxide serve as *antioxidant therapies* in patients with fibromyalgia and CFS, even though both substances are potent oxidants in a test tube. This phenomenon thus demonstrates another aspect of the amazing dual roles of oxygen. In 1998, I published my observations about the apparent paradox of an in vitro (in the laboratory) oxidant serving as a powerful in vivo (in the body) antioxidant therapy in fibromyalgia and chronic fatigue syndrome in *The Journal of Integrative Medicine*.[12] The abstract of that paper is included in the appendix of this book, and the full article is included in the companion volume, *Canary Three: Fibromyalgia Is an Oxidative-Dysoxygenative Disorder (ODD).*

Ozone is a dangerous gas. Ozone is a safe gas. I see most mainstream doctors cringe when they hear about intravenous injections of ozone. They imagine patients collapsing with strokes as bubbles of the gas block small blood vessels in their brains. "How can anyone can be that stupid to inject a toxic gas straight into the blood of a living person?," they ask with indignation. That makes ozone a dangerous gas. "Ozone is *safe*," ozone therapists counter. "Why don't those closed-minded drug doctors simply talk to patients who receive ozone therapy? They will find out that no one keels over after an ozone infusion." That makes ozone a safe gas to inject.

Years ago, I was curious about that controversy. So I thought of a simple experiment and conducted it several times. Immediately after injecting ozone into a vein, I pulled on the plunger of the syringe. What I got back was bright red ozonated blood, not dark vein blood with gas bubbles trapped in it. I found out that ozone diffuses rapidly into the blood and cannot lead to gas bubbles trapped in blood vessels in the brain, or for that matter anywhere else.

Ozone is a useless therapy. Ozone is a valuable therapy. "There is no known scientific evidence that ozone works for anything. If there was any evidence, why wouldn't *The New England Journal of Medicine* publish such evidence?," the drugs doctors tell their patients. That makes ozone therapy quackery. "The scientific evidence of efficacy is not known to *you* because *you* are ignorant of holistic literature," the ozone therapists respond with sarcasm. "There are hundreds of published papers that demonstrate the many clinical benefits of ozone therapies. Why don't you read those papers?" That makes ozone useful.

My personal experience supports ozone therapists. Ozone gives me positive results in the majority of the patients for whom I use that therapy.

Ozone is a toxic free radical. Ozone enhances tissue oxygenation. "Ozone is a powerful free radical," the professors teach medical students. "Free radicals lacerate every living thing in their way. Why would anyone ever damage circulating blood by putting into it a powerful free radical such as ozone? How can twenty, thirty or fifty milliliters of ozone improve oxygen supply to tissues that receive 5,000 or so milliliters of blood *every* minute?," they ask with patronizing smiles. That makes ozone a sharp dagger. "Silly professor stuff!," the ozone therapists hit back. "Why don't those professors simply try it and find for themselves whether or not ozone works? Why don't they get off their high horses and for once do some honest work? Ozone works. We know that. Our patients know that. Those professors can do that as well if only they were serious enough to test ozone therapy." That makes ozone an oxygenator.

Many, but not all, of my patients tell me that ozone therapy lifts their brain fog and they can think clearly. Of course, ozone alone does not cure anything. This is one of the explanations of the paradox of oxidant ozone serving as antioxidant therapy. By improving tissue oxygenation, ozone diminishes oxidosis.

Ozone tightens arteries. Ozone opens up arteries. "Ozone is an irritant, and irritants cause arteries to tighten up, not open up," the academics weigh in the debate. That makes ozone a vasoconstrictor. "Nonsense!" cry out ozone therapists in rebuttal. "Ozone commonly creates a flush effect if given rapidly. That indicates opening up of blood vessels, and not tightening them up." That makes ozone a vasodilator. Many of my patients report a desirable sense of warmth in their tissues after ozone therapy. This is another explanation of the paradox of oxidant ozone serving as antioxidant therapy. By improving tissue blood supply, ozone counters anoxia and oxidosis.

Ozone is useless for viral infections. Ozone is an effective antiviral therapy. "Ozone may have some antiviral activity in a test tube, but it has not been proven effective clinically," the drug doctors argue. When using that argument, they seem not to be troubled by the fact that there they reverse themselves and speak against their laboratory findings. Taken at its face value, that makes ozone useless for viral infections. "Come and we will show you falling viral counts after ozone therapy," the ozone folks challenge. That makes ozone an effective antiviral agent. Of course, drug doctors consider it beneath their dignity to study the clinical histories of patients of ozone therapists.

I see significant drops in the viral counts of my patients with HIV and hepatitis infections after treatment with ozone and/or hydrogen peroxide infusions. This is yet another explanation of the paradox of oxidant ozone serving as antioxidant therapy. Viruses cause cellular injury by causing oxidative cell membrane injury. By reducing the viral load, ozone counters oxidosis.

Ozone is worthless for wounds. Ozone is good for wound healing. Ozone is ineffective for severe immune disorders. Ozone is beneficial in treatment of such disorders, including lupus, multiple sclerosis, vasculitis, and others. Ozone is voodoo treatment for cancer. Ozone is a good therapy to include in a program for controlling cancer. Those controversies have raged for decades.

My view of those debates is this: The academics are right in pure theory. The ozone therapists are right in empirical observations. The trick, of course, is to figure out how oxygen in a ring-around-the-rosie does so many seemingly contradictory things. Ozone rapidly turns into hydrogen peroxide which, in turn, brings to life (turns on) many antioxidant enzyme systems.[20-22] So it is that what I write above for ozone is also true of hydrogen peroxide. Again, I refer the advanced and professional readers to my in-depth discussion of the paradoxical effects of ozone and hydrogen peroxide in *Canary Three: Fibromyalgia Is an Oxidative-Dysoxygenative Disorder (ODD)*.

OXYGEN, OXIDOSIS, AND IMPAIRED CELL ENERGETICS

Many factors in modern life threaten cell energetics and set the stage for illness. *All* such factors do so by causing oxidosis, which interferes with cellular oxygen and the myriad Dr. Jekyll-Mr. Hyde roles of oxygen. In most instances, the cause-and-effect relationship is direct and readily seen, while in others such a relationship is indirect. Those elements are of crucial importance to my discussion of the oxidative-dysoxygenative disorder (ODD) that leads to fibromyalgia, chronic fatigue syndrome, serious environmental illness, the Gulf War syndrome, and malignant tumors. Specifically, cellular oxygen metabolism and energetics are put in serious jeopardy by the following factors:

a. Antibiotics increase oxidative stress.
b. Pesticides are designer killer molecules. (What kills bugs will eventually also kill people. There is simply no way out of that dilemma.)
c. Synthetic hormones jam or damage cell membrane receptors and fundamentally alter the hormone-receptor-gene-product mechanisms.
d. Industrial pollutants increase the oxidizing capacity of the earth as well as of human microecologic cellular and

macroecologic tissue-organ ecosystems.

e.   Radiation pollution directly increases oxidative stress by damaging antioxidant defenses.

f.   Anger and hostility increase oxidative stress. Adrenaline is one of the most potent, if not the most potent, oxidant molecules in the human body.

The central theme of this book is that fibromyalgia is a state of too much oxidation and too little oxygen. I believe the pandemics of fibromyalgia, chronic fatigue syndrome, multiple chemical sensitivity syndrome, and the Gulf War syndrome could have been predicted. Indeed, in *The Canary and Chronic Fatigue,* I predicted the large-scale incidence of the Gulf War syndrome. Two years later, in *RDA: Rats, Drugs and Assumptions*, I wrote about why I made my prediction about that war and how true that prediction came to be.

SUMMARY

In this chapter, I have presented my view of the essential oxygen order of human life and cellular energetics. Oxygen is the most important *nutrient* for human metabolism. It sparks *all* fires of the human metabolism. Oxygen is a molecular Dr. Jekyll and Mr. Hyde without peer. It ushers in life. It terminates life. It orders buildup of molecules while triggering their breakdown at the same time. It is nature's prime antibiotic.

Life is a struggle. Darwin recognized that a part cannot be separated from the whole any more than the whole can be separated from its parts. The struggle for life, then, becomes a struggle in attaining optimal ecologic relationships for continued survival. The essence of that struggle is an *ecologic* balancing act. All living beings must continuously *read* their ecologic conditions and *respond* to their changing environment. This is where oxygen enters the scene again. It is undoubtedly the primary element that determines the human microecologic cellular environment, and therefore cellular energetics.

We are now witnessing the spreading epidemics of chronic fatigue syndrome and fibromyalgia. Both disorders are considered mystery maladies. That need not be so. The cellular energetics are driven, *first and foremost*, by oxygen. To understand chronic fatigue syndrome and fibromyalgia, we must begin with oxygen since both are oxygen deprivation syndromes. In the following chapters, I show how oxygen solves many other riddles in medicine, such as Alzheimer's disease.

References

1. Ali M. Spontaneity of Oxidation in Nature and Aging. Monograph, Teaneck, New Jersey, 1983.
2. Ali M. The agony and death of a cell. Syllabus of the Instruction Course of the American Academy of Environmental Medicine, Denver, Colorado, 1985.
3. Ali M. Intravenous Nutrient Protocols in Molecular Medicine. Monograph. Institute of Preventive Medicine, Bloomfield, New Jersey, 1987.
4. Ali M. Molecular basis of cell membrane injury. In: Syllabus of the Instruction Course of the American Academy of Environmental Medicine, Denver, Colorado, 1990.
5. Ali M. Spontaneity of oxidation and molecular basis of environmental illness. In: Syllabus of the 1991 Instruction Course of the American Academy of Environmental Medicine, Denver, Colorado, 1991.
6. Ali M. Spontaneity of oxidation and chronic disease. In: Syllabus of the Instruction Course of the American Academy of Environmental Medicine, Denver, Colorado, 1992.
7. Ali M. Oxidative coagulopathy. In: Syllabus of the Capital University of Integrative Medicine, Washington, D.C., 1997.
8. Ali M. Hypothesis: Chronic fatigue is a state of accelerated oxidative molecular injury. J Advancement in Medicine 1993;6:83-96.
9. Ali M. Spontaneity of oxidation in nature is the root cause of all illness. In: RDA: Rats, Drugs and Assumptions. pp. 199-304. 1995. Life Span Press, Denville, New Jersey.
10. Ali M. The Canary and Chronic Fatigue. 1994. Life Span Press, Denville, New Jersey.
11. McNamara JO, Fridovich I. Did radicals strike Lou Gehrig? Nature 1993;362:20-21.
12. Ali M. Oxidative regression to primordial cellular ecology (ORPEC): evidence for the hypothesis and its clinical significance. J Integrative Medicine 1988;2:4-55.

13.   Ali M. Amenorrhea, oligomenorrhea, and polymenorrhea in CFS and fibromyalgia are caused by oxidative menstrual dysfunction. J Integrative Medicine 1998;3:101-124

14.   Ali M. Ali O. Fibromyalgia: An oxidative-dysoxygenative disorder (ODD). J Integrative Medicine 1999;3:17-37.

15.   Ali M. Darwin, oxidosis, dysoxygenosis, and integration. J Integrative Medicine 1999;3:11-17.

16.   Koller PT, Bergmann SR. reduction of lipid peroxidation in reperfused isolated rabbit hearts by diltiazem. Cir Res 1989;65:838-41.

17.   Vatner SF, Patrick TA, Knight DR, et al. Effects of calcium channel block er on responses of blood flow, function, arrhythmias, and extent of infarction following reperfusion in conscious baboons. Cir Res 1988;62:105-8.

18.   Muller CA, Worthington MG, Thandroyen FT. Antiarrhythmic and metaboliic effects of indoramin during acute regional ischemia and reperfusion in isolated rat heart.

19.   Rassmussen H, Bordier P. The Physiological and Cellular Basis of Metabolic Bone Disease. Williams and Wilkins, Baltimore, 1974.

20.   Kullik I, Storz G. Transcriptional regulators of the oxidative stress response in prokaryotes and eukaryotes. Redox Rep. 1994;1:23-29

21.   Storz G, Tartaglia LA. OxyR: A regulator of antioxidant genes. J Nutr. 1992;122:627-630.

22.   Greenberg JT, Monach P, Chou JH, et al. Positive control of a global antioxidant defense regulation activated by superoxide-generating agents in Escherichia coli. Proc Nat Aca Sci. USA, 1990;87:6181-6185.

▣▣▣▣▣▣▣▣▣▣▣▣▣▣▣▣▣▣▣▣▣▣▣▣▣▣▣▣▣▣

For me, the fundemental oxygen order of human biology is the most elegant example of nature's order of economy.

▣▣▣▣▣▣▣▣▣▣▣▣▣▣▣▣▣▣▣▣▣▣▣▣▣▣▣▣▣▣

Chapter 6

Oxygen:
The
Great
Communicator

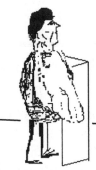

Oxygen Is *the* Information Molecule
of the Human Frame

Some might argue that hormones are the communicating molecules of the body. That, of course, is true. Hormones, by definition, are molecular messengers. Others might counter that genes are the molecular carriers of information. That is also true. However, as I explain in the earlier chapters, an oxygen order governs human biology and covers all the intelligence systems of the body. Indeed, hormones and genes function well only when oxygen metabolism is well preserved. Thus, I consider oxygen as the primary intelligence system while the DNA, RNA, hormones, proteins, and enzymes represent secondary information systems of the body. I support my view at several different levels in this book. At the most basic level, I hold that hormones, proteins, and enzymes carry information only to living cells and no cell can live without oxygen. Similarly, DNA and RNA cannot transmit information to dead cells.

OXYGEN DIRECTS THREE GREAT COMMUNICATION SYSTEMS OF THE BODY

The human frame is a marvel of biology. How does a cell talk to its neighbors? How does a cell read its microenvironment and respond to it? How does it learn about the needs of individual cells in other parts of the body? How does it know what happens in parts of the body far removed from it? How do the body's fifty trillion cells cooperate with each other to maintain perfect health in a baby? And how do those trillions of cells work together to restore health after a life-threatening infection in which every cell of the body gets badly hurt? How do cells in one part of the body know others somewhere else are injured and face death? I see the hand of oxygen in all such happenings. Indeed, it seems certain to me that future research will reveal many more ways by which oxygen serves both as the main messenger and the principal player in all those events.

Oxygen does not earn its title of a great communicator in my opinion simply because it provides the living environment in which information can be sent and received. Oxygen is *the* information molecule. This is the main theme of this book. In this chapter, I present information about how oxygen governs communications in three major systems of the body:

1. The circulating blood.
2. The circulating lymph.
3. The cell membranes.

Furthermore, I show how oxygen not only directs the flow of information in each of those communication systems but also serves as the principal medium of transfer of intelligence from one type of cell to another, from one type of tissue to another, and from one body organ to another.

In two seemingly simple acts of clotting and unclotting blood, oxygen masterminds healthful aging.

The above may seem a wild statement to many. However, a few moments of reflection on what clotting and unclotting involves will make the meaning of my statement clear. The prevailing view that clotting in the circulating blood occurs only in phlebitis and a few other disorders is extremely limited. Furthermore, the view that clotting involves a small number of clotting factors is equally inadequate. In reality, clotting involves, directly or indirectly, *all* substances in the circulating blood (including enzymes, minerals, vitamins, proteins, fats, sugars, and organic acids). In addition, *all* cells in the circulating blood (red blood cells, white blood cells, blood platelets as well as cells lining the blood vessels) actively participate in the clotting process. Neither does the prevailing thought recognize that *all* substances in the plasma (the fluid part of the blood) as well as *all* types of blood cells are also directly or indirectly involved in the unclotting process.

OXYGEN THROWS MOLECULAR SWITCHES

Proteins fold and unfold all the time. This flexibility is made possible by hinge-like bonds among their atoms. An average protein containing 500 amino acids has about 5,000 atoms, many of which participate in rotation at the bonds. It is amazing that any given protein flexes and unflexes in such determined ways that its overall functions are preserved. That may be to serve as a scaffold for other molecules or to swim within the cells or in the tissue fluid to spring to action as an enzyme when needed. A special class of proteins called *allosteric* proteins can take two or more stable forms. Such proteins shift back and forth between their states, thus serving as *molecular switches*. However, to perform that switch function allosteric proteins need a partner that brings forth its energy field (weak or strong electrostatic forces, hydrophobic interactions and others). Several substances can act as partners to activate the hinges of protein molecules (such as methyl, acetyl, or phosphoryl groups). Of importance to my subject of oxygen and aging is the fact that *oxygen within the molecule* can also change the structure—and function—of allosteric proteins.[1] Specifically, oxygen atoms combine with calcium in the vicinity to activate the hinge mechanisms of bonds between atoms. It is one of the great marvels of the intelligence of oxygen that its atoms within the protein molecules seem to know when they need to turn its molecular switches to change the protein structure, thus altering its function to respond to its molecular ecology.

Lipid peroxidation—the process by which fats are broken down for digestion and absorption—is also oxygen-driven and involves similar molecular switches operated by oxygen. Lipid peroxidation is also the process by which butter and oils turn rancid. Oxygen determines whether fats are metabolized or turned into toxic fats. Such is the versatility of oxygen! Oxygen-driven molecular switches are also involved in both the normal and abnormal metabolism of sugars and starches.

OXIDATIVE COAGULOPATHY

There is little, if any, interest in the many and fundamental roles of oxygen in clotting and unclotting of blood in the general physician community. Indeed, the basic notion of the presence of microclots and microplaques in the circulating blood will be most unsettling for most physicians. That is so because in medical schools we were taught that blood does not clot in circulation except in a small number of blood clotting disorders, such as phlebitis and widespread cancers. However, the microclot and microplaque formation that I describe and illustrate (see Figures 1-10) can be readily seen by anyone with even limited experience with high-resolution phase-contrast microscopy.

The basic idea of oxidative coagulopathy is simple: Excessive oxidative stress increases the extent of clotting-unclotting events in the blood. In 1997, following extensive studies of blood slides, my colleague, Omar Ali, and I introduced the term oxidative coagulopathy in an article published in *The Journal of Integrative Medicine*.[2] We observed that oxidative agents of *all* types operating in the circulating blood cause *cumulative* oxidative injury to all blood plasma and cellular components, increasing the clotting tendency of the blood. When seen with a high-magnification (x 15,000) microscope, the blood slides of healthy persons show normal features given in Table 1 (see endnote #1 for details of microscopy).

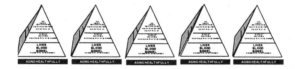

Table 1. MICROSCOPIC FEATURES OF HEALTHY BLOOD SMEARS

1. Clear plasma.
2. Round red blood cells with smooth surfaces.
3. White blood cells that move slowly like amoebae.
4. Blood platelets seen singly or in small clusters.
5. Minute fast-moving fat particles.
6. Few cells with spiked, crinkled, or otherwise irregular outlines.
7. Uncommon bacteria and other types of microbes.
8. Rare zones of solidified (congealed) plasma, loose microclots, and compact microplaques.

Table 2. MICROSCOPIC FEATURES OF OXIDATIVE COAGULOPATHY [2]

1. Deformities of red and white blood cells.
2. Zones of solidification (congealing) of plasma.
3. Clumping and breakdown of blood platelets.
4. Needle-like protein precipitates.
5. Lumpy soft plasma clots.
6. Microclots.
7. Microplaques.

Oxidative coagulopathy is not a matter of mere theoretical interest. My colleagues at the Institute and I consider clotting-unclotting events in the blood of great clinical importance. Specifically, we consider examination of the blood as a centerpiece for assessing health, as well as for evaluating the extent of oxidative stress in the sick and those interested in aging healthfully.

Every fat molecule turned rancid by oxygen-driven oxidation sends a different message to every other molecule, every cell, and every tissue in its vicinity. Every molecular switch in a protein turned by oxygen does the same. And so does every denatured molecule of enzyme, hormone, and sugar. This is the true significance of oxidative coagulopathy.

We consider the study of blood as *the single* most valuable procedure for assessing the efficacy of plans for healthful aging. We recognize that the examination of a drop of blood with a suitable microscope provides:

1. The best assessment of the integrity, or lack thereof, of the bowel and liver ecosystems. A clean blood field shows that the bowel ecosystem is not badly battered and the liver detox is working. Thus, the blood leaving the liver and entering the general circulation is cleansed of microbes as well as toxins.
2. The best assessment of whether the brain, heart, muscles, and other body tissues are receiving clean, well-oxygenated blood or not.
3. The best assessment of whether the brain, heart, muscles, and other body tissues are being exposed to toxins (from

damaged blood cells, microclots, and microplaques).

4. The best assessment of whether the hunter immune cells are effectively eating up the microbes in the body or the microbes have the upper hand.

5. The best assessment of whether the antibody-forming immune cells are healthy and can function properly.

6. The best assessment of whether the immune cells can effectively cope with cancer cells or not. Evidently dead and dying immune cells cannot fight cancer cells.

7. *In essence, at any given time it gives the best assessment of whether a person is in a state of healthful aging or whether he is in accelerated aging.*[3-5]

Figure 1:

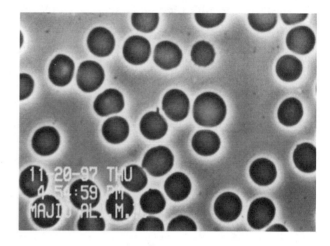

Figure 2:

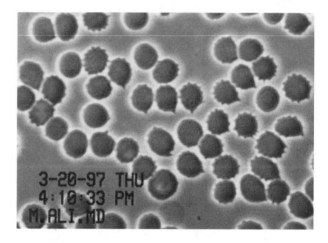

Legends to Figures 1 and 2: Figure 1 shows the microscopic appearance of healthy red blood cells. Note the background made up of plasmais clear and free of any microclots. j of a healthy person. Figure 2 shows early changes of oxidative stress on red blood cells many of which have spiked surfaces. Some cells at 5 o'clock position are pear-shaped.

Figure 3:

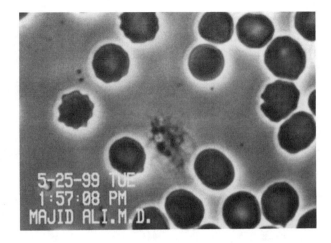

Figure 4:

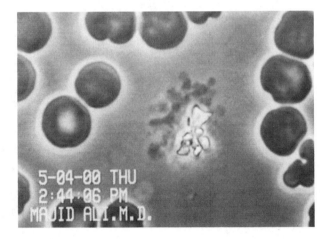

Figures 3 illustrates a small "soft" microclot (in the center field) which represents one of the early changes of oxidative coagulopathy. The black and white bodies enmeshed in the microclots are primordial life forms (see chapter 7 for detailed description of such forms. **Figure 4** shows another example of a soft microclot formed in vicinity of several microcystals. Microcystals are composed of oxalates, urates, and other substances, and frequently trigger microclot formation.

Figure 5:

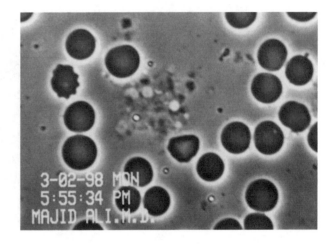

Figure 6:

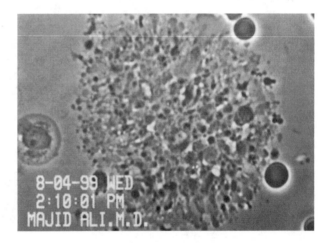

Figures 5 illustrates a larger soft microclot in the center field with some "smudges" representing solidified patches of plasma. Most red blood cells in the field have a smooth outline. Two such cells are deformed. **Figure 6** shows a much larger microclot that covers nearly two-third of the field. An immune cell is seen at 9 o'clock position.

Figure 7:

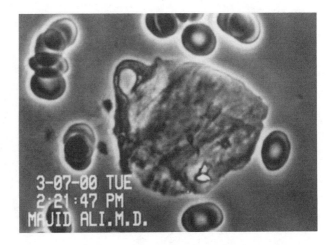

Figure 8:

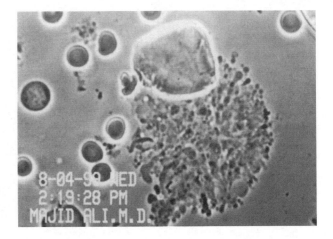

Figures 7 illustrates a well formed, compact microplaque that nearly fills the middle third of the field. Two small bright microcystals are seen within the microplaque at about 6 o'clock position. **Figure 8** shows a large microclot juxtaposed to a smaller microplaque.

Figure 9:

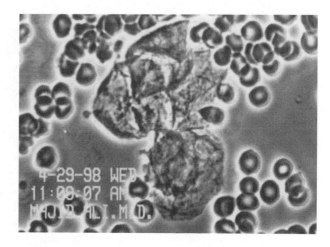

Figure 10:

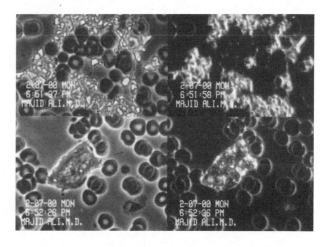

Figures 9 illustrates a large, irregularly shaped microplaque with sharp margins, and a "layered" structure. **Figure 10** shows a composite photomicrograph with two dark field views (left) and two phase-contrast views (right). The upper frames show clusters of crystals while the lower ones s microplaque (center field).

CUE AND CUD

For patient education, I often use the terms CUE and CUD to explain oxidative coagulopathy to our patients. CUE stands for **c**lotting-**u**nclotting **e**quilibrium in health and healthful aging while CUD stands for **c**lotting-**u**nclotting **d**ysequilibrium in disease and premature aging. The term CUE emphasizes the fact that blood clots and unclots all the time. It amazes me to see looks of disbelief on the faces of many doctors when they first hear me describe the clotting-unclotting continuum to them. They forget that there are *several* clotting (thrombogenic) and unclotting (fibrinolytic) mechanisms in the body. For reasons that are not clear to me, they seem to think that such events in circulating blood are of concern only in cases of phlebitis, some bleeding disorders, and some cases of cancer. The disbelief on their faces turns into confusion when I show them pictures of microclots and microplaques in the blood of patients with chronic fatigue syndrome, fibromyalgia, cancer, and other disorders. Then I ask them to think why *all* types of oxidative stress should not cause oxidative clotting. Why should adrenergic hypervigilance, tobacco smoke, very high blood sugar, toxic organic acids, viruses, bacteria, and yeast *not* cause cumulative and excessive oxidative stress and clotting? It is fascinating how hard we doctors fight new knowledge only because it contradicts what we were taught in medical schools decades earlier. *Unlearning is so much harder than learning.*

The circulating blood carries information from one cell to the other, from one part of the body to the other. That explains how the bone marrow in *all* parts of the body responds to an infection in one toe, how an intestinal virus infection can bring along an asthma attack, and how a battered bowel ecosystem can lead to severe brain fog. There are no known hormones that explain *all* such communications between different parts of the body. So, how does that happen? Oxygen solved that riddle for me some years ago. Oxygen amplifies all signals of oxidative stresses of all types in the circulating blood. (Recall the discussion of spontaneity of oxidation in nature in the preceding chapters.)

OXIDATIVE LYMPHOPATHY

Oxidative lymphopathy (lym-phop-athy) is my term for a process by which lymph becomes oxidized, rancid, thick and *gluey*. Lymph is the pale fluid that bathes cells and drains waste materials and toxins from cells. Such fluid stagnates in tissues, preventing the free flow of oxygen-rich blood, and causing cellular toxicity. I introduced this term in 1998 in an article in *The Journal of Integrative Medicine* to focus on issues of stagnant lymph in tissues.[5] I refer the advanced and professional readers to that article for an in-depth discussion of this subject.

The basic concept of oxidative lymphopathy evolved as a logical extension of my studies of oxidative coagulopathy in the blood. The lymph fluid, like blood, contains enzymes, minerals, fats, proteins and toxic organic acids. Oxidative stressors cause congealing and clot formation in lymph just as they cause clotting in the blood. The lymph also contains many cells, though not in such larger numbers as in the blood. Such cells are also damaged by oxidative injury. Thus, the basic mechanisms of oxidative injury in the blood and lymph are identical. Beyond that there is no valid reason to think that in states of excessive oxidative injury—such as fibromyalgia, chronic fatigue, severe immune disorders, and cancer—oxidative damage to enzymes, hormones, proteins, fats, and sugars will not occur in oxidized lymph as it does in oxidized blood.

I must point out that while clotting-unclotting events in the blood can be seen directly with a suitable microscope, I have not yet made similar direct observation on oxidized lymph. Obtaining a sample of lymph requires putting a tiny catheter in a lymph channel. That procedure is not justified since the information obtained by such a study can be more easily obtained by the examination of a blood sample. However, there is much indirect evidence for oxidative lymphopathy.

In my experience, one of the most effective therapies for painful and tender trigger points in chronic fatigue and fibromyalgia is injection in such tissues of several drops of a solution containing equal parts of 50% glucose and 2% procaine. Glucose stimulates an inflammatory reaction that "flushes out" oxidized, curdled, and stagnant lymph from the trigger point regions. Glucose also stimulates collagen production and healing. Three other therapies are effective for relieving trigger point pain, though only for short periods of time unless all underlying issues are addressed with a comprehensive plan that reverses the underlying oxidosis, acidosis, and dysoxygenosis. Those therapies are: (1) deep massage of tissues involved with trigger points; (2) water therapy in which the patient walks in a pool with water reaching the neckline; and (3) acupuncture therapy. Again, it is proposed that the first two therapies relieve myalgic pain by mechanically removing oxidized and stagnant lymph containing oxidatively coagulated and denatured lymph proteins, lipids, and sugars. The mechanism of action of acupuncture remains obscure.

How do hunter immune cells of the body know there are invader microbes around, ready to cause serious infections? In common bacterial infections, the immune cell count in the blood increases rapidly. How do those cells know they are required to increase in their numbers? In serious blood infections (septicemia), the immune cell count is usually dangerously low. How do they know when to divide and when not to? In most infections, hunter immune cells mount ferocious attacks on microbes. How do they know when to attack with full vigor and when to avoid the encounter? Just as oxygen governs all communication in the circulating blood, it also governs all communication in the circulating lymph.

TYPE C LACTATE ACIDOSIS

A sprinter collapses with exhaustion at the finish line. A child stops breathless in the middle of a street. A lion stops his ballistic charge on an antelope abruptly. A fibromyalgia patient makes the mistake of running after a bus and then cannot get out of bed for days. All such events occur when lactic acid builds up rapidly in the muscles. That is called lactic acidosis. It develops when not enough oxygen is available to break lactic acid into water and carbon dioxide. Thus, oxygen determines when a sprinter must collapse and when a lion must terminate his ballistic charge.

Lactic acidosis is divided into two types: (1) Type A, which develops when disorders of the lung and heart lead to insufficient oxygen; and (2) Type B, which occurs in metabolic conditions, such as uncontrolled diabetes and liver failure. As a part of my studies of clotting-unclotting events in the blood and lymph, I also proposed a third, Type C, in which I see evidence of dysoxygenosis without the feature of respiratory (Type A) or metabolic (Type B) disorders. The importance of Type C lactic acidosis is that it indicates dysfunctional oxygen metabolism in the absence of heart and lung disorders as well as metabolic conditions such as diabetes and liver failure. I also consider buildup of excess acidity (cellular acidosis) a hallmark of premature aging. I refer the advanced and professional readers to reference # 5 for additional discussion of this important issue.

OXIDATIVE CELL MEMBRANE DYSFUNCTION

A cell membrane separates internal order inside a cell from external disorder. It permits entry of what is needed inside (nutrients) and facilitates discharge of what is unneeded (waste). It keeps what is outside the cell from flooding the cell innards. It prevents hemorrhaging out of what is inside the cells. It converts physical changes in the fluid that bathes it (lymph) into chemical changes within. To do all that, cell membranes have many different types of communication molecules called receptors.

As in the case of the blood and lymph channels, the nature of cell membrane communication is widely misunderstood. Most people think of cell membrane channels and cell membrane receptors when they think of communication between cells. The basic question of the *initial* triggers for channel operations (closing and opening) and receptor activation received little, if any, consideration.

Cell membrane receptors are generally classified in the following five basic types: (1) mechanoreceptors, which detect and respond to mechanical factors; (2) thermoreceptors, which detect changes in temperature (cold and heat); (3) nociceptors, which are involved in pain sensation; (4) chemoreceptors, which respond to chemicals; and (5) electromagnetic receptors, which are poorly understood and include light-sensitive receptors. I hold that the functions of *all* such receptors are regulated first and foremost by oxygen, though I recognize that evidence for that in some areas is lacking at this time. Again, it seems safe to predict that future research will reveal many additional roles of oxygen in the function of cell membrane channels and receptors. Certainly, I have not been able to discover any evidence to the contrary.

COMMUNICATION IN THE MATRIX

3M oxidopathy is my term for a state of oxidative damage to matrix, membranes, and mitochondria. Matrix is the cement that holds cells together. Membranes are coverings of cells and their inner structures. Mitochondria are tiny power batteries of the cells. Since all three are continuously exposed to oxidized (rancid) blood and lymph, it should not surprise us that the oxidative coals in the blood and lymph (microclots) will also sear the matrix, membranes, and mitochondria. Indeed, the literature on patterns of injury to matrix, membranes, and mitochondria is voluminous, and the thread that runs through all of those events is oxygen-driven oxidative injury.

When a child falls and lacerates his hand, how do the cells on the edges of the wound know they have to multiply rapidly and cover the open wound? When an adult loses blood in an auto accident, how do the cells in the bone marrow know that many red blood cells have been lost and they must actively divide to make up for the lost cells?

After menstrual flow ends, how do the cells lining the cavity of the inner know they must rapidly multiply to cover the raw, denuded areas left open by the lost cells? I do not believe anyone can answer any of those questions except by citing the many roles of oxygen in the matrix-membrane communications.

OXYGEN IN NITRIC ACID

Nitrogen is an inert gas. That is the first thing I was taught in school. I was also taught that 80% of air we breathe is nitrogen and this gas simply moves in and out of lungs and in and out of blood without really doing anything. I suppose such an innocent view of things in nature has its place in schools.

But when nitrogen hooks up with oxygen, miraculous things happen. One atom of nitrogen attached to one atom of oxygen makes nitric oxide, one of the important molecular messengers of the body. Nitric acid helps a nerve cell to talk to other nerve cells as well as immune cells. It prevents clumping of platelets—the blood corpuscles that stick to each other to begin the process of clotting. It affects the production of tumor necrosis factor in immune cells. That is one of the way it goads immune cells to attack cancer cells and kill them. It is the molecular messenger of erection of the penis. It is an oxidant and in that role functions as a detox molecule. In its January 21, 2000, issue, *Science* reported the efficacy of nitric acid as an effective antimicrobial agent, especially against long-standing fungal infections.[6]

Like oxygen, nitric oxide is a molecular Dr. Jekyll Mr. Hyde. It regulates the function of cells lining the blood vessels and, in that role, it provides a counterbalance to excess adrenaline in stressful states. Thus, it protects the heart. In its August, 1995, issue, *Nature Medicine* carried an article showing that nitric oxide under certain conditions actually damages the heart cells. So it also injures the heart.

SUMMARY

In summary, oxygen is the great communicator that governs all information systems in the circulating blood, lymph and cell membranes. All molecular events taking place in those systems are, first and foremost, regulated by oxygen. Specifically, that includes opening and closing of cell membrane channels, functions of cell membrane receptors, and activities of membrane-associated enzymes. To cite one example, the processes by which a hunter immune cell swallows and digests a microbe are *all* triggered by oxygen-driven oxidative bursts taking place at the cell surface. Similarly, oxygen governs the transfer of information in the matrix, the ground substance that serves as the cells' scaffold. Neither hormones nor genes can perform their information-gathering and information-transporting functions without optimal oxygen functions. Chronic fatigue, fibromyalgia, and chemical sensitivity are examples of many syndromes in which the basic problem is dysfunctional oxygen metabolism. Accelerated aging is another example.

References

1. Loewenstein WR. The Touchstone of Life. 1999. Oxford University Press. Oxford, England. pp 68.
2. Ali M. AA Oxidopathy.
3. Ali M. Spontaneity of Oxidation in Nature and Aging. Monograph, Teaneck, New Jersey, 1983.JIM
4. Ali M. Spontaneity of oxidation in nature is the root cause of all illness. In: RDA: Rats, Drugs and Assumptions. pp. 199-304. 1995. Life Span Press, Denville, New Jersey.
5. Ali M. Oxidative regression to primordial cellular ecology (ORPEC): evidence for the hypothesis and its clinical significance. J Integrative Medicine 1988;2:4-55.
6. Pennisi E. Yet another role for nitric oxide. Science 2000;287:419-20.

Endnote #1:

For our studies, we used a special type of microscope that magnifies the images of living cells 15,000 to 18,000 times. It is fitted with phase-contrast optics that throws light at the microscopic slides at an angle in such a way as to illuminate many parts of cells that are not seen well with bright-light optics commonly used in the hospitals. We established the oxidative nature of such changes by reversing the early changes with addition of antioxidants, such as taurine, and vitamins A and E.

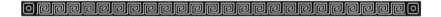

In two simple acts of clotting and unclotting, oxygen exerts the most profound influence on human health and the aging
process. In those two acts, I see the hand of
oxygen in the workings of every enzyme,
every hormone, every receptor, and every
mediator.

Chapter 7

Oxygen, Primordial Life Forms and Aging

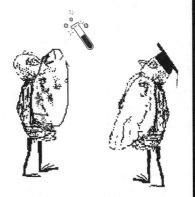

Primordial life forms (PLFs) is my term for a large family of microbes that hates oxygen, loves acid, and thrives on decaying and dead organic matter.[1] I see the primordial forms in the blood of *all* my patients with chronic disorders in which oxidosis leads to dysoxygenosis, including fibromyalgia, chronic fatigue syndrome, Lyme disease, lupus and other severe immune disorders, and cancer.[2-5] Later in this chapter, I include several pictures of PLFs that I commonly encounter. I also present my view of how PLFs affect human health and the aging process.

Human life span is profoundly influenced by man-microbe harmony or the lack of it. Bacteria, viruses, and yeast cause acute and chronic infections and sometimes lead to untimely death. That needs no further comment. The opposite of that—microbes enhancing health and increasing longevity—has also been recognized by many enlightened physicians interested in the aging process. For example, for centuries many physicians in different countries recognized the healthful benefits of microbes that turn milk into yogurt and frequently advised thier patients to consume yogurt. There is yet another aspect of this subject: The matter of certain oxygen-hating, acid-loving microbes that cause dysfunctional oxygen metabolism and lead to premature aging. This subject is rarely, if ever, addressed in discussions of aging. And yet this is of paramount importance for both a deeper understanding of aging and for designing plans for healthful aging.

THE FAMILY OF PLFs

The large family of PLFs includes various forms of stealth microbes, mycoplasma, nanobacteria, bacteroides, yeast (including bakers' and brewers' yeast, *Candida, Penicillium*, and others), uncharacterized yeast-like organisms, and many other microbes. PLFs are easily visualized with high-resolution (x 15,000) phase-contrast microscopy [6] but not with ordinary microscopes with magnification of up to 1,000 used by hospital pathologists. Furthermore, most PLFs cannot be observed in blood smears examined after the staining procedures commonly used in hospitals (chemical processing or "fixing" in technical language, with alcohol or other preservatives).

The reason most doctors are unfamiliar with PLFs is that they do not study living cells with high-resolution microscopy.

This is the first essential point I make in this chapter.

MICROBIAL BIODIVERSITY

Though we doctors generally ignore the issue of microbial biodiversity, biologists often recognize the vastness of the microbial world. Consider the following quote from a recent issue of *Nature*:

Recent advances in the application of molecular genetics approaches have emphasized our potentially huge underestimate of microbial diversity in a range of environmental [conditions].[7]

A huge underestimate! That is the second important point I make here. Most doctors seem to have little, if any, interest in that huge underestimate. Even the infectious disease specialists appear to ignore the vast range of microbial diversity. They limit their work to a relatively small number of microbial species that get written up in their journals.

THE IMPORTANCE OF THE CELLULAR "SOIL"

A desert is bone dry for months. Then one day it rains. A few days later, the desert comes to life with delicate shoots and celebrates with colors a day or two later. That teaches us something about the seed-soil relationship. The seeds of those flowers laid dormant for months until the soil ecology changed. We physicians seldom recognize the relevance of such basic ecologic relationships in our clinical practices. I devoted a recent article to the core issue of the seed-soil ecologic relationship.[8] That article, in a slightly adapted form, is reproduced in the chapter "Oxygen Settles the Great Pasteur-Bechamp Debate." Here, I make a simple point:

The seeds of PLFs germinate rapidly when the "soil" of the cells changes.

That is the third important point. I am also certain that with time the core importance of the PLF overgrowth in triggering and perpetuating the suffering of human canaries will be recognized. Human canaries must learn about the relationship between antibiotic abuse and PLF overgrowth, not only for understanding the true nature of their illness and suffering, but also for designing intelligent treatment plans for recovery.

Simple-minded plans of doctors of "killing bugs" with broad-spectrum antibiotics without nutritional and ecologic therapies can be extremely dangerous.

That is the fourth point. Mindless use of antibiotics without addressing the relevant ecologic issues destroys the antioxidant and enzyme defenses of the sick long before drugs can destroy the last bug. I know this because I have seen hundreds of healthy persons turned into human canaries by such mindless abuse of antibiotics. The same is true of holistic doctors who claim they can "eradicate yeast" by their antifungal drugs and other anti-yeast therapies. No doctor can eradicate yeast from the bowel without first eradicating the patient.

While the world of PLFs is vast, the clinically useful concept of PLF overgrowth is easy to understand. In the simplest words, too much oxidation causes dysfunctional oxygen metabolism (dysoxygenosis) which, in turn, creates excess acidity. Dysoxygenosis and acidosis then feed the fires of excess oxidation, so completing the cycle that feeds upon itself to create primordial cellular conditions. That produces a soil rich in nutrients for PLF overgrowth. Next, PLFs produce their toxins that further feed the oxidative fires. Antibiotics do not work against PLFs. Indeed, antibiotics kill many health-promoting microbes and so encourage further multiplication of PLFs.

ECOLOGIC DEVASTATION CAUSED BY SUGAR, PESTICIDES, AND PROCESSED FOODS

Sugar feeds PLFs. My colleagues and I see evidence of that with high-resolution microscopy every working day. The oxygen metabolism of human canaries is often so stressed that ordinary eating of desserts during holidays throws them in tailspins.

Sugar increases the number of microclots and microplaque that form as components of changes of oxidative coagulopathy. I first recognized that phenomenon in a diabetic patient. His blood smear was "clean," with well-preserved cells and clear plasma when his blood glucose level was 128 mg/dL. A few days later, he returned feeling "bad." His blood was then very "dirty," with changes of oxidative coagulopathy, such as clumped cells, zones of congealed plasma, and many microclots and micro-plaques. His blood sugar was 390 mg/dL.

Sugar increases the rancidity of lymph in human canaries by feeding the fires of oxidative lymphopathy. Though I have not yet observed that phenomenon directly, I presented extensive indirect evidence for that in an article published in *The Journal of Integrative Medicine.*[1] Here is a revealing quote from one of my canaries with fibromyalgia:

> "Dr. Ali, please don't laugh at me when I tell you that sugar turns into glue in my muscles. Does that make any sense?"
>
> "Laugh at you?," I replied with a smile at him. "Does that make sense? You have said in one sentence what I am trying to say in over 500 pages in my fibromyalgia book."

Sugar feeds PLFs in the bowel. PLFs enter the blood in large numbers and trigger oxidative coagulopathy. Sugar also directly speeds up microclot formation. Simmering coals of microclots then light up a thousand oxidative fires wherever they reach. In the lymphatic channels, the fluid also begins to form microcurdles. Oxidized, thickened, and toxic lymph then stagnates in the muscles, causing soreness and weakness. *Glue in the muscles!* How can anyone be more eloquent than that? Those who suffer see things more clearly. If only we physicians would pay more attention.

The dangers of prolonged and low-dose exposure to pesticides and oxidized rancid fats in processed foods may not be so obvious to us. But the damage they do to human canaries is just as bad. Here is a practical tip: When you see a "cholesterol-free" label on a canned food, avoid it. It probably does not contain any natural cholesterol. But most likely it contains highly rancid oxidized fats. A patient recently showed me a sugarless "power" bar. I cringed when I read the label. The bar was loaded with coconut oil and other processed oil. *Some health food!*

It is a little-known fact that sugar in excess binds many healthy proteins and fats and turns them into substances that do not fit well in the metabolic pathways. Beyond that, sugar in excess directly depresses the immune system.

There are many simple explanations of why children who live on sugar and antibiotics get sicker and sicker with time.

This is the fifth point in this discussion.

DYSFUNCTIONAL OXYGEN METABOLISM

Oxygen fascinates me. By now, readers must know about my passion for this life-starting, life-ending, ultimate molecular Dr. Jekyll-Mr. Hyde of human biology. In an article recently published in *The Journal of Integrative Medicine,* I have presented many faces of this greatest of all spin masters.[9] Here is something else about oxygen that both fascinates and puzzles me and which I have not written about yet:

All physicians know people cannot live without oxygen. Yet, there is little interest in understanding normal oxygen metabolism in health and how it might become dysfunctional in illness. Even when they administer oxygen to their patients in intensive care units, they do not seek a deeper knowledge of this element. I have never read an article in mainstream medical literature that recommends nasal oxygen for human canaries, those suffering from fibromyalgia, chronic fatigue syndrome, multiple chemical sensitivity syndrome, and other oxidative-dysoxygenative disorders. The essential message for human canaries here is this:

The crucially important subject of dysfunctional oxygen metabolism caused by the overgrowth of primordial life forms must not be dismissed as mere speculation.

That is the sixth point. Literally, the lives of the chronically ill persons, including *millions* of young Americans suffering from such disorders as fibromyalgia, chronic fatigue syndrome, and many severe forms of autoimmune disorders, depend on normalization of their dysfunctional oxygen metabolism.

Before I describe the patterns of PLF overgrowth and illustrate that with microscopic pictures of PLFs, I present some important information to provide a framework of further discussion of this essential subject.

THE CASE OF VANISHING MICROBES

Over thirty years ago, as a young surgeon in Pakistan and later in England and the United States, I first encountered the problem of the vanishing microbes. On many occasions, I sent samples of pus from abdominal abscesses to the hospital laboratory. Days later I received reports back stating that no organisms could be cultured from the samples. If there were no microbes there, where did the pus come from?, I remember wondering. When I asked the microbiologist in the hospital about the missing microbes, I received no satisfactory explanation. Under the pressure of attending to a ward full of very ill patients, the problem of the vanishing microbes was usually overshadowed by the "unvanishing" problems of sick bodies and festering wounds.

Some years later, as a young laboratory director, I found myself on the other side: Then it was my turn to face the difficult problem of explaining the case of vanishing microbes to my surgeon-friends at the hospital. Nearly every day, they sent me samples of purulent fluids from infected tissues from all parts of the body. In many cases, the culture plates showed no growths and we sent back reports indicating the same. Such reports frustrated my surgeon-friends, as they had me years earlier. They had to take care of their patients, who were obviously very sick. They wanted to know the identity of the microbes that caused those infections. They needed to know the sensitivity to antibiotics of those bugs so they could prescribe the appropriate antibiotics. The laboratory reports with a "no organisms grown" stamp irked them. When pressed for an answer, I would mumble something about bacteroides and other bowel anaerobes in the samples not growing well in the laboratory. I fully understood then that my answer was incomplete. So did they. Once a surgeon-friend saw one such report indicating no growth and gave vent to his angst thusly: "There are weeds in my lawn and I can't stop them from growing no matter what I do. I wonder if I sent a sample of that weed to your laboratory, could your staff grow it?" Of course, the ability to smile at such gibes from irate surgeons is a part of the job description of every chief pathologist. So I dutifully smiled at such displays of exasperation.

The irritation of surgeons on some such occasions was easy to understand. They went on to prescribe highly toxic antibiotics anyway. How could they ignore purulent matter in the bellies of the persons they had recently operated on? Then there was another matter that troubled them much. Without proper culture and sensitivity data, the use of potent and toxic antibiotics poses serious malpractice problems for doctors. (There were many things in the area of nutrition and metabolism they should have done for their infected and toxic patients in addition to the use of antibiotics. But, the American hospital doctors are convinced that nutrition is irrelevant to the care of the sick hospitalized patients. They never *ever* permit nutritional therapies in our hospitals.)

I knew the real problem of negative bacterial culture reports for pus samples was of the limitation of the state of the art in microbiology technology. My bacteriology staff could not manufacture a culture of microbe on demand just to appease the surgeon. With passing years, I finally solved the problem of vanishing microbes. There was only one solution: As far as criticism of surgeons was concerned, I learned to simply ignore the whole issue.

ROCK-EATING AND OXYGEN-HATING MICROBES

My academic curiosity about the vanishing microbes, however, persisted. I knew that certain types of oxygen-hating microbes survive under extremely harsh conditions. As far back as the 1920s, microbiologists had recovered anaerobic (non-oxygen-breathing) microbes from wells 2,000 feet or more deep.[10] Those early reports were dismissed as errors in the research methods used. Decades later, research with samples from hot springs and deep vents in the floor of oceans revealed certain anaerobes thriving at temperatures of over 230 degrees Fahrenheit (hotter than boiling water). Equally surprising were the findings that certain microbes thrived on radioactive stones. Further research revealed that many of such microbes do not depend on organic matter seeping down from the earth's surface. Rather, such microbes are "rock-eaters," surviving on geologic elements such as iron, sulfur, manganese, and hydrogen. More amazing reports followed. Some scientists estimated that the total mass of living beings in the hard rock of the earth's crust might even exceed that on the surface (including marine life). Such estimates were based on the counts of microbes found in the topsoil that contained as many as a billion microbes in a pinch of dirt deep in the rock.

Not only is the number of microbes living in the earth's rock surprising, the diversity of those non-oxygen-breathing microbes is more amazing. As many as 11,000 strains (types) of microbes have been found to exist as far deep as two miles into the earth's core of rock. If 11,000 strains of oxygen-hating microbes exist in the guts of the earth, how many might exist in the guts of people and animals?, I wondered.

THE SICK MADE SICKER BY ANTIBIOTICS

I made an interesting discovery when I returned to clinical medicine after more than 25 years of research and practice of pathology. I saw sick people who had become *clearly sicker* after receiving multiple courses of antibiotics. I discovered that most of my patients with fibromyalgia, chronic fatigue syndrome, Lyme disease, and immune disorders had received extended courses of antibiotics before I saw them. The more I studied such patients, the more convinced I became that long-term antibiotic therapy had done serious damage. Within a few years I accumulated files of hundreds of what I call Lyme cripples. Those are unfortunate persons who had developed disabling chronic fatigue syndrome and fibromyalgia after receiving massive doses of oral and intravenous antibiotics. The antioxidant, enzyme, and immune defenses of such persons clearly had been crippled by antibiotics. Why didn't the antibiotics work for them? I asked myself. The infectious disease specialists told me that was due to drug resistance. That answer was simply too simplistic for me. I had performed autopsies on many persons who had died *after* receiving massive doses of antibiotics that were found to kill the cultured microbes in the laboratory tubes. I had run a microbiology lab for far too many years to accept a superficial answer like that. So, what was the mystery of antibiotics making the sick sicker?

In health, oxygen prevents PLF overgrowth. In disease, PLF overgrowth causes dysfunctional oxygen metabolism.

A wide world of primordial microbes opened before me as I began to study blood samples of my patients with a high-resolution microscope fitted with phase-contrast optics. The vanishing microbes did not vanish any more in the blood samples examined with such a microscope. In the blood smears of fibro, fatigue, and Lyme canaries, I saw hordes of the stealth microbes. Those who had received the most antibiotics generally showed the highest number of primordial microbes, some pale and others dark, some moving slowly and others that moved quickly, microbes of all shapes, and all patterns of breeding. I describe my observations concerning primordial microbes in a series of articles.[1-5]

In 1998, my microscopic work led me to introduce the term PLF because such microbes have primordial metabolic characteristics, i.e., they hate oxygen, love acid, and thrive on decaying organic matter. In their metabolic preferences, PLFs are identical to the early microbes that evolved during the primordial period. PLFs exist in the bowel, blood, and other body ecosystems in health. The oxygen concentration in healthy tissues inhibits the growth of such microbes and so prevents disease states caused by their overgrowth. In dysfunctional oxygen metabolism, PLFs rapidly grow in number and produce a large amount of enzymes and toxins that injure tissue in many ways. A particularly serious effect of such toxins is to block or poison enzymes that are necessary for the transport and utilization of oxygen in tissues. The lack of oxygen allows PLFs to multiply rapidly and a larger number of PLFs that results from the lack of oxygen further blocks the transport and utilization of oxygen. Thus, a destructive cycle is established in which less oxygen means more PLFs, and more PLFs mean even less oxygen, and so on.

The hunter immune cells in the circulating blood efficiently kill microbes only in the presence of optimal concentrations of oxygen. I observe direct microscopic evidence of that when I examine the blood smears of patients with good circulation and oxygenation. In fibromyalgia and chronic fatigue syndrome, the hunter immune cells become sluggish—or are killed—whenever I see microscopic changes of oxidosis and dysoxygenosis.

PLFs thrive when the tissues are under increased oxidative stress, are oxygen-starved, have increased acidity, and are rich in decaying and dead organic matter. Those, of course, are the conditions of oxidosis, dysoxygenosis, and acidosis.

Oxygen inhibits PLFs in health and PLF overgrowth disrupts oxygen metabolism in disease. I consider this as one of my most important insights in forty years of the study of medicine.

Those facts, as I wrote earlier, are of utmost concern to all fibro and fatigue canaries, for learning the fundamental health problem as well as for planning its reversal.

THE PEOPLE-PLF HARMONY

People and PLFs learned to peacefully coexist a long time ago.[11] In the basic scheme of people-PLF harmony, people provide PLFs with suitable living quarters. PLFs, in turn, provide people with their digestive enzymes and nutrients. That arrangement serves both sides well. What holds that relationship together is oxygen. In essence, the oxygen-using life forms protect the non-oxygen-using life forms from oxygen toxicity. PLFs complete digestion of foods, though that fact is seldom given due consideration in discussion of health and disease. PLFs also produce vitamins, fatty acids, and other nutrients for their own use, and then share them with their keepers. The hosts and guests lived in harmony.

Milk spoils within several hours. Cheese lasts for months. How did the ancients learn the art of turning milk into cheese? Grapes decompose in two or three days when left on a kitchen table. Wine can age for years. How did they find a way to ferment grape juice to make wine? We eat yogurt but rarely think about how the ancients figured out that microbes could curdle milk. We eat bread and pay little attention to how anyone ever figured out that putting microbes into the flour would cause bread to rise. At ball games, we drink beer. How does barley get turned into beer? Who left us the legacy of knowledge of employing microbes to enrich our foods? Obviously we owe the gift of that knowledge to the earlier people. They understood that something in the air spoils foods and those foods could be preserved and enriched if that something could be managed. That something, of course, was (and is) oxygen.

All early peoples had skills for processing foods with natural methods. In 1998, I went to Istanbul to present my theory of how dysfunctional oxygen metabolism causes PLF overgrowth. During that trip I saw some Mesopotamian jars estimated to be about 3,000 years old. Then I read about a yellow pigment found in some of those jars that on chemical analysis turned out to be tartaric acid, a substance produced by many PLFs. I find that acid in large amounts in the urine of most of my fatigue and fibromyalgia canaries. Those jars are among the earliest artifacts that prove that the people of Mesopotamia knew the art of winemaking. Egyptian hieroglyphics dating as far back as 2,500 years describe methods of making beer. At about the same time, the Chinese also figured out how to turn grapes into fermented delicacies fit for their emperors. The case of an Assyrian tablet is more interesting. It attempts to explain how Noah managed the animal dung in his crowded ark. The tablet suggests that he carried a magical mash to his ark to biodegrade the copious amounts of waste produced by his stock. *Clever stuff*!

So, the story of people-PLF harmony goes a long way back.

COOKING WITH LOW OXYGEN

The ancients were skilled in the art of cooking with low oxygen. All human canaries need to learn something about that because knowledge of "low-oxygen cooking" is even more important for them. The ancients did such cooking so that their foods would keep longer, to enhance the taste, and to improve digestibility. The canaries have a much more important reason to do so: Their digestive enzymes are often badly damaged and their bowels cannot tolerate the SAD (Standard American Diet). Low-oxygen cooked (predigested or partially digested) foods are essential for them. I make specific recommendations about food choices in the chapter, "Guidelines for Healthful aging."

First, some explanation about low-oxygen cooking. The ancients practiced many methods of "cooking" with microbial cultures and plant enzymes. All such methods, in one way or the other, involved protecting foods from oxygen in the air. Without regulating exposure to oxygen, milk cannot be turned into cheese, nor grapes into wine. The microbial cultures they employed for enhancing and predigesting their foods consisted of various types of PLFs that could grow only in carefully controlled conditions of exposure to oxygen. Without those conditions, milk turns sour and spoils, and grapes decompose and disintegrate.

We do not know whether or not the ancients recognized that there were living microbes in their food cultures. It is doubtful anyone could have imagined the teeming microbes in those cultures before Leeuwenhoek invented the microscope. Nor is there any known record of knowledge of oxygen prior to discovery of that elemental gas by Joseph Priestley and Carl Wilhelm Scheele in 1774.[12] But many among the earlier peoples were astute observers. Some of them must have intuited that the cultures contained some form of life that preserved their foods in so many ways without spoiling it. Some of them must also have figured out something in those cultures could not work if not protected from something "bad" in the air. Indeed, their art of enriching foods could not have advanced so highly without deep intuitive insights into the conditions of their food culture methods. The terms "oxygen" and "PLF" evidently would not have been familiar to them, but a conceptual model of life in their cultures and killing capacity of bad air must have evolved in their minds.

KEEPING OXYGEN ON LEASH

The story of soybeans makes for an illuminating case study. Soybean is an excellent source of minerals such as magnesium, calcium, molybdenum and others. It has a rich content of phytohormones and some very healthful oils. I have observed some extraordinary benefits of low-oxygen cooked (fermented) soy products for patients with irritable bowel syndrome, ulcerative colitis, Crohn's colitis, and related chronic inflammatory bowel disorders. And, of course, soybean has high-quality proteins. It comes close to being a perfect food. But there is something more to it.

Soybean is a seed. Like all other seeds, it is rich in enzyme inhibitors. Here is another masterstroke of nature. Seeds are nature's tiny parcels of future life. They must be preserved. They must be protected not only from the hazards in their environment but also from the enzymes within them. These enzymes are designed to cause autodigestion and breakdown. So Nature gave them outer shells and inner molecular safety in the form of enzyme inhibitors. People in China and other countries of the Far East seem to have intuitively known about those nutritional aspects of soybean, even though little has come down to us about their insights in these matters in a written form. Why else would they hold fermented soy foods in such high esteem? Also, they seem to have recognized the problem of enzyme inhibitors in soybean. Why else would they be so inventive about the antidigestive (enzyme inhibitor) aspects of soybean? Why else would they prepare soybean dishes in so many ways with the specific result of neutralizing and predigesting it?

The ancient Chinese mastered the art of neutralizing enzyme inhibitors and predigesting soybean with several fungus enzymes, mostly from the *Aspergillus* species. They closely regulated the influence of oxygen during fermentation. There is, however, a critical difference between cooking soybean (and other foods) with heat and cooking them with enzymes and low oxygen: Cooking with heat destroys life enzymes, while cooking with enzymes increases the life enzyme content of foods.

Tofu kan, yuba, and *tofu p'i* were the names given to soybean dishes prepared with low-oxygen cooking. Their specific purpose was to increase digestibility of soybean and enhance its nutritional value. They must also have understood that by using the "digestive juices" of foods, they were conserving their own digestive juices. So our concept of lifetime enzyme reserves would not have been unfamiliar to them. *They were prudent about their own lifetime enzyme reserves.* The Chinese also used soybean curd to prepare another dish called *kabitofu.* The people in the Philippines called their favorite partially digested soybean dish *toya.* The well-known *tofu* is a "cheese" made up of partially digested soybean. *Natto* is the name given to a similar product. For many centuries, people of Java treated their soybean with enzymes and named their dish *tempeh.* The Japanese were not to be left behind in this competition for saving their life span enzymes. They perfected *miso,* a fermented soybean food used as porridge at breakfast. The Japanese also experimented with other grains and made *miso* with barley and rice.

The principle of predigesting foods with natural substances to enhance its nutritional value (conserving the life enzyme bank account in our jargon) is not the sole cultural heritage of people of the Far East. Yogurt was the prime predigested food of ancient India. Cheeses were the predigested foods of early Europeans. They prepared their cheese to enhance its nutritional value and for specific taste goals by treating it with specific bacterial enzymes.

Predigestion of food is an old discovery of man. In almost all of his cultures and in all eras of his history, man has used the principle of predigesting his food by borrowing digestive enzymes from other forms of life. Today we find some of its early applications repulsive, even barbaric. Jivaros Indians of the Amazon River basin prepared *nijimanche* by thoroughly chewing the yucca bark and spitting it into large jars where its digestion by amylase enzymes of the saliva continued for hours. They treasured this drink for its nutritional value. We do not need to adopt their specific methods, but we must recognize the relevance of their insights into the matters of food digestion to our health today.

The methods of food "packaging" of those earlier peoples appear repugnant to our delicate taste and sensibility today. Little do we realize that they, in their "barbaric primitiveness," were much truer to their food than we who hide toxic foods in elegant packaging.

Soybean is the current favorite for preparing predigested foods among people interested in their food and health. It is unfortunate that our food industry does not see the intuitive wisdom of the ancients and build upon it for healthier foods with abundant life span enzymes. The ancients perfected the art of preparing healthful predigested foods and drinks. We can both adopt and adapt their methods. Enzyme foods and beverages can be prepared in many aesthetically pleasing ways.

THE DISCOVERY OF DARK PLFs

With high-resolution microscopy, soft, pale round-to-ovoid bodies are commonly observed in the blood smears of chronically ill patients (Figures 1-4). Such bodies often show budding, a term used in microbiology for the process of multiplication (Figures 5,6). It may be seen as a mother microbe delivering a baby microbe. Such bodies do not reflect light in darkfield examination (Figure 7,8). The explanation of that phenomenon is that sugars in their cell membranes absorb light. Unlike PLFs, the red blood cells appear as brightly lit because fats in their cell membrane reflect light.

Until recently, holistic doctors believed that such soft, pale bodies represent *Candida* species. They did not have any scientific evidence to support their belief. The mere fact that those bodies appear dark in darkfield *cannot* be accepted as the proof of their being *Candida.* I know *all* microbiologists will agree with me on that. In 1995, the author and colleagues succeeded in positively identifying *some* such organisms as *Candida* species with immunoperoxidase staining.[13] I published the color photographs (the first ever, to my knowledge) of such microbes in *RDA: Rats, Drugs and Assumption.*[14]

In most chronically ill patients, the peripheral blood also contains dark round-to-ovoid bodies. Such bodies often assume stellate or spidery configurations (Figures 11 and 12). For several years, the author uncritically accepted the prevailing opinion among microscopists who perform such studies that those dark bodies represent cellular debris, damaged and shrunken corpuscles, or mycoplasma. However, recently the author had the opportunity to complete careful morphologic studies of the blood smears containing such dark bodies over extended periods (up to 72 hours) of time, and observed them to grow in unmistakable yeast-like morphologic forms described as PLFs.

Figure 1

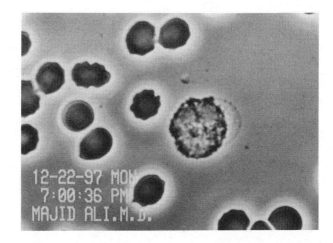

Figure 2

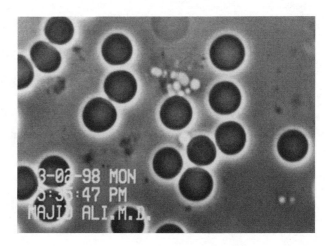

Figure 1 shows a larger white blood (immune) cell with a light-colored inside and several smaller, darker red blood cells, some with crenated borders. The background representing plasma is clear. **Figure 2** shows many dark red blood cells and a cluster of smaller pale, round budding PLFs (upper central field).

Figure 3

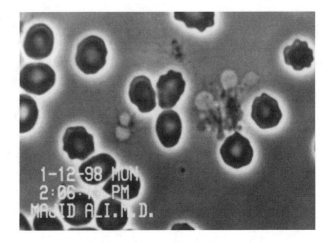

Figure 4

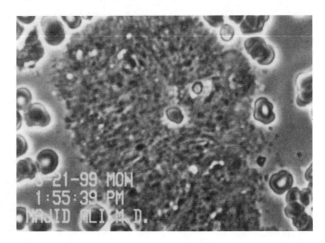

Figure 3 shows a cluster of larger pale and several smaller dark PLFs (right side) and a second grouping of two pale and a third dark PLFs (left side). **Figure 4** shows a large colony of pale and dark PLFs surrounded by small clusters of clumped and deformed red blood cells. Note two shrunken red blood cells trapped within the colony of PLFs.

Figure 5

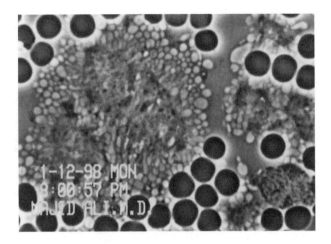

Figure 6

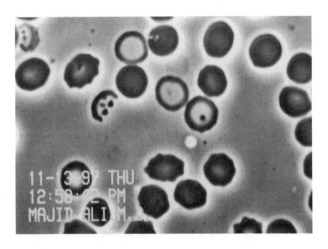

Figure 5 shows five clusters of larger pale and several smaller dark PLFs. The central zones of each colony show compacted microclots. PLFs cause microclot formation, just as culture turns milk into yogurt. Red blood cells included in the picture show normal appearance. **Figure 6** shows dark PLFs in three red blood cells (one PLF each within two red blood cells (right of the center field) and upper left corner) and two PLFs in damaged red blood cells (left of the center field). A single pale PLF is seen near the center of the picture.

Figure 7

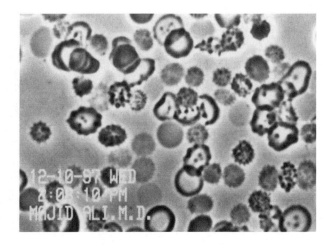

Figure 8

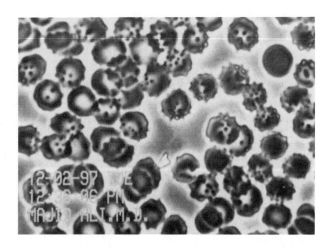

Figure 7 shows many red blood cells containing multiple PLFs. Some PLFs float outside the cells in open plasma (one o'clock position). **Figure 8** shows one or more dark PLFs in the majority of red blood cells. Note the irregularities of cell membranes, indicating oxidative stress in most cells.

Figure 9

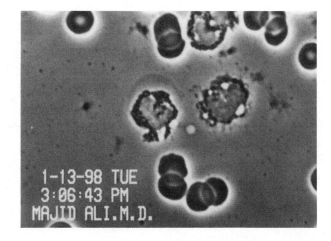

Figure 10

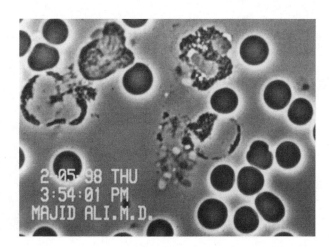

Figure 9 shows three white blood cells (scavenger cells) with engulfed pale PLFs. In health, such scavenger cells swallow and digest PLFs and so clear the blood of microbes that largely reach there from the bowel. **Figure 10** shows four white blood cells. Two white blood cells in the right field are invaded by clusters of pale and dark PLFs. Continued observation of such cells usually shows their death and disintegration. The blood sample belonged to a person with fibromyalgia/fatigue complex. *The predator becomes the prey.*

Figure 11

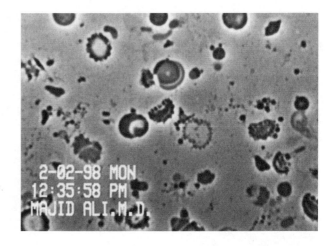

Figure 12

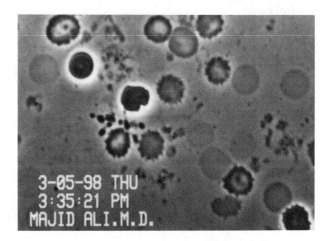

Figure 11 shows active multiplication of dark PLFs. In the center field, a row of PLFs is seen emerging from a damaged red blood cell, while PLFs at the periphery of a second cell produced the appearance of a beaded bracelet. **Figure 12** shows dark PLFs aligned in strings (left center field).

Figure 13

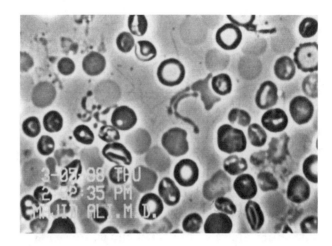

Figure 14

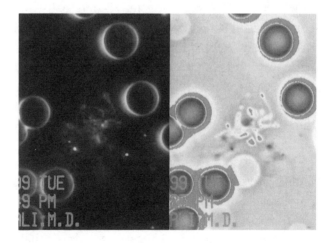

Figure 13 shows active multiplication of dark PLFs arranged in starfish configuration in the right central field and as long curved bodies in the left central field. **Figure 14** Phase-contrast (right) and dark field (left) views of the same cluster of pale PLFs showing active germination (growth of mycelia forms).

DARK PLFs ARE HARDER TO CONTROL
THAN PALE PLFs

I have observed the following: (1) the dark bodies floating free in the plasma as well as those found within the corpuscles are in reality PLFs, which can be readily identified as such by their motility and patterns of luxuriant growth when the smears are examined continuously from the time of drawing the blood to 72 hours; (2) the dark PLFs are more prevalent and cause oxidative coagulopathy to a greater degree than do the pale PLFs; (3) dark PLFs may be seen in more than 50 percent of red blood cells in severely immuno-compromised patients; (4) the growth of dark PLFs in budding, non-budding, and hyphal forms is unequivocally more pronounced in the peripheral parts of the smear where the erythrocyte membranes show more advanced evidence of oxidative damage; and (5) the heavy growth of PLFs in the blood was markedly reduced with therapies that improved tissue perfusion, facilitated lymphatic drainage, controlled tissue acidosis, and included antifungal pharmacologic agents such as Nystatin, fluconazole, and others.[15] However, dark bodies representing intracellular PLFs could still be seen within blood corpuscles after treatment.

For months after I became convinced that dark PLFs are much harder to control than pale PLFs, I kept this finding to myself. (I often do that with new observations to see if any of my associates will validate my observation independently.) Then one day Judy Juco, M.D., one of the senior physicians at the Institute, asked me if I had noticed the higher degree of virulence of the dark PLFs. I told her I had. Some months later, my good friend, professor Robert Bradford of Capital University, also told me he had encountered greater difficulty controlling dark PLFs.

How amazing! Oxygen orchestrates the whole drama of death. Oxygen in health is nature's prime antibiotic. And oxygen in disease is nature's prescription for not prolonging the process of dying. Oxygen is efficient in health as well as in dying.

INFECTIONS FROM WITHIN: THE ORPEC STATE

The notion of an "infection from within" may appear ridiculous to many in medicine. But I consider it another one of my important insights.

In 1997, I read a report in *Science* that sent a shudder down my spine. In that report, the genetic map of bakers' yeast was compared with the then-known gene pool of mammals, including humans.[14] The comparison revealed that mammalian cells and yeast cells have in common more than 30% of their genes. Furthermore, the common genes also share common functions, so that what a gene did in mammals also performed a similar function in the yeast. For years I had known that animals share many genes. What stirred such excitement in me that day was a moment of clarity: If yeast genes *exist within our genetic pool*, then should we not see the overgrowth and infections of yeast as "infections from within"? Would that also not be true of all other types of primordial life forms? For the first

time in my life and all in a flash, I saw the novel possibility of a
microecologic-genetic model of illness.

**PLF infections occur from within because their
genes pre-exist in human beings.**

That simple idea, of course, flew in the face of everything that
I had been taught about infectious diseases, first in medical school,
then in my surgery and pathology residency programs, and later
during my years of directing a microbiology laboratory. Yet, that
simple idea was too powerful to be ignored. It has strong explanatory
power, as I show later in this chapter, for many of my microscopic
observations that could not be explained in any other way. (I did not
then fully realize that that *was* the basic argument in the Pasteur-
Bechamp debate which I discuss at length in a later chapter.

MICROBIAL PLEOMORPHISM

Every medical school student is taught about the phenomenon
of microbial pleomorphism. Simply stated, pleomorphism means
more than one morph (shape) of a microbial species. The primary
importance of bacterial pleomorphism is that change in form often
results in change in virulence of that microbial species. Another
important consideration is that changes in form often cause difficulty
in identification.

**Thus, pleomorphism carries a double whammy,
becoming more dangerous and escaping
recognition at the same time. In other words,
pleomorphism often creates stealth organisms.**

There, of course, was nothing new there. Almquist, a Swedish microbiologist, first observed and described the phenomenon of bacterial polymorphism involving typhoid organisms. An astute observer, he also recognized that as the microbes changed their appearance, they also changed in their function (ability to cause disease). That was followed by a vigorous debate lasting for two centuries about what else pleomorphism meant. Notable players in that debate were the Frenchmen Pasteur and Bechamp, the Swede Almquist; the Germans Weismann and Underlein, the French-turned-Canadian Naessens, the Japanese Kikuo Chishima, and the Americans Livingston and Mattman. I was aware of that debate. (See the chapter, "Oxygen Settles the Great Pasteur-Bechamp Debate.") But, to my knowledge, none of them had written anything about gene sharing as the basis of microbial pleomorphism. What shook me hard in the *Science* report describing the gene pool in common among the yeast and mammalian cells was the possibility of a genetic explanation of the various pleomorphic phenomena observed and documented by the various authors.

That insight led me to propose my theory of *Oxidative Regression to Primordial Cellular Ecology (ORPEC).*[11]

The basic concept of the ORPEC theory is simple: It holds that the cellular states of oxidation and oxygenation determine how the shared genes express themselves.

As an analogy, the soil in a backyard holds seeds of grass as well as weed, and the condition of the soil will determine whether we see a beautiful lawn of grass or a field overgrown with weeds. In clinical terms, the ORPEC theory offers a novel microecologic-genetic model that fully explains symptom complexes of many chronic disorders, such as chronic fatigue syndrome, fibromyalgia, Gulf War syndrome, and cancer. In a lengthy article published in *The Journal of Integrative Medicine* in 1998,[11] I presented extensive microscopic, chemical, and clinical evidence to support the ORPEC theory. That article is reproduced in full in the companion volume, *Canary Two: Oxygen and Fibromyalgia.* I recommend that advanced and professional readers peruse that article for all the scientific facts that support the theory.

The ORPEC theory challenges the following three most rigidly held beliefs of prevailing drug medicine:

1.   That infections are always caused by microbes invading the body from the outside.
2.   That for a given microbe to be accepted as the cause of disease, it must be cultured in the laboratory.
3.   That infections caused by microbes can be cured by the use of the antibiotics to which such microbes are sensitive.

The crucial importance of my view will be readily seen by the mothers of children who live on antibiotics for recurrent ear infections and sore throats. The more antibiotics their children take, the sicker they get. Many women with unending attacks of cystitis and yeast infections will also see the truth in my statement. Each course of antibiotics sets them up for the next infection. The cases of men with recurrent prostatitis, bronchitis, diverticulitis, and other infections are similar. All such children, women, and men must realize that their infections come from *within,* and not from outside.

A DEAD DEER BLOATS UP

Some time ago, I saw the body of a bloated deer, a road kill left by some motorist hours earlier. That was the first time I fully recognized how malicious oxygen is to the primordial microbes and how intensely those microbes hate oxygen.

How does the abdomen of a deer killed by a motorist bloat up? When the deer stops breathing, it stops pulling in oxygen. Within minutes, the oxygen in the body of the deer is used up. The lack of oxygen triggers many mechanisms designed to recycle the tissues of the dead deer as quickly as possible. In essence, all those mechanisms unleash the three killer furies of oxidosis, dysoxygenosis, and acidosis. Oxygen is nature's main weapon against primordial microbes.

Take out oxygen, PLFs go rampant.
Absent oxygen, enter the killer furies!

Those are the best conditions for PLFs to take off, multiply at a rapid rate, ferment the contents of the bowel, produce large quantities of gas, and bloat the deer's abdomen. And, of course, that is not where the fast-breeding PLFs and killer furies rest. Within days, what is left behind of the deer is mere skeleton. Later, other types of PLFs take over and turn bones into calcium, magnesium, and phosphate dust. For persons who have had a brush with cancer or who harbor tumors now, I might add that the killer furies that shatter the antioxidant, enzyme, and immune defenses of a person with spreading cancer are the same as fibro furies: oxidosis, dysoxygenosis, and acidosis.

Trillions of microbes in the bowel of the deer did not threaten its health as long as the deer was breathing. Oxygen inhaled by the deer kept the genes of the primordial microbes in check. But that changed when the deer was killed. What determined the deer's cellular state? *At the most fundamental level, it was oxygen.* And that, in essence, is the oxidative regression to primordial cellular ecology.

The lesson for persons with cancer here is the same: At the most fundamental level, it is oxygen that determines whether their immune cells win over cancer cells or whether cancer cells defeat the immune cells.

GRASS DIES, WEEDS FLOURISH

A man taking great pride in his lawn seeds, feeds, and weeds the grass regularly to maintain it in a manicured state. A drought forces the township to ban the use of municipal water for watering lawns. In several weeks, the velvet green grass is replaced with overgrown weeds that overwhelm the grass. In this analogy, the drought turned the soil ecology from one that nourished grass to one that strongly favored weeds. As the soil ecology changed, so did the growth sustained by it. In the ORPEC state, the physiologic oxygenative, alkaline, and nontoxic cellular ecology is oxidatively converted (regresses) into an anoxic, acidotic, and toxic primordial state. The primordial ecology so produced favors the activation and perpetuation of primordial DNA sequences of PLFs (including those of yeast) that remain dormant in physiologic (well-oxygenative and alkaline) conditions, as evidenced by the absence of their active proliferation in the freshly prepared peripheral blood smears of healthy volunteers. The human DNA sequences involved in inflammatory and healing responses, by contrast, are at a clear disadvantage in anoxic and acidotic primordial conditions.

INNATE AND ADAPTIVE DEFENSES
Defensins and Tolls

Nature is a master of balancing acts. It blesses every life form with two types of arsenals against other life forms that threaten its existence: an innate (ready-made) defense system and an adaptive (rising to the occasion) defense system. I include below a brief section about hundreds of known natural antifungal, antimicrobial, and anti-PLF substances produced and deployed by our oxidative, enzymatic, and immune defenses to fight off infections from without as well as within. Even though I limit myself to simple details, some readers may find some terms tedious. Those readers may simply skip this section.

The innate immune defense system includes a family of hunter immune cells in the circulating blood as well as in tissues which directly attacks the invading microbes, kills them, swallows them, and digests them. In essence, the microbes serve as its fodder. It also includes natural killer immune cells that produce "microbial poisons" called cytokines that paralyze or kill microbes. The adaptive defense system, by contrast, includes the antibody-forming immune cells and some specific cell membrane docking sites (the T-cell receptors).

Nature creates PLFs and grants them the ability to survive under harsh conditions. It arms PLFs with toxic organic acids so those life forms are not completely defenseless against the hunter cells. Under certain conditions, their toxins paralyze and kill the immune cells. *The predator becomes the prey.* Nature also gives the hunter immune cells some survival advantages. One such advantage is the ability of human cells to make antimicrobial agents called defensins.[15-18]

Defensins are two families of natural antibiotics (peptides, in chemical composition) found in people, mammals, insects, and plants. In humans, the first family, designated *a*-defensins, is produced by the hunter immune cells of the circulating blood (neutrophils) and certain cells lining the bowel wall (Paneth's cells). The second family, called *b*-defensins, is produced by the cells in the skin, kidneys, and the bronchial tubes. During the last twenty years, hundreds of antimicrobial peptides have been discovered in human cells, marine life, and plants. Defensins are produced by the human cells when they come in contact with microbes and PLFs.

The fruit fly (*Drosophila*) protects itself against certain fungi by producing an antifungal peptide ("little protein") called drosomycin. The production of this antifungal substance is under the control of a fruit fly protein called Toll.[19] Thus, nature gave the humble fruit fly a powerful way of taking a toll on fungi and PLFs. Similarly, many plants produce antifungal proteins. (I suppose I can call them *"plantimycins."*) So nature also blessed lowly plants with their own antifungal drugs. Recently researchers discovered that we humans also have a family of toll proteins that help us manufacture our own antifungal (and, undoubtedly, anti-PLF substances). At the time of this writing, five members of this family have been recognized. It is safe for me to predict that future research will reveal the existence of many such proteins and antifungal and anti-PLF agents produced by them.

Where there is a disease, there is a bug.
Where there is a bug, there is a drug.

My purpose in including the above brief comments about defensins and toll defense substances is simply to make the following essential point: Those in medicine who think they can *cure* infections by prescribing antibiotics are misguided. Antibiotics can give us an edge in our battle with microbes, but that is all. In the man-microbe struggle for peaceful coexistence, each is blessed with many tools. The diversity of defenses of both is stunningly broad. It is silly to think that we can eradicate *all* the Lyme spirochetes, mycoplasma, stealth microbes, and other less commonly known microbes. The same is true of holistic physicians when they claim they can "root out" yeast with their therapies. We physicians should take the lead from marine biologists, who are discovering many "new" diseases that are killing marine life species on a large scale. They use such terms as extinction on "massive scales."[20] The message here is simple:

We must learn to coexist with PLFs as our forefathers did for millennia or be banished by our killer antibiotics. We must learn to harness our natural antibiotics-like defensins to seek a peaceful coexistence with PLFs.

LIMITATIONS OF THE CULTURING METHODS

The bowel ecosystem teems with life. It has been estimated that the bowel contains as many as fifty trillion microbes. That means, roughly speaking, there may be more than one microbe in the bowel for every cell in the body. I have concluded from my microscopic studies that the bowel flora described in microbiology textbooks represents but a very small part of the total microbial population in the gut.

The reason why medical laboratories fail to grow PLFs from clinical samples is that the culture media used do not create the ecologic conditions for PLF growth.

This is the seventh essential point in this chapter. PLFs, as I indicate earlier, grow rapidly in the presence of dead and decaying organic matter and conditions of excess acidity and absence of oxygen. Those are not the conditions offered by the culture media used in most medical laboratories.

A case in point: Researchers at Mayo Clinic recently discovered fungal infections to be a major factor in hard-to-treat sinusitis. Only now have the culturing techniques become advanced enough to discern that. There is no doubt in my mind that in the future many more types of PLFs will be recognized and characterized, including a variety of stealth microbes and nanobacteria which cannot be grown under ordinary laboratory conditions at this time.

SUMMARY

The human aging process is deeply influenced by primordial life forms (PLFs). Such forms hate oxygen, love acidity, and thrive on sugars and decaying matter. Present-day microbes which share the metabolic characteristics of PLFs are designated as primordial microbes and include the commonly recognized bacteroides and other bowel anaerobes, mycoplasma and related stealth microbes, nanobacteria, yeast and yeast-like organisms. The human bowel ecosystem teems with diverse microbial populations. Undoubtedly, the recognized bowel flora represents but a small number of primordial microbes.

Premature aging occurs when the ecologic conditions in the bowel, blood, and other major ecosystems of the body shift to those of oxidosis, dysoxygenosis, and acidosis (the three furies). Such ecologic changes favor the growth of PLFs over those of human defense cells. The PLF overgrowth, in turn, fans the flames of the three furies, thus setting up destructive cycles. The more intense the primordial conditions, the greater the PLF overgrowth. The larger the number of PLFs, the more advanced the degree of primordial regression.

The problems created by oxidative regression to primordial cellular ecology and PLF overgrowth have four clinical faces: (1) overgrowth in the bowel, blood, and other body ecosystems; (2) allergy to PLFs; (3) PLF toxicity; and (4) "infections" caused by PLFs. All four factors feed upon each other. For those reasons, I consider the overgrowth of primordial microbes in the bowel as one of the two fundamental issues in my ecologic thinking about the bowel ecosystem. The other major issue is that of food incompatibilities and related digestive-absorptive problems. For healthful aging, all of the above issues must be addressed effectively and for a sufficiently long time to achieve ecologic restoration and health. Drug therapies, while essential for acute disease, do not address any of the real underlying issues that threaten human health.

References

1. Ali M. Ali O. Fibromyalgia: On oxidative-dysoxygenative disorder (ODD). J Integrative Medicine 1999;3:17-37.
2. Ali M, Juco J, Fayemi A, et al. Efficacy of ecologic-integrative management protocols for reversal of fibromyalgia. J Integrative Medicine 1999;1:48-63.
3. Ali M, Ali O, Fayemi AO, et al. Efficacy of an integrative program including intravenous and intramuscular nutrient therapies for arrested growth. J Integrative Medicine 1998;2:56-69.
4. Ali M. Amenorrhea, oligomenorrhea, and polymenorrhea in CFS and fibromyalgia are caused by oxidative menstrual dysfunction. J Integrative Medicine 1998;3:101-124.
5. Ali M. Of doctors and gardeners. Aging Healthfully 1999;1:1-4.
6. Ali M, Ali O. AA Oxidopathy: the core pathogenetic mechanism of ischemic heart disease. J Integrative Medicine 1997;1:1-112.
7. Nature 1998;392;801
8. Ali M. Oxygen order of human biology. J Integrative Medicine (in press).
9. Ali M. Darwin, oxidosis, dysoxygenosis, and integration. J Integrative Medicine 1999;1:11-16.
10. Krajick K. To hell and back. Discover. July 1999, pp 75-82.
11. Ali M. Oxidative regression to primordial cellular ecology (ORPEC): evidence for the hypothesis and its clinical significance. J Integrative Medicine 1988;2:4-55.
12. Gilbert DL, Colton CA. Reactive Oxygen Species in Biological Systems. 1999. Kluwer Academic / Plenum Publishers. New York. pp 9.
13. Ali M.RDA: Rats, Drugs and Assumption, 1995. Life Span, Denville, New Jersey.
14. Botstein D, Chervitz SA, Cherry JM. Yeast as a model organism. Science 1997; 277:1259-1200.
15. Ganz T. Defensins and host defenses. Science 1999;286:420-1.
16. Tang Y, Yuan J, Osapay G et al. A cyclic antimicrobial peptide produced

in primate leucocytes by the ligation of truncated a-defensins. Science. 1999;286:498-502.

17.   Medzhitov R, Preston-Hurlburt P, Janeway CA Jr. Human homologue of the Drosophilia Toll protein signal activation of adaptive immunity. Nature 1997;388:394-7.

18.   Yang RB, Mark MR, Gray A, et al. Toll-like receptor-2 mediates lipopolysaccharide-induced cellular signalling. Nature 1998;395:284-8.

19.   Modlin RL, Brightbill HD, Godowski PJ. The toll of innate immunity on microbial pathogens. N Eng J Med 1999;340:1834-5.

20.   Harvell CD, Kim K, Burkholder JM, et al. Emerging marine diseases-climate links and anthropogenic factors. Science 1999;285:1505-1510.

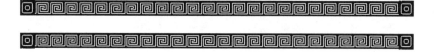

A desert is bone dry for months. Then it blooms after rain. That, in the simplest words, is the seed-soil relationship. In the bowel, whether seeds (microbes) contribute to health or threaten it is determined by the ecologic conditions that prevail there. In the blood, oxygen determines whether PLFs flourish or become fodder for the hunter immune cells there.

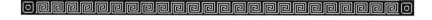

"We are all agreed that your theory is crazy. The question which divides us is whether it is crazy enough to have a chance of being correct.'

Niels Bohr, Nobelist physicist.

Chapter 8

The History of Oxygen and Dysfunctional Oxygen Metabolism

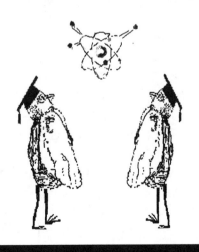

By now the reader should be fully familiar with the first six of the seven major insights that led me to recognize that oxidosis leads to dysoxygenosis and to formulate my dysoxygenosis theory of aging. Briefly, in 1983, in my first monograph concerning oxygen, *Spontaneity of Oxidation in Nature and Aging*,[1] I described my first two insights about oxygen and oxidation. The first insight gave me a recognition that oxidation in human biology occurs by itself, without an external clue and without expenditure of energy, and led me to propose my spontaneity of oxidation theory of aging. That means that spontaneity of oxidation provides the *fundamental* mechanism that initiates and perpetuates molecular and cellular injury in the aging process. The second insight gave me a clear view of the many Dr. Jekyll-Mr. Hyde roles of oxygen, and how oxygen turns many other elements into other forms of Dr. Jekylls and Mr. Hydes.[2] The third insight opened windows to the world of dis-ease, the zone between absence of health and presence of disease.[3] The fourth insight gave me a fresh perspective between the worlds of psychology and spirituality.[4] Spirituality dissolves anger and heals while psychology feeds our addiction to recycle past anger and, when that is not enough, to precycle feared, future misery. The fifth insight concerned ecologic harmony among the various body ecosystems that determines the state of health or absence of it, and the realization that the bowel, blood, and liver ecosystems formed the base trio of the Pyramid of Trios of the Human Ecosystems.[5] The sixth insight allowed me to recognize oxygen as the primary determinant in the competitive struggle of life between the oxygen-loving human cells and the oxygen-hating primordial life forms.[6]

The seventh insight concerns the recognition that excessive oxidative injury (oxidosis) leads to dysfunctional oxygen metabolism and forms the molecular basis of aging. In 1998, I presented evidence for my hypothesis in an article published in *The Journal of*

Integrative Medicine.[7] I devote this chapter to an in-depth discussion of the last insight since it forms the basis of my dysoxygenosis theory of oxygen.

ABNORMAL CELLULAR OXYGEN METABOLISM

Dysfunctional oxygen metabolism (DOM), as I wrote earlier, is my term for abnormal cellular oxygen metabolism. It is not merely a lack of oxygen, which is called anoxia in medical terminology. This is an important distinction.

The insight that dysfunctional oxygen metabolism is the molecular basis of accelerated (premature) aging through my work with a very large number of air-hungry fibro canaries and my studies with their blood and urine samples led me to conclude that their air hunger was neither imagined nor caused by a lack of oxygen due to disorders of the lung, heart, or blood (anemia). Rather, their basic problem was *dysfunctional* oxygen metabolism developing at a *cellular* level so that they could not properly *metabolize* oxygen, which they did breathe in. That was a major insight for me.

Anoxia is a lack of oxygen in tissues in conditions when oxygen metabolism itself is *normal*. For example, during an asthma attack, a person is short of breath and air-hungry because his bronchial tubes are in spasm and he cannot breathe in enough air. That condition creates anoxia. The *cellular* oxygen metabolism in asthma is normal, hence as soon as the bronchial spasm ends, the patient breathes easily and his air hunger disappears. The asthma sufferer looks completely normal within minutes of taking an inhaler treatment. There is no dysfunctional oxygen metabolism. That is not the case in fibromyalgia. If a fibro canary runs even seventy yards to catch a bus (assuming that he can do so), he may not be able to get out of his bed for a few days. That is so because oxygen metabolism in fibromyalgia is dysfunctional.

As I wrote earlier in this volume, persons with fibromyalgia commonly complain of air hunger or oxygen hunger. Many of my fibro canaries had consulted pulmonologists (lung specialists) for air hunger before they saw me. Their blood oxygen levels and other lung function test results were reported as "within normal limits." They were then told there was nothing wrong with them. Their pulmonologists had concluded that those fibromyalgia patients had only imagined their air hunger. In other words, they were malingerers—the old all-in-the-head theory. But, of course, those fibro canaries were not imagining their air hunger. When the fibro canaries heal with proper treatment, the symptoms of air hunger or shortness of breath clear up, indicating that the symptom of air hunger is a component of the total picture and is not merely imagined.

When proper laboratory tests are done, the fibro canaries often show clear evidence of abnormal oxygen metabolism. For example, tests for urinary organic acids show increased amounts of lactic acid and related compounds. That indicates incomplete metabolism of sugars, proteins, and fats due to impaired oxygen metabolism. Again, following successful treatment of fibromyalgia, such tests become normal. Studies of blood samples with high-resolution microscopy also correlate well with both the clinical improvement and normalization of urine tests.

I coined the term oxidative-dysoxygenative disorder (ODD) for dysfunctional oxygen metabolism and described the various aspects of ODD in a series of articles published in *The Journal of Integrative Medicine.*[7-11] The abstracts of those papers are included in the Appendix of this volume and the full articles are reproduced in the companion volume, *Canary Three: Fibromyalgia Is an Oxidative-Dysoxygenative Disorder (ODD).* To provide a framework for a clear presentation of dysfunctional oxygen metabolism, I include below a brief review of the four periods of the history of oxygen on the planet Earth. That historical perspective sheds additional light on the ORPEC state discussed in the preceding chapter and shows how progressive oxidative stress leads to the production of the oxidative-dysoxygenative state.

****

The Four Periods
of History of Oxygen

The history of oxygen on the planet Earth can be briefly stated to have gone through four stages:

1.   An oxygen-free primordial state.
2.   A period of accumulation of free oxygen in the atmosphere, rising to 30 to 35 percent of the air.
3.   A period of decreasing concentration of free atmospheric oxygen, the level falling to 21 percent and lower at present.
4.   A period of *cellular* dysoxygenosis (dysfunctional oxygen metabolism) in oxidative-dysoxygenative states, such as fibromyalgia, chronic fatigue state, and cancer.

In this chapter, I present basic aspects of each of the four periods that are important for understanding oxygen metabolism in health and dysfunctional oxygen metabolism in fibromyalgia.

THE FIRST PERIOD:
AN OXYGEN-FREE PRIMORDIAL STATE

Scientists generally agree that during the primordial period, oxygen occurred only as a component of various compounds. No oxygen existed as free gas in the air because all oxygen released from oxygen-containing compounds was immediately trapped by the organic matter in the oceanic water as well as that on the earth's surface.

Scientists also generally agree that the atmospheric conditions during the primordial era (primordial ecology, in my terminology) were strongly reducing. Reduction, I explain in the first chapter, is the opposite of oxidation. Thus, the early single-celled microbes (PLFs, in my terminology) came on the scene during a period of absence of free atmospheric oxygen. Since primordial microbes were not exposed to oxygen toxicity, those single-celled organisms developed, lived, and multiplied without learning to cope with oxygen. In other words, primordial microbes had no defenses against oxygen. At present, the commonly used term for microbes that grow in the absence of oxygen is anaerobic microbes (or anaerobes). Like their primordial ancestors, the anaerobes that live in human and animal bowels are also defenseless against oxygen.

This is the scientific basis of my statement that oxygen is Nature's primary antibiotic.

It is also easy to understand from the above comments that when oxygen concentration falls in the tissues, the anaerobes there will flourish. Thus, the two main lessons from the study of the first period of history of oxygen are: (1) oxygen prevents growth of primordial microbes in health; and (2) The lack of oxygen promotes the growth of primordial microbes.

THE SECOND PERIOD OF RISING ATMOSPHERIC FREE OXYGEN

In the second period, plants began the process of photosynthesis, in which the green pigment of plants (chlorophyll) turned the sunlight into the energy of chemical bonds.[12] In the process, the plants took in carbon dioxide from the air and released free oxygen into the air. At first, all oxygen, when released, was rapidly absorbed by oxygen-binding substances in the oceans and on the earth's surface. Later, oxygen released during photosynthesis began to accumulate in the air as free oxygen, first slowly and later much more rapidly. Oxygen is a powerful oxidizer and a potent antimicrobial agent. For those and other reasons discussed in the preceding chapters, rising levels of oxygen posed a serious threat to primordial microbes (PLFs) that were defenseless against oxygen. They could not cope with oxygen, since they had neither been exposed to oxygen nor had they learned to protect themselves from its toxicity. Thus, PLFs were ill-prepared to face oxygen toxicity in ever-increasing degrees. They had the following three possible choices:

The primordial bugs could die out.
The primordial bugs could hide out.
Or the primordial bugs could branch out.

PLFs die out. It is completely safe to state that a large population of primordial microbes could not survive increasing oxygen toxicity and simply died out. A simple laboratory experiment can be conducted today to demonstrate that fact clearly. Samples of pus taken from abdominal abscesses and cultured in the laboratory media without oxygen sometimes grow anaerobic ("oxygen-hating") microbes. If such a culture is then put into a petri dish and exposed to room air containing oxygen, the microbes die within hours. Indeed, that explains why in our hospital laboratories accidental exposure of culture samples to oxygen in the room air leads to the death of microbes and negative culture reports. This is the reason why the laboratory staff diligently avoid any contact between such microbes and oxygen.

PLFs hide out. It is also safe to state that many of those primordial microbes escaped oxygen toxicity by hiding in niches where atmospheric oxygen did not reach. For example, deep crevices in the earth's crust offered PLFs protection from oxygen. With time, many of those microbes searched and found other oxygen-free or oxygen-deficient environments. For example, with passing time various animals appeared on the scene. The large bowels of those animals contained decaying matter with little or no free oxygen. The ecologic conditions in those bowels offered PLFs safe harbors to thrive and multiply rapidly. The anaerobic microbes of today, such as those grown from infected wounds and bowel abscesses, are undoubtedly related to PLFs of the primordial era. Present day examples of such microbes include mycoplasma, stealth organisms, nanobacteria, yeast, yeast-like organisms, bacteroid species, and other such bacteria.

PLFs branch out. Lastly, it is safe to state that some oxygen-hating primordial life forms branched out (adapted to their changing ecologic conditions) and developed methods for coping with the toxicity of free oxygen. Without such branching out (adaptation), today we would not have any oxygen-utilizing cells, such as those of humans and animals. Indeed, that was a masterstroke of microbial engineering. Those oxygen-hating primordial microbes not only learned how to neutralize oxygen, but also found ways to harness the energy of oxygen. Mitochondria are the tiniest bodies within human and animal cells that metabolize oxygen to produce energy. Among mitochondria researchers, there is complete agreement that mitochondria are derived from primordial microbes that acquired the ability to metabolize oxygen.

Scientists estimate that dinosaurs ceased to live about 65 million years ago.[13] The dinosaur that often causes most excitement is *Tyrannosaurus rex,* a name that stands for tyrant lizard king. This meat-eating dinosaur weighed up to 10,000 pounds (as much as seventy men, each weighing 140 pounds). It ran at speeds up to 30 miles an hour, faster than any athlete today. How much energy did a monster like *T. rex* need to run at such a speed? How could such a dinosaur breathe in enough oxygen to produce such high amounts of energy? Some hyperventilation state! (Are stories of such feats by dinosaurs mere figment of imagination? Not so. Such information must not be seen as mere conjecture. Twenty-one complete skeletons of *T. rex* have been unearthed and painstakingly studied by scientists. Our present knowledge of those dinosaurs is based on those studies.)

There is an interesting aspect of that second period of the history of oxygen that is seldom, if ever, discussed by doctors. During an era called the Carboniferous Period, the oxygen concentration in the air rose as high as 30 to 35%.[14] As plants grew in number and their capacity for releasing free oxygen into the air increased, oxygen rose to levels much higher than that in the air today (about 21%). Thus, there was a much higher concentration of oxygen in the air for *T. rex* to inhale during its mad rush of a feeding frenzy. If that dinosaur were to breathe today's air, it would have to breathe nearly twice as fast as it did then to inhale an equivalent amount of oxygen. Or, in other words, its required labor of breathing would have been 40% more. That is not a small extra effort for a huge animal that lived on hunted meat. It would have starved to death if its prey could run faster than it could.

THE THIRD PERIOD
OF FALLING LEVELS OF ATMOSPHERIC OXYGEN

The drop in atmospheric oxygen concentrations occurred slowly over a long period of time. The extent of that drop has been estimated with many different methods. For instance, measurements of the ratios of heavy oxygen 18 and light oxygen 16 isotopes in plankton fossils have revealed the global ice volume and the concentration of oxygen in the air. Light oxygen isotopes evaporate more readily than do the heavy oxygen isotopes and the differences in their relative concentrations are evident in plant matter. Air bubbles trapped in ice contain samples of gas concentrations from periods of time millions of years ago. Measurements of those gases also give clues to relative concentrations of oxygen, carbon dioxide, and other gases, such as methane. Analysis of such tiny samples of air have enabled researchers to determine that concentrations of carbon dioxide and methane have risen by 25 and 100 percent respectively during the past one hundred years.[15] Of course, oxygen levels in the air fell to make room for such increases of those two gases.

What might be the meaning of a near 40 percent drop in the

concentration of oxygen? I never wondered about that until I traveled to Kenya's Serengeti National Park. Standing in a roof hatch of a van, I watched two mammoth African bull elephants escorting a herd as the driver slowly moved to within about fifty feet of the animals. I stood in awe of the size of the bulls. Then my mind drifted to the subject of size in the animal kingdom and ended up with the mental images of dinosaurs. Two questions arose before me:

Why Did Dinosaurs of Yesteryear Become So Big?
Why Don't Elephants of Today Become That Big?

With questions like those, my mind usually drifts to the subject of oxygen. I recognized that my myopic eyes see everything through the prism of oxygen. Yet, the questions persisted. It was tempting to look for a simplistic oxygen-related explanation. Can oxygen solve that mystery as well? (I can almost see some readers chuckle.)

Common sense told me that oxygen should be the most important ecologic factor in the growth and the size of various animal species. But I was not aware of any direct evidence to support such conjecture. Indeed, scientists who had considered that matter had thought otherwise. Animals tend to be larger in areas closer to the poles. That is called polar gigantism. In the past, it was assumed that was due to lower temperature and slower metabolism of such animals.[16] That assumption did not seem unreasonable. Still, that left me, obsessed as I am with oxygen, feeling empty. Amazingly, that changed only two months before the time of this writing.

Some giant insects lived in the Carboniferous Period when the oxygen concentration in the air was nearly twice what it is today (30-35%).[14] Why did those giant insects become extinct? Again, it is tempting to speculate that giant insects died out when the oxygen level in the air fell. Less available oxygen could not support the giant bodies of those insects. (Ridiculous! I can hear some readers protest loudly. Doesn't this disciple of Darwin know anything?, they may ask. Aren't there hundreds of ecologic factors to be considered? Aren't there big and small animals everywhere? Doesn't his obsession with oxygen blind him to everything else?)

Something very interesting was reported a few months ago. Belgian researchers analyzed data for 1,853 animal species from 12 sites worldwide, extending from polar to tropical and freshwater to marine.[17] They took into account many variables, and confirmed that oxygen is the most important ecologic factor in determination of the size of a species. One of their many observations that support their conclusion is that oxygen dissolved in the hemolymph of certain marine life forms increased from tropical to polar ecosystems. (Hemolymph is mixed blood and lymph fluid in some marine life forms.) It has been proposed that if global oxygen levels decline, giant amphipods may be the first species to disappear.[17] Oxygen solubility in water increases as salinity decreases. If the predictions about global warming were to come true and the massive bodies of frozen water in the Arctic and Antarctic were to melt, it would be expected to reduce the salinity of ocean water. Such a change in salinity could possibly improve oxygenation of water and increase availability of oxygen to marine life.[18]

THE FOURTH PERIOD OF CELLULAR OXYGEN DEFICIENCY AND DYSFUNCTIONAL OXYGEN METABOLISM

The twentieth century has been an age of chemical avalanches. Pesticides, herbicides, synthetic hormones, and industrial pollutants have produced a total chemical load that has seriously threatened the oxygen metabolism of people, animal, and plants. In the United States, we are regularly exposed to an estimated 65,000 different chemicals. Radiation pollution has been an underestimated threat. Chronic anger, resentment, and hostility have further increased oxidative stress. Thus, our century has been a period of progressive oxidative stress on human biology.

Oxidosis affects all human ecologic systems. The oxidizing capacity of the entire planet Earth is increasing for a variety of reasons. Thinning of the ozone layer is increasing oxidant stress. And so is the greenhouse effect of rising levels of carbon dioxide in the air. Industrial environmental pollutants and pesticides are oxidizing. Indoor pollution is reportedly greater than outdoor pollution in many cases. Sugar overload is prevalent in all countries, and excess sugar intake increases oxidant stress. Antibiotic abuse is pervasive and antibiotics, as necessary for acute infections as they might be, damage the normal bowel flora, cause proliferation of PLFs, and so serve as powerful oxidizing agents. Chronic dehydration has become an epidemic problem, and lack of optimal hydration is oxidizing because it results in accumulation in the body of organic acids and toxic reactive species. Excess acidity in our external and internal environments is oxidizing. The external factors include pesticides and herbicides, industrial pollutants, and toxic metals. The internal factors include stress, sugar overload, processed food, and PLF overgrowth. Lactic acidosis is common in chronic illness such as fibromyalgia and chronic fatigue syndrome, and it is oxidizing. Synthetic hormones are oxidizing, albeit indirectly, by interfering with hepatic detoxification pathways. And, finally, the pervasive adrenergic hypervigilence caused by anger and violence are powerfully oxidizing.

In a larger sense, the significance of the ORPEC state described in the preceding chapter goes far beyond the issue of pandemics of fibromyalgia, CFS, Gulf War syndrome, chemical sensitivity syndrome, hyperactivity/attention deficit disorder in children, severe autoimmune disorders such as multiple sclerosis, and disseminated cancer. The growing menace of progressive, unrelenting oxidative stress on our internal and external environments casts long shadows over the future of humankind.

For emphasis I repeat that all of the oxidative factors mentioned above threaten cellular oxygen metabolism, create an oxidative-dysoxygenative dysfunction, and accelerate the aging process. The resulting dysfunctional oxygen metabolism leads to fibromyalgia and chronic fatigue syndrome, serious environmental illness, and the Gulf War syndrome. Below, I list seven major oxidative factors and give brief explanations of how oxidative-dysoxygenative aging stress is caused by each of them:

1.   "PLF Oxidosis" (too much oxidative stress caused by PLF overgrowth);
2.   Dehydration oxidosis;
3.   Lifestyle stress oxidosis;
4.   Damaged foods oxidosis;
5.   Antibiotics oxidosis;

6. Pesticides and herbicides oxidosis;
7. Toxic metals, chemical pollutants and radiation oxidosis.

1. PLF OXIDOSIS, ODD, AND AGING

I consider PLF oxidosis as the *most* important hazard in the genesis of dysfunctional oxygen metabolism. I make that bold statement because that is a conclusion I cannot escape from my high-resolution study of nearly five thousand patients with fibromyalgia, CFS, Lyme disease, severe immune disorders, and cancer. I state the evidence of my view in the following simple sentences reproduced from the preceding chapter on primordial life forms:

1. *The sicker the patient, the dirtier the blood.*
2. *The larger the number of PLFs in the blood smears, the greater the oxidative stress on the cells and blood plasma.*
3. *The healthier the sick become with treatment, the cleaner their blood becomes.*
4. *Severe oxidative stress is seen in some conditions without PLF overgrowth, but PLF overgrowth is not seen without oxidative stress on blood cells and plasma.*

My associates at the Institute, professors Alfred Fayemi and Judy Juco, have studied a large number of blood smears with high-resolution microscopy. I showed them a draft of this page and asked them if they disagreed with any of the above statements. Both of them fully agreed with me.

Some readers may ask how I can be sure that PLF overgrowth causes excess oxidative stress. In other words, what is my proof that PLF oxidosis is real? The answer to that question is in the last of the above four statements. PLF overgrowth was *always* associated with oxidosis of blood in my patients. However, I did not always see PLF overgrowth in every case of blood oxidosis. In other words, oxidosis can exist in the absence of PLF overgrowth, for example, in very early stages of acute viral and bacterial infection. In the later stages, such infections suppress the immune system and PLF overgrowth occurs as a consequence of immune suppression. For advanced and professional readers interested in this subject, I recommend an article entitled "Oxidative Regression to Primordial Cellular Ecology" published in *The Journal of Integrative Medicine*[6] in 1998 and reproduced in the companion volume, *Canary Three: Oxygen and Fibromyalgia.*

2. DEHYDRATION, DOM, AND AGING

All human canaries are severely dehydrated unless they drink up to three to four quarts of water a day. The degree of dehydration is always obvious from the dry states of their skin and tongue. "My eyes, there is a desert out there!" a fibro canary said once. I see clear evidence of dehydration in the blood samples of most of my fibro canaries. I observe crystal formation in most blood smears, a clear signal of dehydration. Such signs of dehydration disappear when those canaries learn to keep themselves well hydrated (see the chapter, "Guidelines for Healthful Aging."

Though the oxidative-dysoxygenative effects of dehydration in the cells of human canaries are difficult to measure directly, studies with plants shed much light on this subject.[19-21] For example, experiments with peas exposed to dehydration[19] (water stress) have shown the following changes:

a. Up to 78% reduction in photosynthesis (the process by which plants use sunlight to build their food and release free oxygen in the air).
b. Up to 80% depression of activities of antioxidant enzymes, including catalase and those of vitamin C-glutathione.
c. Increased oxidative damage to oils (lipid peroxidation) and oxidative disfigurement of proteins.

In plants, reduced photosynthesis leads to excess excitation energy, which is converted into free radicals.[22] The plants, of course, have their free radical scavenging systems that in health neutralize such oxidants. However, those scavenging systems also depend on an ample water supply to function well. Thus, dehydration carries a double jeopardy for the plants. In human cells, dehydration causes dysfunctional oxygen metabolism in the same way.

3. ANGER, LIFESTYLE STRESS, DOM, AND AGING

Acute stress causes rapid release of adrenaline and its sister "stress molecules" from the adrenal glands. Adrenaline is one of the most potent, if not the most potent, oxidant molecules in the human body. I call such a state of excess adrenaline "adrenergic hypervigilence." In its most acute form, adrenergic hypervigilence produces what I call the Fourth-of-July chemistry. I use that analogy to explain that acute adrenergic hypervigilence creates unpredictable patterns of fireworks in the body. The agitation and hyperexcitability in the tissues caused by such fireworks can affect any or all parts of the body. Anger and hostility also increase oxidative stress in the same way.

Adrenaline and its sister molecules (together called catecholamines) trigger oxidative pathways in the body in different ways. First, such molecules undergo spontaneous oxidation (auto-oxidation) and produce many secondary oxidants. Second, adrenaline and its sister molecules are converted into a host of oxidants by an enzyme system called the mixed oxidase system. Adrenaline is also changed into organic radicals by the action of superoxide.

For a detailed discussion of this essential issue, I refer the interested readers to *What Do Lions Know About Stress?,* in which I provide much practical information in the following three chapters:[23]

1.   "Stress and the Fourth-of-July Chemistry";
2.   "Anxiety, Lactic Acid, and Limbic Lions";
3.   "Adrenergic Hypervigilance, Mitral Valve Prolapse, Dysautonomia, and Chronic Fatigue Syndrome."

4. OXIDIZED FOODS, DOM, AND AGING

Foods, like people, have their life spans and age and spoil with oxidative injury. The ancients recognized this and recommended that foods be eaten fresh. They must have recognized that foods contained some healthful components that were lost when foods became stale. Today we recognize those components as natural antioxidants, such as vitamins C and E, carotenoids, flavonoids, glutathione and others. We now recognize that foods become stale when they lose their natural antioxidants and can no longer resist oxidation and decay by oxygen in the air, as well as by many natural and man-made environmental oxidants, such as nitrates and sulfates.

The ancients also recommended moderation in eating. What could be the redox (oxidative-antioxidative) basis of that recommendation? I cite one example. Most fish oil fatty acids have antioxidant effects. However, when taken in excess, such oils facilitate oxidation by becoming pro-oxidative.[24] That is another fascinating example of molecular duality in nature. In nature, there is a delicate play of oxidants turning into antioxidants and vice versa. Even in experiments, the point at which an antioxidant takes on pro-oxidant functions can be very hard to predict.[25,26]

Sometimes I hear food enthusiasts claim that if only they could convince people to take enough of a particular food, they can cure this or that disease. Some antioxidant enthusiasts even claim that if only they could pour enough antioxidants into the body, they could not only control disease but "anti-age" themselves. Nature seems to have no respect for such foolishness. (I suspect such enthusiasts really do know that they cannot anti-age themselves or anyone else, but know they can sell their favorite antioxidants by making those claims.)

5. ANTIBIOTIC OXIDOSIS, DOM, AND AGING

Antibiotics increase oxidative stress by several direct and indirect mechanisms, including the following:

a.   Most antibiotics promote overgrowth of PLFs, which increases oxidative stress by causing leaky gut syndrome as well as oxidative coagulopathy.

b.   Some antibiotics decrease the reserves of glutathione in the liver. Glutathione, of course, is the quarterback antioxidant of the antioxidant defenses of the liver.

c.   Some antibiotics reduce the amount of taurine in the hunter immune cells. Taurine is a powerful antioxidant and a cell membrane stabilizer.

d.   Some antibiotics are known to turn many species of microbes into their cell-deficient forms that, in many cases, are far more virulent. Microbes trigger oxidative bursts simply by contacting the surfaces of red blood cells, hunter immune cells, cells lining blood vessels, and cells in other tissues.

e.   Many antibiotics are metabolized in the liver where, as is the case with most synthetic chemicals, drugs trigger oxidative chain reactions.

Many of my fibro canaries told me they had lived on sugar and antibiotics for years before they came down with fibromyalgia. That happened because their pediatricians and family doctors simply had not learned how to diagnose the underlying immune deficits and manage common infections with immune-supportive therapies and treatment of hidden allergies, without employing antibiotics. Nor had they considered it important to warn the mothers of the children against the serious adverse effects of sugar.

Beyond the issue of antibiotic abuse by doctors, who are ignorant about natural ways of treating infections, is the matter of daily exposure of children to *massive* amounts of antibiotics in their food. The following simple calculation reveals the true threat of antibiotic oxidosis we face. The total yearly amount of antibiotics fed to poultry and cattle that reach the dining tables in the United States has been estimated to be about twenty million pounds. That comes to more than an ounce of antibiotics for every U.S. citizen. An ounce equals about 30,000 milligrams. Most antibiotics are prescribed in doses of 100 to 1,000 milligrams per day. For example, for common infections, the usual dose of doxycycline is 100 milligrams daily and that of ampicillin is 250 milligrams three times a day for five to seven days. Thus, common infections are treated with 500 to 3,500 milligrams of antibiotics. Now compare the two quantities, 30,000 milligrams in food and a median value of 2,000 milligrams for treating an infection.

An equally important issue is that of a short-term, high-dose antibiotic use for acute infections versus year long, very low-dose exposure. It is well established that microbes mutate and become resistant to antibiotics more quickly and frequently with continuous low-dose therapy. Thus, antibiotics taken via foods are much more dangerous than those taken for infections. Is this merely a matter of theoretical interest? Not so. Ceftiofor is commonly fed to cows and pigs and is very similar to ceftriaxone used to treat *Salmonella* infections in people. Not unexpectedly, a ten-fold increase in ceftriaxone-resistant *Salmonella* was reported at the 1999 Interscience Conference on Antimicrobial Agents and Chemotherapy.[27] Similarly, virginiamycin, an antibiotic added to chicken feed for the last 25 years, has led to an increase in the number of vancomycin-resistant microbes in human stool and chicken meat samples.

It is safe to predict that the oxidative-dysoxygenative hazard of antibiotics will continue to grow. It is not likely that antibiotists of drug medicine will learn about natural alternatives to drugs any time soon. Nor does it seem probable that antibiotists of the meat industry will discontinue feeding their animals potent antibiotics.

6. PESTICIDE AND HERBICIDE OXIDOSIS, DOM, AND AGING

Pesticides are designer killer molecules. What kills bugs will eventually also kill people. There is simply no way out of that dilemma. All pesticides kill pests (insects) by blocking or inactivating their respiratory enzymes. An example of that is destruction of the enzyme cholinesterase. It turns out that the cholinesterase enzyme of insects is identical to that in people. The reason pesticides kill pests efficiently but do not seem to have immediate toxic effects on people is because there is so little of pests to be killed but so much of humans to be destroyed. It is only a difference of size and time.

Most herbicides in common use kill plants by excessive production of toxic oxygen forms (reactive oxygen species, ROS). Increased activity of oxidants so produced overwhelms plants' antioxidant defenses.[28] For example, paraquat, a commonly used herbicide, penetrates the plant protoplast and directly oxidizes the plant substances, diverting electrons from photosynthesis to produce reactive free radicals. (In scientific terms, paraquat accepts electrons from the compounds formed as the result of photosynthesis and passes those electrons to oxygen, so turning safe oxygen in the air into toxic superoxide.) At the same time paraquat reduces the production of an essential antioxidant called NADPH. Thus, the plant faces the double jeopardy of too many oxidants and too little antioxidants. Some other herbicides, such as monuron, block electron transport in the chloroplast by interfering with steps involved with substance Q. Again, of importance to the oxidative-dysoxygenative hazards are the close similarities between the plant and human electron transport pathways.

7. CHEMICAL AND TOXIC METAL OXIDOSIS, RADIATION OXIDOSIS, DOM, AND AGING

Toxic metals, such as mercury and arsenic, increase oxidative stress by several mechanisms. For example, glutathione is the quarterback molecule of the antioxidant system in the liver, and mercury destroys it by ripping apart its sulfhydryl groups.[29] Some arsenic compounds paralyze respiratory enzymes and "chemically suffocate" cells. Cellular suffocation causes severe oxidative stress. Synthetic hormones cause oxidative stress in many direct and indirect ways. Such substances jam or damage cell membrane receptors (hooks) that cells use to catch natural hormones as those molecules swim by in the fluid that bathes cells. The result is that natural hormones are unable to reach their destiny. Beyond that, synthetic hormones fundamentally alter the hormone-receptor-gene-product mechanisms.[30] Industrial pollutants increase oxidizing capacity of the earth as well as of human microecologic cellular and macroecologic tissue-organ ecosystems.[31] Radiation energy causes direct oxidative stress by literally bouncing electrons from various molecules. Recall that the term oxidation means loss of electrons. Radiation of various types also increases oxidative stress by damaging cellular antioxidant defenses.[32]

FROM OXIDOSIS TO DYSOXYGENOSIS

In this section, I summarize seven sets of biochemical observations that show how oxidosis leads to dysoxygenosis. I limit myself here to the bare facts and avoid describing chemical reactions that are involved in oxidosis causing dysoxygenosis for the fear that the general reader will find it too cumbersome. I refer the advanced and professional readers to an in-depth discussion of this subject in my article, "Fibromyalgia: An Oxidative-Dysoxygenative Disorder (ODD)," published in *The Journal of Integrative Medicine*[7], which is also reproduced in full in *Canary Three: Oxygen and Fibromyalgia.*

First, excessive oxidative stress in fibromyalgia causes overproduction of many toxic organic acids* which blocks the actions of enzymes of oxygen metabolism, both by creating excess acidity that inhibits enzyme activity and directly inactivating enzymes.

Second, PLF overgrowth in fibromyalgia results in production of large amounts of toxins. Many PLF toxins** and mycotoxins

---

* Examples of such acids include arabinose, furan compounds, beta alanine, pyrrolidine compounds, and others.

**For example, tartaric acid is a PLF toxin that is frequently excreted in large amounts in the urine of the fibro and fatigue canaries. The production of that toxic organic acid diminishes rapidly when PLF overgrowth is controlled with treatment. That indicates excessive production of tartaric acid due to PLF overgrowth. Tartaric acid directly inhibits conversion of fumaric acid to malic acid.

(toxins produced by molds) directly block specific steps in oxygen metabolism, either by blocking oxygen enzymes or altering the raw materials on which those enzymes act.

Third, a condition of too much acid within the cells (called intracellular acidosis) develops in fibromyalgia for several reasons discussed in this chapter and elsewhere in this book. The buffers in the circulating blood and lymph try to neutralize such excess acidity, creating a condition of too much alkalinity in the blood. This is called compensatory alkalosis and is produced when the response of blood and lymph buffers overshoots the mark and retains excess alkalinity. Alkalosis directly reduces the oxygen-carrying capacity of the blood.

Fourth, dehydration is always present in unreversed fibromyalgia and interferes with both oxygen transport to tissues as well as oxygen utilization in the cellular metabolism. Dehydration directly slows down oxygen enzymes. It also contributes to dysoxygenosis by other mechanisms, such as increasing acidity as well as toxins in the cells.

Fifth, digestive-absorptive dysfunctions are encountered in nearly all patients with fibromyalgia and lead to nutritional deficiencies of both functional and numerical types. Oxygen metabolism directly depends on many members of the vitamin B complex, and deficiency of those vitamins interferes with activities of enzymes and coenzymes of oxygen metabolism.

Sixth, the capacity of the liver to detoxify pesticides and related synthetic chemicals in the liver is diminished in fibromyalgia. When the liver fails to quickly neutralize pesticides, the uncontrolled activity of such chemicals poisons oxygen enzymes.***

***For example, organophosphates block an enzyme called cholinesterase, which is essential for insects to breathe. It turns out that human cholinesterase is very similar to insect choline esterase and is paralyzed in the same way.

Seventh, toxic metal overload is often seen in the fibro canaries. Toxic metals such as mercury and arsenic, even in minute amounts are much more toxic to the fibro canaries than healthy subjects. Heavy metals further depress the activities of enzymes involved in oxygen transport and utilization.[****]

Again, I refer the advanced and professional readers to a detailed discussion of this subject in *Canary Three, Fibromyalgia: An Oxidative-Dysoxygenative Dysfunction.*

SUMMARY

Human ecologic systems are under increasing oxidative stress. Such stress is caused by an ever-increasing number of oxidants in our internal and external environments. The oxidants of the internal environment include toxins produced by normal metabolic activity, the PLF overgrowth, acidosis, and damaging chain reactions triggered by oxidative coagulopathy and oxidative lymphopathy. The oxidants of the external environment include pesticides, herbicides, synthetic hormones, industrial pollutants, and different forms of radiation. All such oxidants further feed the oxidative flames of the internal factors. Together, all internal and external oxidants poison oxygen enzymes and lead to dysfunctional oxygen metabolism.

The ORPEC and ODD states, in my view, are the two most important pathways by which chronic disease is caused. A careful

[****] Mercury compounds literally rupture sulfhydryl groups of glutathione and related sulfur-containing antioxidants as well as detox molecules.

study of both states makes the following four conclusions inescapable:

1. The prevailing notion that microecologic cellular and macroecologic tissue-organ ecosystems are not relevant to the care of the sick must be rejected.

2. The prevailing notion that infections are caused only by microbes invading the body from outside the body must be challenged. Many chronic syndromes, such as fibromyalgia, chronic fatigue syndrome, chemical sensitivity syndrome, and others can be neither understood nor successfully treated without addressing issues of oxidative regression to primordial cellular ecology. Fibromyalgia can be neither understood nor successfully treated without addressing issues of oxidative regression to primordial cellular ecology.

3. The prevailing notion that the sick can be treated only with blockade medicine must be discarded. Notwithstanding the value of beta blockers, channel blockers, and enzyme inhibitors in suppressing symptoms, the blocker drugs simply cannot restore damaged ecosystems of the body.

4. The prevailing notion that integrative management protocols, including nutritional, herbal, immune-enhancing, and redox-reducing therapies, are not scientific must be dismissed silly.

For the coming century, we must either learn to think ecologically or prepare to watch helplessly as our drug therapies miserably fail to restore the health of hundreds of millions of chronically ill persons. Without enlightened ecologic thinking, we are doomed to wallow in ignorance as we encounter a growing number of pandemics of "mysterious" maladies for which all drug medicine can do is to come up with a bunch of meaningless, nonsensical diagnostic labels.

References

1.   Ali M. Spontaneity of oxidation in nature is the root cause of all illness. In: RDA: Rats, Drugs and Assumption, 1995. Life Span, Denville, New Jersey, pp. 199-304.
2.   Ali M. Oxygen: The Molecular Dr. Jekyll and Mr. Hyde. In RDA: Rats, Drugs and Assumption. Page 200-208. 1995 Life Span, Denville, New Jersey.
3.   Ali M. Absence of Disease Is Not Always Presence of Health. The Cortical Monkey and Healing. 1989. pp 9-11.The Institute of Preventive Medicine, Bloomfield, New Jersey.
4.   Ali M, energy-over mind In: The Ghoraa and Limbic Exercise. 1993. pp 9-10. Life Span, Denville, New Jersey.
5.   Ali M. The bowel and blood are open ecosystems. In RDA: Rats, Drugs and Assumption. Page 409-462. 1995 Life Span, Denville, New Jersey.
6.   Ali M. Oxidative regression to primordial cellular ecology (ORPEC): Evidence for the hypothesis and its clinical significance. J Integrative Medicine 1988;2:4-55.
7.   Ali M. Ali O. Fibromyalgia: An oxidative-dysoxygenative disorder (ODD). J Integrative Medicine 1999;3:17-37.
8.   Ali M. Oxidative Theory of cell membrane and Plasma damage. In RDA: Rats, Drugs and Assumption. Page 281-303. 1995 Life Span, Denville, New Jersey.
9.   Ali M. Ali O. AA oxidopathy: The core pathogenetic mechanism of ischemic heart disease. J Integrative Medicine 1998;1:6-112
10.   Ali M. Darwin, Oxidosis, Dysoxygenosis, and Integration. J Integrative Medicine 1999;1:11-16
11.   Ali M, Ali A. Oxidative coagulopathy in fibromyalgia and chronic fatigue syndrome. Am J Clin Pathol 1999;112:566-567
12.   Stadman J. Protein oxidation and aging. Science 1992;257:1220.
13.   Erickson GM. Breathing life into Tyrannosaurus rex. Scientific American. September, 1999. pp 41-49.Ali M, energy-over mind Ghoraa
14.   Graham JB, Dudley R, Aguilar NM. Nature 1995;375:117-120.
15.   World Resource. 1988-89. Global systems and cycles. pp 11.
16.   Atkinson D. Sibly RM. Trends Evol Ecol. 1997;12:235-239.
17.   Chapelle G, Peck LS. Polar gigantism dictated by oxygen availability. Nature. 1999;399:114-5.
18.   Bazikalova AY. Lake Baikol Amphipods. Proc. Baikol Limnol Stn Acad Sci. USSR 11, 1-440, 1945.
19.   Moran JF, Becana M, Iturbe-Ormaetxe I, et al. Drought induces oxidative stress in pea plants. Planta 194;3:346-52.
20.   Price AH, Atherton N, Hendry GAF. Plants under drought stress generate active oxygen. Free Radical res Commun. 1989;8:61-66.
21.   Smirnoff N. The role of active oxygen in the response of plants to water deficit and dessication. New Phytol. 1993;125:27-58.
22.   Baker CJ, Orlandi EW. Sources and effects of reactive species in plants. In: Reactive Oxygen Species in Biological Systems. Edi: Gilbert DL, Colton CA. 1999. Kluwer

Academic / Plenum Publishers. New York. pp 489.

23. Saito M, Nakatsugawa K. Increased susceptibility of liver to lipid peroxidation after ingestion of a high fish oil diet. Int. J. Vitam. Nutr. Research. 1994;64:144-151.

24. Gilbert DL. The role of pro-oxidants and antioxidants in oxygen toxicity. Radiation Research Suppl. 1963;3:44-53.

25. Gilbert DL. Introduction: Oxygen and life. Anesthesiology. 1972;37:100-111.

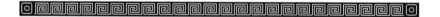

Nature put nearly fifty trillion oxygen-loving cells in the human body so we can live healthy. It also put nearly 50 trillion, mostly oxygen-heating, microbes in the bowel so that it can clear away the bodies after we die. Oxygen preserves the ecologic balance for the two types of cells.

Chapter 9
Oxygen Settles the Great Pasteur-Bechamp Debate

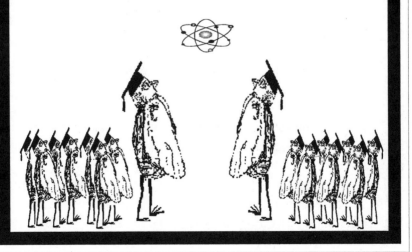

Oxygen, the ultimate spin doctor, is also a great peacemaker. In this chapter, I show how oxygen settles the important and long-standing Pasteur-Bechamp debate.

Louis Pasteur, a 19th-century French chemist, introduced the germ theory and stated that specific infections are caused by specific microbes invading the body from outside. He further believed microbial species were fixed (monomorphism)[1-3]. Antoine de Bechamp, his opponent and a prominent microbiologist of the French Academy of Science, believed infections were caused by organisms that develop from within the body and that such organisms underwent radical changes under different conditions (polymorphism, pleomorphism). Pasteur and Bechamp showed nothing but disdain for each other's view. Thus began the great Pasteur-Bechamp debate. Pasteur's *without* versus Bechamp's *within* view of the origin of diseases controversy persists.

My view that oxygen settles that debate may be simply stated as follows:

When oxygen metabolism is optimal, Pasteur's microbes from outside play more important roles in causing disease. When oxygen metabolism is dysfunctional, Bechamp's life forms multiplying from within the body become more important.

I draw the above conclusion from a large number of personal clinical and experimental observations. To fully understand the above simple statement, we need to be familiar with the essential oxygen order of human biology, which has been discussed at length for the professional readers in a series of articles.[4-14] In this chapter, I include a brief history of pleomorphism and an examination of the work of many pioneers in the fields of pleomorphism and the study of life forms in the circulating blood. The immediate relevance of this material to my oxygen (dysoxygenosis) theory of aging becomes apparent later in this chapter.

During the 150 years after Pasteur, most mainstream doctors accepted Pasteur's dogma as an article of faith. Indeed, many of them scoffed at the very idea of microbes developing from within. Many researchers and clinicians, on the other hand, championed Bechamp's cause and openly laughed at the blind faith of mainstreamers. To this day, the Pasteur-Bechamp debate among persons with interest in the ecology of the blood has been usually lively, sometimes bitter, but always inconclusive.

A peculiar aspect of the Pasteur-Bechamp debate is that the leaders in Bechamp's camp ("Bechampists") have been passionate microscopists while Pasteur's disciples ("Pasteurists") have shown little, if any, inclination to use their microscopes to study the patterns of microbial growth in the blood. The ideas of Bechampists often seemed radical to their peers, but they used their microscopes with great care and persistence. In clinical medicine, they focused on changing the internal conditions of the body. The Pasteurists, by contrast, completely neglected issues of blood ecology and committed themselves to killing microbes with chemicals. Their attitude was all the more remarkable because they considered themselves scientists and took great pride in the scientific method in medicine. Yet, they refused to use their microscopes to validate or refute the findings of Bechampists. What could be more scientific than to observe directly with a microscope what populates the blood of their patients? That question never seemed to trouble them.

By the middle of the twentieth-century, the main body of physicians had forgotten about both Pasteur and Bechamp. Oddly, Pasteur's name survives for reasons quite removed from his seminal work linking microbes with human disease. The milk industry adopted his method for treating milk and dubbed it pasteurization. Thus, children learn of Pasteur's name when they are taught the difference between good milk and sour milk. The wine industry also co-opted Pasteur. His name comes in handy when telling stories about how wines are aged. Fresh air, we are told, is an enemy of wines. The difference between death and glory in drinking can be minutes of exposure of wine to oxygen in the air, so counselled the French enologist, Emile Peynaud. Of course, the man behind all such insights about wine was Pasteur. In 1863, he was asked by Napoleon III to find out why so much of his choice wine from the Mediterranean was going bad. The great Pasteur did not disappoint the emperor. He figured out that the culprit was air (oxygen, in the present context). And so it is that Pasteur's name lives on in our class rooms as well as in our vinyards.

Bechamp did not have the fortune to have any such method named after him. With uncommon exceptions, doctors only pay lip service to the history of medicine. They have been too preoccupied with antibiotic chemistry to pay any attention to the matters of terrain (integrity of the microecologic cellular and macroecologic tissue-organ ecosystems, in my terminology). Medical schools have turned out generations of antibiotic enthusiasts with total commitment to an ever-growing list of antibiotics. They have had neither any use for the great medical controversies of bygone years nor an interest in understanding the pertinent ecologic issues. They ridiculed all ideas of natural restorative therapies based on the basic Bechamp concept of diseases arising from within. Professors in medical schools in the United States and elsewhere never bothered to learn anything about the great Pasteur-Bechamp debate. How could their students be expected to know even Bechamp's name?

But pleomorphism did not die. A handful of diehard bacteriologists and physicians continued their search. Some of them developed remedies derived from their special "cultures." That created a commercial reason for keeping the names of the pioneers alive long after they became inactive or passed away. The great benefit of such commercial activity was that some important books were reprinted and translated so that valuable original works were saved from extinction.

Then came the epidemics of fibromyalgia, chronic fatigue syndrome, chemical sensitivity syndrome, and infections by the so-called stealth microbes that could not be controlled no matter how hard the antibiotists tried and how many killer antibiotics they used. Many caring physicians in different parts of the world began to search for answers outside the "box" of the prevailing dogma of symptom-suppressing pharmacologic therapeutic regimens. That led to a widespread resurgence of interest in pleomorphism.

Now we need to revisit the old Pasteur-Bechamp debate. But it must be done in light of the newer knowledge of genetics and the essential roles of oxygen in preserving man-microbe harmony. In this chapter, I show that Pasteurists and Bechampists argued ineffectively because they failed to understand the many roles of oxygen in man-microbe interrelationships. As in all other areas of disagreement about the cause of disease, oxygen effectively settles the Pasteur-Bechamp debate. It validates where Pasteur and Bechamp were right, and where both men went wrong.

TWO ESSENTIAL QUESTIONS ABOUT
MICROBIAL PLEOMORPHISM

Microbial pleomorphism is a phenomenon in which microbes change their shapes under different conditions ("pleo" derived from the Greek word *pleon* meaning more; and morphs, meaning shapes). From reading the chapter, "Oxygen and Primordial Life Forms," many readers might wonder what relationship, if any, microbial pleomorphism might have with my theory of primordial life forms (PLFs). Here again, oxygen explains the relationship between the phenomena of microbial pleomorphism and PLF overgrowth.

Champions of both Pasteur's monomorphism and Bechamp's pleomorphism agree that microbes *do* change their shapes under different conditions. At the heart of the debate is what pleomorphism really means. There are two issues there:

1.   Can pleomorphic forms arise from within the body?
2.   Can microbes change from one species to another, from bacteria to fungus to parasite?

Based on my understanding of the genetics and the many seemingly contradictory roles of oxygen in health and disease, the following are my simple answers to the above two questions:

1.   Pleomorphic living bodies (primordial life forms, in my terminology) do arise from within the blood cells.
2.   Microbes do not change into different species of bacteria, fungi, and parasites.

Thus, in my view, people in both Pasteur's camp and Bechamp's group are right, but only partially.

Mainstream doctors hold that microbes do not arise from within, and that when microbes do change, that affects only their appearance and not their nature. Most holistic and integrative physicians interested in pleomorphism will answer both above questions with a forceful "yes." Notwithstanding the revolution unfolding in the so-called alternative medicine, there is a wide gulf between the views of mainstream doctors and holistic physicians on the above two issues. The main point of the present chapter is that both groups are partially right and the ongoing confusion results from their failure to understand the many paradoxical roles of oxygen and their unfamiliarity with the oxidative-dysoxygenative phenomena discussed in the chapter, "The History of Oxygen and Dysfunctional Oxygen Metabolism." I will briefly cover the main arguments of both groups and return to the matter of how oxygen settles the Pasteur-Bechamp debate later in this chapter.

Returning to the two questions, I will first address the second question because it requires simple answers and because those answers pave the way for more effectively answering the first question. Furthermore, I believe the first question concerning the matter of microbes arising from within could not be effectively presented without a historical review of the work of the great microscopists of the past who concluded, as I did from my own studies, that microscopic bodies with features of life *do* arise from within the blood cells.

MICROBES DO NOT CROSS SPECIES BOUNDARIES

Ernst Almquist, a nineteenth-century Swedish microbiologist, first observed that typhoid microbes may look different under different conditions, but they do not change into some other microbial species. The microbes remain typhoid bacilli. The altered forms revert back to their original form when their ecologic conditions return to the prior state.

I cite a simple experiment to illustrate the point. *Proteus* species (a microbial species that is frequently present in the human bowel) can be grown in a culture medium in the laboratory under different sets of conditions so that bacteria grow in pleomorphic forms. That culture can then be exposed to sound waves and the microbes broken up (ultrasound homogenization) so that bacteria turn into an organic soup and no whole bacteria survive. Next, the microbial soup can be divided into 100 portions and the samples sent to 100 good laboratories in 100 different countries, asking the laboratories to identify the microbial species by using antibodies specific for various bacteria. Almost all laboratories will correctly identify the *Proteus* species. Such an experiment clearly established the distinctness of that *Proteus* species regardless of how many different forms it might take. Similar experiments have been performed. For example, in actual studies, *Proteus* species were cultured for thousands of generations over a period of about ten years. At the end of that period, all microbial samples were clearly identified as *Proteus* species. None of those microbes had morphed into fungi or parasites.

PREGNANT CATS DO NOT DELIVER PUPPIES

Another line of strong evidence that supports the view that bacteria do not change into fungi and parasites is the specificity of their DNA. Simply stated, one has to reject the entire field of genetics before one can make a case for some particles within the body turning into bacteria, then into fungi, and then into parasites. The celebrated case of O.J. Simpson has made one thing clear: Most people in the world now do have some basic understanding of how human beings can be distinguished from each other. What is not common knowledge is that microbiology laboratories have routinely used DNA techniques for identifying many microbial species. Thus, the very notion of pleomorphism proposing that particles in cells turn into bacteria, fungi, and parasites seems to be utterly incompatible with the genetic specificity observed by everyone every day. Roses do not grow on pine trees. Eagles do not emerge from hens' eggs. Pregnant cats do not deliver puppies.

A SCIENTIST HAS NEITHER A DOGMA NOR ANY PARADIGM

Science is purity of observation. An accurate scientific observation should not be open to debate, although all conclusions drawn from it may be. Thus, a true scientist knows that an observation once accurately made, stands on its own. It needs no support from anyone. The fact that roses do not grow on pine trees is not open to question. Many holistic physicians steadfastly cling to the notion of microbial pleomorphism turning cellular particles into bacteria, fungi, and parasites. It puzzles me when I hear them express their strong belief in pleomorphism and yet consistently sidestep the core issue of DNA specificity of microbial life. Bacteria are as different from fungi as dogs are from donkeys. Fungi are as different from parasites as frogs are from fruit flies. Those facts are not open to debate.

And yet, I cannot ignore the diligently documented microscopic observations of researchers in pleomorphism concerning appearance and multiplication of bodies with features of living beings which I call primordial life forms. This matter deserves a careful consideration. But first we must return to Pasteur and summarize the work of several important pleomorphism researchers.

PASTEUR'S SHEEP AND ANTHRAX MICROBES

Pasteur is generally credited with the germ theory of illness. But, as we have seen in the chapter, "Oxygen and Primordial Life Forms," he was not the first to think of that theory. Indeed, the idea of a *contagium animatum* as the cause of disease had germinated in the minds of some very ancient writers[15]. More than two centuries before Pasteur, Anton van Leeuwenhoek, the inventor of the microscope discovered his "animalcules." Beginning around 1676, he sent a series of letters to the Royal Society of London in which he described microbes he had found in water, wet organic matter, and scrappings of his own teeth. We know the microbes from his teeth as Streptococci. Amazingly, neither he nor anyone at the Royal Society saw the link between his animalcules and disease. Thirteen decades earlier and more than three hundred years before Pasteur, one Girolamo Fracastoro predicted that *seminaria,* his term for an unseen microbe, will be found to explain the cause of disease[16].

Pasteur was led to his germ theory by a beer brewer of the French city of Lille, where he was Professor of Chemistry. The beer brewer was distressed by the "mysterious" disaster that spoiled his beer and turned it into a distasteful slimy liquid. The curious professor examined samples of spoiled and good beer, and discove monomorphism in medicine. A natural extension of that idea is the now prevailing dogma: Where there is a disease, there is a bug. Where there is a bug, there is a drug.

The infatuation of the disciples of Pasteur with the bug-drug thinking was fanned by research in antibiotic chemistry. The discovery of penicillin was hailed as the ultimate control of man over the world of bugs. That, as it turned out, was silly thinking. Amazingly, it still persists among many doctors, mostly because they failed to learn about natural ways of controlling common infections. That is ironic, because Pasteur himself believed that microbes cause disease when the *terra* (terrain) is suitable. How could he, the developer of a vaccine against anthrax, have failed to grasp the point? Is the very efficacy of vaccination not the *absolute* proof that internal condition determines the outcome when microbes invade the body?

BECHAMP'S MICROZYMES

Bechamp is credited with the idea that some preexisting particles within the human body develop into disease-causing agents under certain conditions. He claimed to have seen minute particles in the blood which he believed were of vegetative origin and which he called *microzymes*[17]. Next, he proposed that microzymes multiplied, changed their shapes, and grew into microbes under certain conditions, thus causing disease. That phenomenon of microscopic bodies changing their form and function was called pleomorphism. Bechamp fought hard against Pasteur's monomorphism of fixed microbes causing fixed diseases. However, Bechamp's voice was drowned out in the sea of the germ theory, except among some elite in medicine who kept the mono-pleo debate alive, but only as an intellectual exercise.

As far as I can determine from what is known of Bechamp's views, he believed that his microzymes were the source (seeds) of the larger microbes that caused disease under certain conditions. He did not believe that microbes, once fully developed, could change their species.

HIPPOCRATES' PHYSIS AND DEMOCRITUS' ATOMISM

In a sense, the nineteenth-century Pasteur-Bechamp debate was but a new twist to the older seed-soil debate of physicians of earlier times. The supporters of the seed (*without)* theory always searched for outside seeds (external causes of disease) while the proponents of the soil (*within)* theory looked for changes in the soil that favored the sprouting of those seeds (internal factors that created the condition suitable for a disease to take hold). In a larger sense, the Pasteur-Bechamp debate can be traced to the one between Hippocrates and Democritus nearly 2,500 years ago. The Greek physician, Hippocrates, who came to be known as the father of medicine, believed in *physis*, which to him meant the innate healing nature of the human body[18]. He taught his pupils to look inside the body for answers to the problems of sickness. Democritus, a contemporary of Hippocrates, disagreed. Democritus believed the human body was composed of tiny particles, which he called *atoms*. According to his theory of *atomism*, diseased tissues are incapable of healing themselves.

The Hippocratic concept of the inner healing nature of the human body needs no support today. Who has not seen four friends get exposed to a virus and show four different patterns of illness and healing? The first has a touch of sore throat for a day. The second develops cough and mild fever, and heals without any treatment. The third contracts a flu-like illness with muscle pain and fatigue that lasts for a few weeks in spite of antibiotic therapy. The fourth develops disabling fibromyalgia or chronic fatigue syndrome that lasts for months.

Over forty years ago, I was taught that damaged heart muscle and brain nerve cells cannot regenerate. Like other medical students in my class, I held on to that belief for decades. Now even persons without a medical background know that such cells do regenerate and heal. Hippocrates is proven right again.

BEALE'S MEDUSA HEADS

In 1864, L.S. Beale, an English microbiologist, published a startling picture that showed peculiar bodies emerging out of red blood cells. Those strange "organisms" escaped from the red cells as delicate filaments and thrashed vigorously in all directions, like "Medusa heads."[19] (In Greek mythology, Medusa was the monster with snakes rising from her head and thrashing around to frighten anyone that had the courage to look at her.) The bacteriologists of Beale's time were astonished by the pictures. They tried to establish Beale's organisms as spirochetes (the family of microbes that cause syphilis, Lyme disease, and other diseases). The classification as spirochetes was rejected, since Beale's organisms did not show the corkscrew motility characteristic of spirochetes. Nor did the thread-like structures emerging from the blood cells show any terminal hooks that spirochetal microbes display. Having failed to pin down Beale's peculiar organisms, the bacteriologists dismissed them as pseudospirochetes. So it turned out that Beale's important discovery was ignored by microbiologists for 136 years.

ALMQUIST'S PLEOMORPHIC TYPHOID MICROBES

In 1881, Ernst Almquist, a Swedish student of the famous German bacteriologist, Robert Koch, was the first to observe and document the phenomenon of microbial pleomorphism[20]. He discovered that the blood of patients suffering from typhoid fever contained both motile and nonmotile forms. The motile forms were elongated and rod-like, while the nonmotile microbes had oval bodies. He also documented that motile microbes behaved and grew differently from the nonmotile organisms. In 1905, Koch won the Nobel Prize for his work with tuberculosis, and seems to have lost interest in pleomorphism. Though Almquist recorded his observations carefully, his work went largely unrecognized. Indeed, many pleomorphism researchers who followed Almquist failed to take into account his work while describing their own observations. While presenting my theory of oxidative-dysoxygenative dysfunction at the 1999 meeting of the Danish Society of Orthomolecular Medicine in Copenhagen, I asked for a show of hands of persons who knew who Almquist was. Only one among the many Swedes present in the lecture hall raised his hand. Pleomorphism has a neglected history.

Almquist's profound understanding of pleomorphism is evident from his following words penned in 1922:

Nobody can pretend to know the complete life cycle and all the varieties of even a single bacterial species. It would be an assumption to think so.

In closing the above brief comments about Almquist's original work on pleomorphism, I must point out that there is no indication (known to me) that Almquist ever considered the possibility that his pleomorphic typhoid microbes or any other microbial species can cross into another microbial species when changing their appearance. He did not record any observations that suggested to him that bacteria can change into fungi or parasites.

METCHNIKOFF'S TUBERCULOSIS MICROBES

In the latter half of the nineteenth-century, Elie Metchnikoff, a Russian biologist, conducted an interesting experiment. In his famous experiment, he poked a wood splinter into the body of a crab, took it out after several hours, and examined the splinter with his microscope. He found white blood cells sticking to the wood surface in large numbers. He concluded that those cells were trying to break down and dispose of the wooden matter, since it was foreign to the body of the crab.[21] In other words, the cells were engaged in a scavenger function. That opened the world of cellular immunity for everyone. For his work, he was honored as the father of cellular immunity.

Metchnikoff was an ecologic thinker. In 1888, he also investigated the relationship between environmental conditions and microbial growth. He observed microbial pleomorphism and recorded the development of different forms of microbes under different sets of conditions and contributed to the early knowledge of that growing field. Specifically, he described abnormal branching forms of mycobacterium and noted that such microbes behaved differently from the rod-like tuberculosis bacilli that are seen in the tissues of patients with tuberculosis.

In the context of pleomorphism, the considerations of the immune functions of Metchnikoff's scavenger cells are more important than his findings of pleomorphic mycobacteria. Every time I study the blood smears of a patient, I recognize the profound influence of the phagocytic system on the PLF status. Next to the integrity of oxygen homeostasis, I consider the integrity of this system as *the single important determinant* of the degree of pleomorphism in the peripheral blood. I encounter very few pleomorphic forms (primordial life forms, in my terminology) when the white blood cells (phagocytic polymorphonuclear leukocytes) are well preserved. PLFs flourish in all cases in which a large number of such leukocytes are damaged or dead. For that reason, I consider Metchnikoff a giant in the field of pleomorphism.

It is also noteworthy that Metchnikoff, like Almquist before him, did not believe that his pleomorphic mycobacterium crossed into another microbial species when changing their appearance. To him, pleomorphism meant different forms of the *same* species.

ENDERLEIN'S SPERMIT AND ENDOBIONT

A notable figure in pleomorphism research was the German zoologist, Gunther Enderlein. He conducted extensive microscopic studies of pleomorphic forms during the late 1800s and the early 1900s. Following Bechamp's lead, he claimed to have discovered a very small microscopic body of vegetative origin, similar to Bechamp's microzymes. He called that body *spermit* (little sperm). He went on to propose that all human cells carry spermit, which to him was the seed of common diseases[22,23].

An amazing aspect of the Enderlein theory of pleomorphism was his belief that blood cells of all mammals also contained larger bodies of vegetative origin which he termed *endobiont*. He proposed that endobiont was nonpathogenic in health, but under certain conditions was capable of "upward developing" into larger pathogenic organisms, including bacteria, fungi, and parasites. When endobiont moved upward, the smaller spermit under favorable conditions copulated with the larger forms of endobiont and made them disappear, reminiscent of the way a black widow spider kills her male partner after copulation and often devours him. He designated such spermit-endobiont activity as microbial sexual function and devoted a whole chapter to that subject in his book *Bacterial Cyclogeny* published in 1916. That discovery should have earned him a Nobel Prize. Instead, he was laughed at. I can only imagine how much amusement the notion of microbial sexual escapades might have brought to his opponents. However, that discovery did bring a Nobel Prize, though the winner was not Enderlein. It is a little known irony that Lederberg of Rockefeller University in New York City won the Nobel prize for his rediscovery of microbial sexual reproduction, nearly fifty years after Enderlein had discovered the phenomenon and painstakingly documented it. Lederberg did not acknowledge Enderlein's prior discovery, perhaps because he was unaware of Enderlein's work. But it should not surprise us if it is found that he did know of the prior discovery, since Pasteurists generally do not acknowledge the prior work of Bechampists.

Enderlein made yet another discovery that, in my view, should have earned him a second Nobel prize, just as Otto Warburg won two Nobel prizes between 1931 and 1934 for discovering that a cancer cell does not like oxygen. (The metabolism of cancer cells is largely fermentative in nature [glycolytic, in chemistry terms] and utilizes little or no oxygen.) Enderlein's second important discovery was what he called "prethrombosis" in the circulating blood caused by the various "upward-growing" forms of endobiont. That clearly proves that Enderlein had recognized that his pleomorphic forms were capable of triggering the process of thrombosis in the blood. The profound significance of that observation went unrecognized not only by Pasteurists but also by Bechampist contemporaries.

In 1997, my colleague, Omar Ali, and I introduced the term oxidative coagulopathy for a range of changes in blood cells and plasma that result in congealing of plasma and microclot and microplaque formation in the circulating blood.[6] We conducted various experimental and clinical studies to demonstrate conclusively that microclots and microplaques formed as a result of oxidative injury, and the observed changes in early stages could be reversed by the addition of antioxidants. We also recognized that such formations were also caused by what we considered to be a large family of primordial life forms.[8,11] I am not aware of any record that Enderlein ever thought that his prethrombosis in the circulating blood might be triggered by factors other than his pleomorphic forms. Nor is there any indication that he recognized his prethrombosis to be oxidative and/or dysoxygenative in nature. Nor have I been able to determine whether or not he recognized the obvious relevance of microclots and microplaques to the pathogenesis of coronary artery disease, stroke, Alzheimer's disease, and a host of degenerative disorders characterized by oxidative-dysoxygenative metabolism. But that is exactly what we concluded from our high-resolution microscopic studies nearly eighty years later. I must point out here that Enderlein wrote in German and I have had access only to English translations of his work. However, the English translators do claim to cover all of his *core* ideas.

Enderlein was an accomplished microscopist and an astute observer. His terminology for the various stages of his "bacteria cyclogeny" was extensive and quite different from our much simplified microscopic descriptions of changes of oxidative coagulopathy. *The critical point here is that we were able to confirm all of his microscopic observations.* However, in my view, as I indicate earlier, his conclusion that endobiont changes into bacteria, then into fungi, and finally into parasites can neither be defended on morphologic grounds nor can it be accepted in light of the established knowledge of genetics. I return to this subject later in this chapter.

NAESSENS' SOMATID CYCLE

During the late 1940s, Gaston Naessens, a French biologist and chemist, developed a high-resolution microscope which he dubbed somatoscope. With his somatoscope, Naessens began to study particles in the blood that were regarded as "dross" by his teachers in Lyons. He called those particles somatids (little bodies).[24] Like Beale nearly 75 years before and Enderlein nearly 50 years before him, he observed certain bodies emerge from red blood cells when such cells were stressed with heat. He considered them as stages of what he believed was *the somatid cycle*. Following intensive studies extending over a period of decades, he put forth his theory claiming that his somatid particle is the first stage in a string of microbial transformations that produce larger microbes, including bacteria, fungi and parasites. He designated that string of polymorphic microbes the somatid cycle and proposed that the somatid cycle has three phases in healthy subjects: (1) somatids; (2) spores; and (3) double spores. In the disease state, the three stages transform in a progressive, string-like fashion into the following forms: (1) bacterial form; (2) double bacterial form; (3) rod form; (4) bacterial form with double spores; (5) bacterial form; (6) rod form; (7) bacterial form with double spores; (8) bacterial form with double granular spores; (9) and (10) microbial globular forms; (11) bursting; (12) yeast form; (13) ascospore formation; (14) and (15) mycelial forms; and (16) rich milieu and fibrous thallus.

Naessens believed that his somatids in some sense are precursors of DNA, though such bodies do not contain nucleic acids. He also proposed that cancer grows because malignant cells overconsume nitrogen and create a nitrogen deficiency for the healthy cells.

Putting aside the issue of what the stages of his somatid cycle signify, *the important point here is that the shapes and activities of those stages are the same as those in Enderlein's bacteria cyclogeny or our primordial life forms.* Again, as is the case with Enderlein's cyclogeny, in my view Naessens' pleomorphic forms in no way prove that somatids grow into bacteria, then into fungi, and finally into parasites. That conclusion can neither be defended on microscopic findings nor can it be accepted in light of DNA studies. Again, I return to this subject later in this chapter.

CHISHIMA'S MASTER RED CELL

During 1971 and 1972, Professor Kikuo Chishima, President of the Society of Neo-Haematology of Japan, published his provocative "bio-dialectic" theory[25]. According to that theory, the red blood cell is the primordial cell that can change its form and function as it sees fit. Specifically, Chishima proposed that *all* cells in the body develop from red blood cells. My basic comment about Chishima's work is the same as for the work of Enderlein and Naessens. His observations about the emergence of pleomorphic *life forms* from red blood cells are valid, as were those of Beale nearly one hundred years earlier. However, his work also fails to *prove* that those life forms turn into bacteria, fungi, and parasites. In endnote #1, I include an outline of Chishima's eight principles in his own words for advanced and professional readers.[25]

Professor Chishima attempts to support his theory with several photomicrographs. However, in my opinion, those included in the ninth volume of his book[20] (available to me) fail to support his theory. For example, on page 43, he uses two pictures to make his point that an ovum in a frog's ovary arises from red blood cells. On pages 18,19 (Figure 1), he does the same for spermatozoa in mouse testes. In both cases, he uses the proximity of red blood cells to ova and spermatozoa as an evidence that the germ cells arose from red blood cells. In a series of photomicrographs on pages 20 and 21 (Figures 10-12), he attempts to show that cancer cells arise from red blood cells by demonstrating proximity of cancer cells to red blood cells. I do not believe any pathologist experienced in the histology and pathology of ovaries and testes will accept these photomicrographs as proof of Chishima's theory. Mere proximity of cells must not be accepted as evidence of origin of one type of cell from another. Pathologists regularly see cancer invade the blood vessels and mingle with red blood cells. That by no means indicates that cancer cells arise from the blood cells.

MATTMAN'S STEALTH MICROBES

In 1992, Linda Mattman, an American microbiologist, published her landmark book titled *Cell Wall Deficient Forms: Stealth Pathogens.*[26] In that volume, Mattman summarized her life's work with pleomorphic and cell wall-deficient forms. She conducted an exhaustive survey of work of past and contemporary researchers in the field, and added to that literature many of her own observations. Her *core message* is this:

Pleomorphic microbial forms develop readily under the influence of a large number of agents and readily *revert* back to their original forms when the causative influences are removed.

Mattman also summarized several studies showing pleomorphism involving bacterial and fungal species.[22-25] Many agents, such as yeast extract, mucin, vitamin E, trypsin, and muramidase spermine cause *reversion* of pleomorphic forms to the original microbial forms. Many pleomorphic forms, when cell wall deficient, become even more dangerous. It is noteworthy in this context that penicillin (and other antibiotics in its family) does not kill microbes. Rather, it works by interfering with the synthesis of microbial walls. Thus, penicillin and many other antibiotics favor the formation of yet more dangerous pleomorphic microbes, even though the use of such antibiotics is essential in life-threatening infections.

The essential point here is this: Structural changes can cause profound changes in function. Pleomorphic forms can lose or gain in their pathogenicity and virulence, but such changes do not mean bacteria crossing species boundaries. Specifically, Mattman did not cite a single study, her own or that of others, that documented conversion of bacteria into fungi and parasites.

NANOBACTERIA, STEALTH MICROBES, AND MYCOPLASMA

There is a widespread disillusionment about discovering the underlying cause(s) of several chronic disorders that are spreading in epidemic proportions, including fibromyalgia, CFS, environmental sensitivity syndrome, Gulf War syndrome, and others. In the chapter, "Oxygen, Primordial Life Forms, and Aging," I summarize the result of my own extended microscopic studies of PLF overgrowth in patients with fibromyalgia, CFS, and other chronic disorders. In that and other articles,[8-11] I have discussed the clinical significance of those observations. Many other researchers and clinicians are also beginning to think beyond the limits of conventional microbiology for determining the pathogenic roles of conventional clinical microbiology. Below, I cite four examples.

Olavi Kajander, a Finnish scientist, coined the term nanobacteria for minute particles which he believed represented a newly discovered form of life. He further proposed that nanobacteria represent primitive life on earth. Such bacteria are rounded in shape, measure between 50 and 500 nanometers, and are highly resistant to chemicals and heat because of their hydroxyapatite coat.[27] Nanobacteria do not grow in conventional laboratory culture media, but are believed to cause a variety of human illnesses. For example, the presence of nanobacteria has been reported in over 90 percent of kidney stones. In polycystic kidney disease, bacterial endotoxins were present in cases in which no recognizable bacteria were found with traditional cultures but nanobacteria were found in ten of twelve patients.[28-29]

Mycoplasmas are a very large family of some of the smallest oxygen-hating pleomorphic microbes that lack discrete cell membranes. Such microbes do not grow in commonly used laboratory culture media and require complex testing techniques (DNA PCR [polymerase chain reactions]) for their detection. There are over 100 *Mycoplasma* species, each with multiple strains (subdivisions). These microbes often exist in the oral cavity and the bowel. In the past, mycoplasmas were considered innocent bystander microbes that live outside the cells and sometimes invaded the cells. One species, *Mycoplasma pneumoniae*, causes a chronic type of lung infection called atypical pneumonia (commonly known as walking pneumonia). It is now recognized that these microbes can effectively dodge the host immune defenses and cause chronic immune disorders. Drs. Garth and Nancy Nicholson of the Institute of

Molecular Medicine recently reported positive tests for mycoplasma in fifty percent of their patients with fibromyalgia, chronic fatigue syndrome, Gulf War syndrome, rheumatoid arthritis, and AIDS. [30]

Stealth microbes are another family of microbes that cause serious chronic illnesses, such as fibromyalgia and chronic fatigue syndrome. Like nanobacteria and mycoplasma, such microbes cannot be grown in commonly used laboratory culture media, hence their role in the cause of illness is rarely appreciated by most practitioners. Some Californian researchers reported the detection of stealth microbes in a majority of their patients with chronic fatigue syndrome.

Professor Peter O. Behan and his colleagues at the University of Glasgow have also made important contributions to our understanding of patterns of microbiologic overgrowth and infections in patients with fibromyalgia and chronic fatigue syndrome. Using their technique that employs complementary DNA PCR amplification, he documented the presence of sequences of coxsackie, polio, and enteroviruses in a majority of their patients. [31-32] Similarly, a large number of investigators have made similar observations for Epstein-Barr virus.

LESSONS NOT LEARNED FROM *C. difficile* INFECTIONS

Clostridium difficile, an oxygen-hating microbe, is an interesting case study. It is a common cause of antibiotic-associated colitis [33]. Until 1978, almost no doctor had ever heard of it as a cause of a severe, potentially life-threatening form of colitis. Ten years later, it was reported that nearly one-third of all patients in hospitals in the United States were infected with this microbe.[34,35] Interestingly, of these, one-fourth had the infection before coming to the hospital while the remaining three-fourths acquired it in the hospital. Major outbreaks of colitis caused by this microbe were reported soon after. In persons with chronic colitis, mainstream doctors look for this microbe as obsessively as holistic physicians do for *Candida*. Of course, both groups, in my view, miss the main point: the overgrowth of both species of microbes is a *consequence and not the cause* of changes that make people sick.

Before *C. difficile* was accused, *Staph* infections were blamed for colitis caused by antibiotics. In the 1970s, a new name, "clindamycin colitis" was chosen for such colitis[36]. During the following decade, the use of clindamycin decreased. Yet, the incidence of colitis increased in patients hospitalized for other reasons (including some who went in to have benign breast lumps removed). The obvious conclusion should have been to focus on other *ecologic issues* of the bowel. But, we physicians are not ecologic thinkers, as I point out earlier. Indeed, a recent editorial published in *The New England Journal of Medicine* addressed this issue, recognized that "the epidemic of *C. difficile* diarrhea continues to grow in our health care instititions," and focused heavily on the issue of the choice of antibiotics. Yet, it completely ignored the fundamental *ecologic* (oxidative-dysoxygenative) issues involved in such epidemics[33].

WHAT WE FIND DEPENDS ON WHAT WE LOOK FOR

The important point I make here is this: *In human canaries we will find what we look for.* If anyone performs sensitive micro-ELISA tests for detecting antibodies to *Aspergillus, Mucor, Candida* and other molds, he will find those tests positive in *all* cases of fibromyalgia, as we observed and reported.[39] If someone looks for evidence of infections by herpes, Epstein-Barr, CMV, and other viruses, he will certainly find that to be the case. If he tests for various species of mycoplasma, he will most assuredly find those in a majority of the fibro canaries, as did Nicholsons.[30] I can safely make that prediction. If someone searches for nanobacteria, I am also certain, he will find those microbes in a high percentage of patients with fibromyalgia, as Kajander and his colleagues found in patients with kidney diseases.[29] That prediction is also entirely safe. If the search is conducted for stealth microbes, surely those microbes will be found, as was the case with Californian researchers.

Indeed, that is the reason why I introduced the term primordial life forms. Nanobacteria, mycoplasma, and stealth microbes clearly are examples of pleomorphic, oxygen-hating, acid-loving microbes that multiply rapidly in the presence of dead organic matter. I have no doubt that future research with DNA technology will reveal the presence in the blood and bowel of the fibro canaries of many other specific forms of primordial life.

BRADFORD'S OXIDOLOGY

One of the pioneers in the fields of oxidative phenomena involving the circulating blood today is Professor Robert Bradford of Capital University of Integrative Medicine, Washington, D.C. He and his colleague, Henry Allen, have devoted nearly twenty years to intensive studies of oxidative phenomena occurring in the peripheral blood in health and disease. In their *Oxidology: The Study of Reactive Oxygen Species*,[38] they present a panorama of patterns of oxidative injury involved in the pathogenesis of nearly all major disease categories, including acute and chronic immune disorders and neoplastic diseases. Their work has substantially expanded our understanding of the pathophysiology of intravascular coagulation (see endnote #2). One of the contribution of Bradford and Allen in the field of oxidology concerns an abnormal pattern of clotting initiated by increased oxidative stress that involves activation of sialidase by hydrogen peroxide and the removal of sialic acid from fibrinogen. They have designated that pathway as the Bradford-Allen pathway.[33]

Bradford has also investigated the problem of overgrowth of yeast-like organisms in the peripheral blood of patients with chronic immunologic disorders and malignant neoplasms.[34] In 1994, Robert Bradford, Omar Ali, Madhava Ramanarayanan, and I developed an immunologic method to specifically stain *Candida* organisms with human anti-Candida antibodies.[39]

SOME LESSER KNOWN PLEOMORPHISM RESEARCHERS

It is not possible to include here even passing references to the work of many other pleomorphism researchers. German readers are as likely to know about the work of Weisman as Americans are of Livingston's. Even if the space here were to permit me, I could not do justice to the morphologic observations of many others. *The essential point is that while pleomorphism researchers interpreted their findings differently, the remarkable aspect of their work is the consistency of their core microscopic observations.*

OXIDOSIS, DYSOXYGENOSIS, AND ACIDOSIS: Dying Oysters of Chesapeake Bay

In the chapter, "The History of Oxygen and Dysfunctional Oxygen Metabolism," I present my view that oxidosis, dysoxygenosis, and acidosis are the three principal mechanisms of molecular and cellular injury in all acute and chronic disorders. The disease process is initiated by oxidosis caused by a host of nutritional, ecologic, and immune factors. Oxidosis leads to dysoxygenosis (dysfunctional oxygen metabolism) by several mechanisms. Oxidosis also causes acidosis. Both dysoxygenosis and acidosis further feed the fires of oxidosis. Thus are created destructive and self-perpetuating cycles of molecular and cellular injury. I have marshaled evidence for my view in several publications.[4-14] I illustrate the impact of the oxidosis/dysoxygenosis/acidosis trio with the following text from a previous article:

An important issue of relevance to the oxygen order of human biology is the progressive global drop in the oxygen content of ambient air and oceanic waters. The rising concentrations of carbon dioxide in the atmosphere has drawn much attention in both scientific and lay communities. However, little attention has been paid to the ill effects on humans and wildlife caused by the anoxia and hyperacidity that accompany increasing amounts of carbon dioxide. Marine biologists have identified several areas of hypoxic waters in the world.[40] For example, both man-made and natural causes have rendered the Black Sea anoxic to such a degree that many life forms in it have been seriously affected. In the United States, waters of both Chesapeake Bay and Mobile Bay have become so anoxic as to kill many kinds of fish. In June 1995, thousands of fish were reported to have died in North Carolina's New River sanctuary as a result of anoxia and excess acidity caused by a spill of 25.8 million gallons of hog feces and urine.

An illuminating case study of the ill effects of anoxia and excess acidity in marine biology, and one that is very pertinent to the proposed ORPEC hypothesis, is that of the Eastern oysters of Charleston Harbor. The oysters are normally resistant to a deadly parasite called dermo (*Perkinsus marinus*) and kill the parasite by producing toxic reactive oxygen species. However, under anoxic and acidic conditions, the oysters are unable to employ their oxidative arsenal and become vulnerable to the parasite. This happens when the tidal salt marshes in which the oysters live become hypoxic and acidic. The experimental evidence for this phenomenon was obtained in experiments with oysters. When kept in tanks under normal anoxic conditions for two days, the oysters in anoxic tanks had acidic hemolymph which produced almost no reactive oxygen species. An interesting parallel observation is that blue crabs can make their hemolymph alkaline when exposed to anoxic and acidic stressors, thus enabling them to cope with the damaging effects of both.

There are both theoretical and clinical considerations that suggest that adverse anoxic phenomena such as those described above for marine life also affect patients with fibromyalgia, CFS, severe autoimmune disorders and disseminated cancer. From a theoretical perspective, accelerated oxidative injury leads to both anoxia and acidosis. From a clinical standpoint, I have observed most patients benefit considerably from oxygenative therapies, such as intravenous ozone and hydrogen peroxide infusions, as well as intermittent nasal administration of oxygen (3 liters per minute given for an hour, two to three times during the day). I have discussed this subject at length previously.

The important point I make here is that the killer furies that shatter the antioxidant, enzyme, and immune defenses of a person with chronic fatigue syndrome, fibromyalgia, progressive immune disorders, and spreading cancer are the same: oxidosis, dysoxygenosis, and acidosis.

GENES LEGISLATE LIFE; THE ENVIRONMENT INTERPRETS THE LAWS SET FORTH BY GENES

I include below some general comments about genes and environments before discussing my theory of oxidative regression to primordial cellular ecology (ORPEC). The ORPEC state, in my view, is *the core* issue in how oxygen settles the Pasteur-Bechamp debate.

DNA in genes legislates life; the environmental elements interpret the laws of biology established by genes. DNA in human cells provides the blueprint for approximately 60,000 proteins. These molecules are essential for human life in all its stages: during embryogenesis and early development after birth; during spurts of growth during adolescence; for wound healing; for immune defense and healing responses; for digestive-absorptive functions; for the functional integrity of energy and detoxification pathways; and, finally, for the decay and dying processes. Genes do not drive evolution. Rather, genes are the products of evolutionary changes. If DNA were copied flawlessly each time a cell divided, there would have been no evolution. To evolve is to change, and no change can be maintained for a long time except through a change in DNA configuration (or damage to enzymes involved in its synthesis). Without DNA alterations, today we would have the same DNA as our genetic ancestors over three billion years ago—and the same physical characteristics as single-celled microbes that existed then. When DNA is copied with a mistake, each copying error carries the risk of fatal structural or functional derangements.

PEOPLE AND PLFs SHARED GENES

A subject of core significance in the Pasteur-Bechamp debate is the matter of shared genes of men and microbes. In 1996, the composition of DNA of bakers' yeast was reported.[41] For advanced and professional readers, I include some important additional information in endnote #3. Briefly, it was found that about one-third of the genes of bakers' yeast were identical to human genes. This sharing was much higher for genes with well-established functions.

What does that mean in plain language? It means that our DNA contains a large part of the DNA of PLFs. Those common parts can grow differently under different sets of conditions of the cellular ecology. When oxygen is abundant, acidity is low, and the cells are free of decaying or dead organic matter, the same genes can grow as elements generally *considered* to human nature. On the other hand, when oxygen is lacking, acidity is high, and the cells are rich in decaying or dead organic matter, those very genes can grow as elements that may be regarded as primordial in nature.

OXIDATIVE REGRESSION TO PRIMORDIAL CELLULAR ECOLOGY (ORPEC)

In 1998, I described the phenomenon of oxidative regression to primordial cellular ecology in an article published in *The journal of Integrative Medicine.*[8] This hypothesis suggests an altogether novel microecologic-genetic model of illness associated with PLF overgrowth. The essential concept of the ORPEC state has been validated by my colleagues, Professors Alfred Fayemi and Judy Juco, at the Institute. It calls for a totally new way of thinking about the roles of primordial microorganisms in the pathogenesis of such disorders as fibromyalgia, CFS, Gulf War syndrome, severe immune disorders, and malignant neoplasms.

In health, normal oxygen metabolism does not allow the overgrowth of PLFs within the body and Pasteur's monomorphism prevails. In states of

oxidosis, unrelenting oxidative fires in human canaries create cellular ecologic conditions that are similar to those that existed in the primordial era. Specifically, the cells accumulate toxic organic acids that choke oxygen metabolism and cause dysfunctional oxygen metabolism. Without oxygen, certain human genes (those shared with primordial organisms) favor the growth of PLFs which, in turn, further fans the oxidative flames of the three furies (oxidosis, dysoxygenosis, and acidosis). That undoubtedly is Bechamp's domain.

Again, for the advanced and professional readers, in the Appendix I reproduce the abstract of the original paper describing the ORPEC state published in *The Journal of Integrative Medicine.*[8] I strongly urge such readers to read that abstract.

The core ecologic concept presented in that article is simply stated: No cause of human suffering may be sought in any individual biologic event, divorced from the larger ecologic elements that affect the human condition.

Specifically, the cause of oxidative regression to primordial cellular ecology may not be found in individual oxidative triggers. Rather, the microecologic-genetic shift of the ORPEC state represents the sum total of cumulative oxidative stressors. The clinical significance of the ORPEC hypothesis is that: (1) It provides a sound scientific model for a clearer understanding of the pathogenesis of syndromes associated with accelerated oxidative molecular injury, such as fibromyalgia, CFS, Gulf War syndrome, severe autoimmune disorders and malignant tumors; and (2) It provides a framework for a rational and logical approach for repairing oxidatively damaged cellular ecologies and for restoring health. Notwithstanding the lack of nucleotide sequence and taxonomic data concerning PLFs, the ORPEC hypothesis has strong explanatory power for: (1) the morphologic patterns of growth of PLFs documented in this report; (2) the pathogenesis of clinical syndromes characterized by accelerated oxidative injury; and (3) the sound scientific basis and/or rationale for the empirical efficacy of "anti-PLF" oxygenative, antioxidant, and other therapies employed to restore cellular ecology from the ORPEC state to a physiologic, healthful condition.

TWO ESSENTIAL POINTS IN THE PASTEUR-BECHAMP DEBATE

By now, I have made the following two essential points: First, our ideas of pleomorphism must be fully consistent with the established knowledge of genetics and the *total* lack of evidence that pleomorphic forms can cross the species barrier. Since Almquist made his initial observations concerning pleomorphism, no one has ever shown that. The boundaries set by DNA sequences of individual microbial species cannot be sacrificed in the interest of promoting this or that point of view (or, to sell this or that remedy). Here, we must accept the fundamental and totally valid argument of the Pasteurists in the world of genetics when they insist on verifiable evidence of pleomorphic forms transcending genetic limits.

Second, our ideas of pleomorphism must be consistent with morphologic observations of a large number of preeminent microscopists in the field of pleomorphism. No one should dismiss highly reproducible microscopic findings of pleomorphic life forms simply because he thinks those findings were mere artifacts. The skeptics can express doubt about the validity of microscopic observations if they study five, fifty, or seventy-five patients. But no one who studies the blood of a 1,000 or more chronically ill patients can do that. The sick have dirty blood with undeniable PLF overgrowth. The sicker the patient, the dirtier the blood. When the sick patients get better, PLF overgrowth and the accompanying changes of oxidative coagulopathy clear up. The healthier the individual, the cleaner the blood. It is that simple. No one must dismiss those observations without first conducting diligent and extended studies of freshly prepared peripheral blood smears with high-resolution microscopy with suitable phase-contrast and darkfield optics.

PASTEUR WAS RIGHT. PASTEUR WAS WRONG.

Pasteur was clearly right in his core belief that discrete microbial species cause discrete diseases. That view (the germ theory and monomorphism, in the context of the present discussion) requires no further validation. Strep throat is caused by *Streptococcus* species microbes, and tuberculosis results from infections of tuberculosis microbes (*Mycobacterium*). Lyme disease is caused by the Lyme spirochete (*Borrella burgdorferi*) and shingles by herpes virus (*H. zoster*). No one has ever demonstrated that tuberculosis microbes are capable of causing typical bull's eye skin rash caused by the Lyme organism, nor has *Streptococcus* ever caused skin rash of the type seen in shingles. No one with even the most basic medical knowledge can question that.

Pasteur was also wrong. His rejected Bechamp's view that elements from within (microzymes, in his terminology) can assume pathogenic roles. That was clearly a serious error. His opposition to Bechamp was not based on actual work to validate or refute the microscopic observations of the latter. Indeed, if he had studied freshly prepared blood smears to see whether or not pleomorphic forms could be seen emerging from erythrocytes, he would have seen what other pleomorphism researchers did. Thus, his opposition was purely theoretical and indefensible. He made the same serious mistakes that many professors in medical schools make today about the work of holistic practitioners: They reject observations of others without taking the time to study the natural phenomena themselves.

BECHAMP WAS RIGHT. BECHAMP WAS WRONG

Bechamp was right. The core microscopic observations concerning pleomorphism of Beale, Almquist, Enderlein, and Naessens are accurate and reproducible and fully validate Bechamp's core idea of life forms (microzymes, in his terminology) that exist within the human body in health and multiply under certain conditions to cause disease. As I wrote earlier, accurate physical observations are not open to question; the conclusions drawn from those findings are, and should be, open to debate.

Microscopic studies at the Institute by my colleagues, Professors Fayemi and Juco, and I conclusively show that overgrowth of PLFs (primordial life forms) occurs in the circulating blood in *all* patients with spreading cancer, fibromyalgia, chronic fatigue syndrome, and advanced immune disorders. Specifically, we have documented the emergence of pleomorphic forms from the red blood cells. We also observe advanced changes of oxidative coagulopathy caused by PLFs. Such overgrowth diminishes drastically when such persons regain their health. The sicker the patient, the dirtier the blood. Other groups of researchers, including Bradford's team, have also amply documented the overgrowth of PLFs in their patients and have seen the clear and direct relationship between the severity of clinical illness and degree of oxidative damage to the blood components.

Bechamp was also wrong. His opposition to Pasteur's proposition that anthrax bacilli cause anthrax disease was a serious mistake. It was not based on his actual experiments to validate or refute the latter's work. Indeed, the two men made exactly the same serious error.

ENDERLEIN WAS RIGHT. BUT WAS HE ALSO WRONG?

Enderlein was right. His theory of sexual reproduction in bacteria has been fully validated, including global recognition carried by a Nobel Prize awarded much later for that. His microscopic observations concerning the various pleomorphic forms and their development has been, and continues to be, validated. Indeed, a large number of practitioners in Europe and the United States routinely study the peripheral blood smears of their patients and classify their microscopic observations according to Enderlein's terminology and classification. Only those who have never used high-resolution phase-contrast and darkfield microscopes dismiss Enderlien's masterful descriptions of pleomorphic forms. (Sadly, that happens only too frequently.)

But there is a serious problem with how disciples of Enderlein present pleomorphism and attribute ideas to the great master. The proposal that the vegetative microzymes or spermit can turn into bacteria, then into fungi, and finally into parasites is *totally and utterly* inconsistent with the *genetic distinctness* of various species of bacteria, fungi, and parasites.

But did Enderlein really believe what his disciples today want us to believe? His book, *Bacteria Cyclogeny,* and other papers are difficult to read because of extensive and cumbersome German terminology which does not translate well in English. The key question here is what he really meant by pleomorphism.

Did he claim that pleomorphic forms crossed the species border?
Or did he believe that pleomorphic forms represented many and varied forms of the same microbial species?

From my readings of *Bacteria Cyclogeny*, I cannot ascertain which one was the case. Of course, most proponents of pleomorphism seem to imply that Enderlein believed in the former (that pleomorphic forms crossed the species barrier). If Enderlein indeed did claim that, he must be considered in error.

No one has ever demonstrated that any mycoplasma, bacteria, yeast, or parasite crosses species lines.

That notion of pleomorphism is contrary to the entire field of genetics. But I cannot be certain that Enderlein ever clearly defined that to be the case, as his followers vigorously claim. He only observed pleomorphic forms arise from blood cells and change shapes. And changes in morphology, of course, *must not* be accepted as a proof that bacteria turn into molds and so on. Again, I emphasize that I do not have access to all of Enderlein's writings.

AS SOIL CHANGES, SO DOES WHAT GROWS IN IT. OXYGEN SETTLES THE GREAT DEBATE.

So, what can we make of Beale's Medusa heads today? How may we look at Bechamp's microzymes? How may we regard Enderlein's spermit and endobiont? Or Naessens' somatid? Or Livingston's bodies? Or of nanobacteria, stealth microbes, and mycoplasma? Or of the overgrowth of primordial life forms, which I describe in patients with cancer, fibromyalgia, chronic fatigue syndrome, and autoimmune disorders? Specifically there are four important issues the:

1. Is the Pasteur-Bechamp debate relevant to the ever-enlarging menagerie of mystery maladies of our time, such as chronic fatigue syndrome, fibromyalgia, chemical sensitivity syndrome, and Gulf War syndrome?
2. Is it relevant to how cancer spreads?
3. Is it relevant to the established high level of gene sharing (DNA homology) among microbes and people?

4.   And, finally, is such homology relevant to how people
        turn into human canaries?

Here, in light of the information presented so far in this
chapter on the subject of pleomorphism, is the simple answer:

> **The genes of primordial life forms exist within the
> human body as residues from an earlier
> primordial era. In acute illness, oxygen metabolism
> is normal and Pasteur's germ theory
> (monomorphism) determines the type of infection
> caused by specific microbial species. In chronic
> illness, oxygen metabolism is dysfunctional and
> Bechamp's pleomorphism takes over. Primordial
> life forms overgrow under primordial conditions
> and perpetuate as well as increase the intensity of
> illness caused by oxidosis, dysoxygenosis, and
> acidosis. Thus, oxygen finally settles the great
> Pasteur-Bechamp debate.**

ARISTOTLE'S COAGULUM
AND GOETHE'S BUILDING BLOCKS

Form and function of living beings has always intrigued
humankind. Jain stone carvings unearthed in Pakistan and Northern
India and dated to about 8,000 B.C. symbolize their spiritual beliefs
about the structure of God. The ancient Greeks were more
imaginative. They structured their gods creatively and freely assigned
them functions which they thought befitted their deities. The same is
true of many earlier peoples and cultures.

One of the earliest concrete records of human musings about the origin of life may be attributed to Aristotle, who proposed that semen[42] "arranges and coagulates" the menstrual blood to initiate the formation of the baby. He thought semen disintegrated rapidly, hence did not enter the uterus. Biologists have many bones to pick with the Greek philosopher. They are forever irked by his sweeping statements about people and animals that are at odds with what they know. For instance, they are perturbed by his view that the sperm disintegrates quickly and does not enter the uterus, let alone the egg. So at that level, Aristotle obviously is off the mark. An egg cannot be fertilized without a sperm entering it. Furthermore, the sperm does enter the uterus, fallopian tubes, and, in rare cases, the general abdominal cavity. Consider the example of not uncommon ectopic pregnancy in the fallopian tubes and the very uncommon true abdominal pregnancies in which the fetus grows outside the cavity of the uterus.

But there was more to Aristotle than the petty disputes about the precise anatomic location of fertilization of the egg by the sperm. His notion of the ability of semen to *arrange* and *coagulate* fascinates me. In *De partibus animalium* and *De generations animalium*, he writes about *eidoes,* the form-giving principle (in the semen). He used the analogy of a building plan, something that gives structure to a building but does not become part of the building itself. Consider the following quote from *De generations animalium*:

> **It contributes nothing to the material body of the embryo but only communicates its program of development....It does not become part of the embryo, just as part of a carpenter does not enter the wood he works.**

How prescient! What intuition led Aristotle to his form-giving principle? What better definition of DNA can we give for its form-giving influence on the human frame?

And beyond DNA, I see Aristotle's form-giving principle in the organizing influence of oxygen. (Oxygen appeared on the scene a long time before the DNA molecule learned how to take its double-helix form.) No matter where I go in my search for answers to human illness, I cannot escape the organizing influence of oxygen.

I return to Aristotle's notion of the ability of semen to *arrange* and *coagulate.* The *single* most important microscopic finding in my patients is the *degree of coagulation* of plasma. Tiny plasma clots give me the best assessment of the status of oxygen metabolism. The sicker a patient, the greater the degree of coagulation in his blood smears and "dirtier" the blood. Zones of congealed plasma are the first indication that the patient is not effectively coping with oxidative stress. That is the beginning of oxidosis and dysoxygenosis. The mechanisms of "de-clotting" of plasma are also *primarily* influenced by oxygen. The healthier the patient becomes with *oxygenative* therapies, the fewer the microclots and lesser the degree of related changes of oxidative coagulopathy. That explains why I consider microscopic examination of a drop of patient's blood as the *single* most valuable test for assessing the health of my patients as well as monitoring the success of my therapies. Thus, I see the organizing influence of oxygen in every microscopic field. That may seem an oversimplification to some but that is my main conclusion from my microscopic studies of over 5,000 patients. My microscope reminds me of Aristotle's form-giving principle every working day.

The beginning of the discipline of morphology as the science of the form and structure of plants and animals is usually attributed to Johann Wolfgang von Goethe, the eighteenth-century German poet and polymath.[39] In his search for the basic plan of all life forms, Goethe recognized the prevalence of patterns of repeated segments in plants as well as animals, and put forth his theory that nature employs a building block approach to generating life. *Building blocks*! That is the second important aspect of my work. Like Goethe, I see building blocks everywhere I look. Blocks of oxygen and its radicals. Blocks of DNA sequences. Blocks of redox-restorative molecules. Blocks of digestive-absorptive and detox enzymes. Blocks of neurotransmitters and hormones. Blocks of the body's many ecosystems.

Then I see the hand of oxygen in Aristotle's coagulation as well as in Goethe's building blocks. And then there are moments of clarity about the workings of oxygen, that greatest of all spin doctors of human life. Oxygen is Aristotle's coagulator and arranger. Oxygen is Goethe's block builder. I begin to see the role of Pasteur's microbes from outside in the beginning of disease, when the oxygen metabolism is normal. I now also dicern the core importance of Bechamp's life forms from within as the cause of disease when oxygen metabolism is dysfunctional.

THE HEART OF THE MATTER

Now we come to the heart of the matter in the Pasteur-Bechamp debate. What does this debate have to do with little children who live on sugar and antibiotics, and who get ear tubes put in repeatedly but without much benefit? What is the relevance of this issue to teenage girls who suffer from disabling menstrual syndromes and who are prescribed synthetic hormones that help for a short time but create long-term problems, including the higher risk of breast cancer? What does Bechamp's theory have to teach us about infections arising from within in patients given chemotherapy for whom antibiotics stop working? Or for adults with Crohn's colitis and ulcerative colitis who are given chemotherapy drugs (6MP, cyclosporine, and others) by their gastroenterologists because steroids stop working? Or to older people who keeping getting *H. pylori* infections even though they receive repeated courses of multiple antibiotics? Or, urinary infections caused by *E. coli, Proteus*, and *Pseudomonas* species that do not respond to *any* of the antibiotics, even though such microbes show sensitivity to many antibiotics in the laboratory cultures? Or, young men and women crippled by Lyme microbes *and* massive antibiotic therapy for years? Or, to patients who go to hospitals without *C. difficile* but return home with infection by that microbe and chronic diarrhea? Or, to patients with chronic syndromes of mycoplasma, stealth microbes, nanobacteria, Epstein-Barr and herpes viruses for whom there are no effective therapies? Or, to human canaries caged in the diagnostic labels of chronic fatigue syndrome, fibromyalgia, multiple sensitivity syndrome, Gulf War syndrome, and other related chronic oxidative-dysoxygenative disorders?

By now it must be clear even to the most die-hard enthusiasts of Pasteur's monomorphism that the antibiotic approach simply does not work for any of the patient groups mentioned above. What is missing is Bechamp's notion of diseases arising from *within* which in my terminology is oxidosis and dysfunctional oxygen metabolism.

We can recognize the central role of dysfunctional oxygen metabolism in accelerated and premature aging now or we can wait for another few decades. I predict that the prevailing Pasteur's one-

bug/one-drug model for the clinical disorders mentioned above will not work, regardless of how many advances are made in genetics and antimicrobial chemistry.

A fundamental issue here, of course, is this: Can integrative ecologic-restorative nutritional and herbal therapies and detox procedures that primarily focus on the issues of oxidosis and dysfunctional metabolism promote healthful aging? The answer that my colleagues at the Institute and I give is an emphatic "yes." Our group has published several clinical outcome studies that provide unequivocal evidence for our view. Such studies included patients with disabling fibromyalgia,[11] chronic fatigue syndrome,[43] young women who lost their menstrual function,[37] children who stopped growing after chemotherapy for cancers or steroid therapy for colitis,[44] and patients with failed coronary bypass operations and angioplasty.[45]

In order to present the interrelatedness of the various ecosystems of the human body, some years ago I introduced a simple schema designated The Pyramid of Trios of the Human Ecosystem.[14] I also used that schema to emphasize my clinical perspective that the bowel, blood, and liver ecosystems form the base trio of that pyramid. Finally, that schema provides a conceptual ecologic-restorative model for stematically addressing all the relevant oxidative-dysoxygenative issues of importance for healthful aging. I devote the following chapter to a brief outline of that model.

SUMMARY

Oxygen coagulates. Oxygen arranges. Aristotle's comments about the roles of coagulation and arrangement in the beginning of a newborn's life are also relevant to our discussion of the great Pasteur-Bechamp debate. In performing those two great roles, oxygen reveals the mysteries of microbial pleomorphism. Pasteur is right in that specific microbial species cause specific types of diseases. Bechamp is also right in that life forms can arise from within the body and under certain conditions (primordial, in my terminology) multiply rapidly, produce large amounts of toxic organic acids, and lead to chronic illness that does not respond to antimicrobial therapies.

Oxygen for the human body is the primary determinant of the ecologic struggle that formed the core of Darwin's work. When functional, oxygen provides the basic drive for human metabolism, is the quarterback detox molecule of the body, and is nature's most potent antimicrobial agent. Thus, it is the guardian angel of human health. When dysfunctional, oxygen is oxidizing, acidifying, and dysoxygenative. Thus, it favors the primordial life forms.

I believe monomorphism and pleomorphism are fundamentally not incompatible with each other. Indeed, the two views are complementary. Man and microbe share a majority of their genes.

Gene sharing, in reality, is seed sharing. Thus, the soil of the cells of men and microbes carries many of the same genes. That makes Bechamp right. His vegetative microzymes are today's shared DNA sequences.

A human hunter immune cell loves oxygen, hates excess acid, and shuns decaying and dead organic matter. A primordial life form, by contrast, hates oxygen, loves acid, and thrives on decaying and dead organic matter. Thus, the cellular state of oxidation and oxygenation determines the conditions that favor either the germination of those seeds along "human lines" or along the "microbial lines." That, of course, is the core Darwinian notion applied to human health and disease.

References

1.   Nuland SB. Doctors: The Biography of Medicine, New York, Alfred A. Knopf, 1988, p. 362-364.
2.   Pasteur L. *Correspondance Generale*, collected and annotated by Louis PasteurVallery-Radot. Paris, Flammarion, 1951, 1:21.
3.   Nuland SB. Doctors: The Biography of Medicine, New York, Alfred A. Knopf, 1988, p 362-4.
4.   Ali M. Spontaneity of Oxidation in Nature And Aging. Monograph. 1983. Teaneck, New Jersey.
5.   Ali M. Spontaneity of Oxidation in Nature Is the true cause of Aging in Humans and Root Cause of All Disease. page 199-304, RDA: Rats, Drugs and Assumption. 1995. Life Span Press, Denville, New Jersey.
6.   Ali M. Ali O. AA oxidopathy: The core pathogenetic mechanism of ischemic heart disease. J Integrative Medicine 1998;1:6-112
7.   Ali M. Ascorbic acid reverses abnormal erythrocyte morphology in chronic fatigue syndrome. Am J Clin Pathol. 1990;94:515.
8.   Ali M. Oxidative regression to primordial cellular ecology. Journal of Integrative Medicine 1999; 2:4-56.
9.   Ali M. Darwin, Oxidosis, Dysoxygenosis, and Integration. J Integrative Medicine 1999;1:11-16
10.   Ali M. Darwin, fatigue, and fibromyalgia. J Integrative Medicine 1999;3:5-10.
11.   Ali M. Ali O. Fibromyalgia: An oxidative-dysoxygenative disorder (ODD). J Integrative Medicine 1999;3:17-37.
12.   Ali M. Oxidative Menstrual Dysfunction. J Integrative Medicine 1998; 3:101-124.
13.   Ali M. Under Darwin's Glow (editorial J Integrative Medicine 1999;3:1
14.   Ali M. Of gardeners and doctors: A medicine of human ecosystems for the new millenium. Aging Healthfully 1999;1:1-4.
15.   Nuland SB. Doctors: The Biography of Medicine, New York, Alfred A. Knopf, 1988, p. 363.

16.   Nuland SB. Doctors: The Biography of Medicine, New York, Alfred A. Knopf, 1988, p. 363.
17.   Bechamp A. Compt. rendus hebd, (1866) 451, T66 (1868) 366. T68 (1869) 466.
18.   Jouanna J. Hippocrates, The Johns Hopkins University Press, Baltimore, 1999, p317-248-49.
19.   Beale LS. Observations upon the nature of the red blood corpuscles. Trans Microsc Soc. London 1864:12:37.
20.   Almquist E. Studien uber das Verhalten einiger pathogenen mikroorganismen bei n iedriger temperatur. Zbl. Bakt. I Abt Orig. 1908;48:175-186.
21.   Metchnikoff E. Untersuchungen uber die intracellular verdauung berwirbellosen thieren. Arb Zoologischem Inst Univ Wien 1883;5:141
22.   Enderlein G. Bacterial Cyclogeny. 1916. Translated by Enderlein Enterprises Inc.(by permission of Semmelweis Verlag Experimental Oncology GmbH, Germany). 1999. Preface V-VIII.
23.   Enderlein G. Archiv fur Entwicklungsgeschichte der Bakterien Bd. 1 Heft 1-4, Bd 2 Heft 1, Immunologica Heft 1-6.
24.   Naessens N. Centre d'Orthobiologie Somatidienne de L'Estrie, Inc. C.O.S.E. The Cancer Chronicles Volume 5, No. 5-6, p5-15.
25.   Chishima K. Revolution of Biology & Medicine, Volume 9, Gifu, Japan, Neo-Haematological Society Press, 1972. p4-5
26.   Mattman, LH. Cell Wall Deficient Forms: Stealth Pathogens. CRC Press, Boca Raton, Florida, 1993.
27.   Kajander O. Proc. Nat Acad Sci 1998;95:8274-8279.
28.   Abbot A. Battle lines drawn between 'nanobacteria' researchers. Nature 1999;401:105.
29.   JT. Nanobacteria strike the kidney again. Science News. 1999;155:395.
30.   Nicholson GI. Mycoplasma linked to GWI/CFS/FMS/AIDS. International Council for Health Freeddom. 1999;3:15-16.
31.   Behan P. Behan W. Bell E., The post viral fatigue syndrome, an analysis of the findings in 50 patients. Journal of Infection. 1985;10:211-222.
32.   Behan P. Behan W. CRC Critical Reviews in Neurobiology. 1988;4:2-157.
33.   Gorbach SL. Antibiotics amd Clostridium difficile. N Eng J Med. 1999;341:1690-1691.
34.   McFarland LV. Mulligan ME. Kwok RYY., et al. Nosocomial acquisition of Clostridium difficle infection. N Eng J Med. 1989;320:204-210.
35.   Barlett JG. Chang TW. Gurwith M., et al. Antibiotic associated psedomembranous colitis due to toxin-producing clostridia. N Eng J Med. 1978;298:531-534.
36.   Johnson S. Samore MH. Farrow KA, et al. Epidemics of diarrhea caused by a clindamycin-resistent strain of Clostridium difficile in foru hospitals. N End J Med 1999;341:1645-1651.
37.   Ali M. Amenorrhea, oligomenorrhea, and polymenorrhea in CFS and fibromyalgia are caused by oxidative menstrual dysfunction (OMD-I) J Integrative Medicine 1998;2:101-124.
38.   Bradford RC. Allen H. Oxidology 1997. Bradford Research Institute, San Diego, California.
39.   Ali M. Bradford R. Ali O., et al. Immunostaining of Candida organisims in peripheral blood smears (abstract) 1995, American Academy of Otolaryngic Allergy, SPring Meeting, Palm Desert, California.
40.   Burnett LE. The challange of living in hypoxic and hypercapnic aquatic environment. Amer Zool 1997;37:633-640.
41.   Botstein D, Chervitz SA, Cherry JM. Yeast as a model organism. Science 1997;277:1259-1260.
42.   Loewenstein WR. The Touchstone of Life: Molecular Information, Cell Communication, and the Foundations of Life. 1998. Oxford University Press. Oxford. page 338.
43.   Ali M. Hypothesis: Chronic fatigue is a state of accelerated oxidative molecular injury. J. Advancement in Medicine. 1993; 6:83-96.
44.   Ali M. Ali O. Fayemi A., et al. Efficacy of an integrative program including intravenous and intramuscular nutrient therapies for arrested growth. J Integrative Medicine. 1998;2:56-69.
45.   Ali M. Ali O. Fayemi A., et al. Efficacy of an integrative program including intravenous

and intramuscular nutrient therapies for arrested growth. J Integrative Medicine. 1998;2:56-69.

Endnotes

1. Following are the eight principles of Prof. Chishima his theory in his own words[8]: (1) Red blood corpuscles with polipotency differentiate into all kinds of somatic cells and germ cells, in accordance with their cellular environmental conditions; (2) Reversible differentiation between the red blood corpuscles and the fixed cellular elements [occurs] under different nutritional conditions or the developmental stages; (3) Bacteria and viruses arise spontaneously from organic matter by means of AFD (aggregation, fusion and differentiation); (4) Cells increase in number, mainly by new formation from organic matter but not by the so-called mitotic division; (5) Haematopoietic (blood-cell forming) organ of the red blood cells is not the bone marrow but the intestinal villus in the adult and the placental villus in the embryonic stage; (6) Orthodox genetics contains some basic mistakes. For instance, according to my finding, germ cells such as spermatozoa and ova cells arise newly from the somatic elements, the red blood cell corpuscles; (7) Darwinism involves some important contradictions of the origin of life, the mutation theory, existence of microorganisms (amoebae, bacteria) which remained as they were without evolution, and then negligence of symbiosis (mutual aid) as an important evolutionary factor; and (8) I have presented a new scientific methodology, bio-dialectic instead of formal logic or material dialectic.

2. Bradford-Allen Pathway of Coagulation.[33] According to this pathway, formation of soluble fibrin complexes with cellular and extracellular debris occurs prior to clearance of such complexes from the circulation. They contrast their pathway to the coagulative pathways that involve the established intrinsic and extrinsic coagulation factors and result in the formation of a hard clot composed of insoluble fibrin needles or meshwork. This mechanism provides for control of bleeding and prevention of blood loss. For that reason, the Bradford-Allen pathways, once further validated by biochemical studies of sialic acid activation by bacterial neuraminidase or activated sialidase, will be recognized as a major breakthrough.

3. There is well established high level of homology of nucleotide sequences of mammalian cells and microbial species. For instance, Botstein et al.[36] compared all yeast protein sequences to the mammalian sequences in GenBan, and found a statistically robust homologue among the mammalian protein sequences for nearly 31 percent of all potential protein-encoding genes of the yeast. In 1996, the DNA sequence of Saccharomyces cerevisiae was published.[36] That genome is widely accepted as a highly suitable model for interpreting and comprehending human DNA sequences.[37] It is well established that certain genes in yeast and mammals encode very similar proteins.[38] Some homologues encode for proteins of molecular systems such as ribosomes and cytoskeletons. A notable example is the presence in yeast of two close homologues (RAS1 and RAS2) of the mammalian ras proto-oncogene. Yeast organisms lacking both homologues are not viable. In 1985, Kataoka et al.[39] expressed in yeast the mammalian H-ras sequence, with the remarkable result that the viability of yeast was restored, indicating not only conservation of sequence but also preservation of biologic function. After publication of the complete DNA sequence of the yeast, they considered this high homology figure an underestimate since databases do not yet contain all the mammalian sequences. Intriguingly, they noted that yeast genes with homology to mammalian sequences are much less likely to have no experimentally verifiable functions; however, the potential role of such sequences in multiplication of

PLFs has not been explored.

4. In clinical states characterized by chronically accelerated oxidative stress, enzyme systems involved in oxygen transport and utilization, redox regulation, and acid-base equilibrium are severely impaired. Such oxidative states include fibromyalgia, chronic fatigue syndrome (CFS), Gulf War syndrome, severe immune disorders, and malignant neoplasms. It is proposed that normal "oxygenative" cellular ecology in such states undergoes an "oxidative regression to primordial cellular ecology" (ORPEC) in which state progressive anoxia, acidosis, excess reactive oxidative species, and accumulation of certain organic acids create cellular ecologic conditions that closely simulate the primordial state. The ORPEC state results in rapid multiplication in blood and tissues of pleomorphic anaerobic organisms with yeast-like morphologic features, which are designated "primordial life forms" (PLFs) for lack of precise nucleotide sequence and taxonomic data. PLFs are readily observed with high-resolution phase-contrast and darkfield microscopy in freshly prepared and unstained smears of peripheral blood. Strong homology among yeast and mammalian DNA sequences indicates that the genetic codes for PLF growth may already exist in human cells and that organisms observed in this study may not indicate an infection from an outside source. Rather, the clinical syndromes associated with PLF proliferation may represent a novel "microecologic-genetic" model of illness. Organic acids and other toxins produced by the growing number of PLFs further feed the oxidative flames of the ORPEC state, thus generating oxidative cycles that feed upon each other and are damaging to antioxidant and oxygenative enzyme systems of the body.

The proposed ORPEC hypothesis draws its primary support from the microscopic findings presented in this paper when these are considered in light of the following: (1) the fundamental "oxygen order" of human biology; (2) the history of oxygen during the primordial era; (3) the primordial cellular ecology as reconstructed from the origin-of-life studies; (4) morphologic evidence of accelerated oxidative injury to all components of circulating blood (oxidative coagulopathy), and to cell membranes, intracellular matrix, and cell organelles such as mitochondria (AA oxidopathy); (5) oxidative oxygenative dysfunctions (pathologic states characterized by impaired cellular oxygenation and caused by oxidative injury); (6) a high level of homology among yeast and mammalian nucleotide sequences (reflecting conserved primordial nucleotide sequences) that may lead to de novo growth of PLFs under primordial conditions; (7) phenomenon of gene swapping in nature that may enlarge the cellular genetic pool ; (8) oxidative 3 C (complement, coagulation, and capsases) cascades that contribute to and perpetuate primordial conditions; (9) evolving concepts of mycosis and PLFs; (10) increased urinary excretion of certain organic acids that provide biochemical evidence of overgrowth of yeast and PLFs in patients in the ORPEC state; and (11) clinical syndromes of accelerated oxidative molecular injury.

Chapter 10

A Menagerie of Mystery Maladies for the Millenium

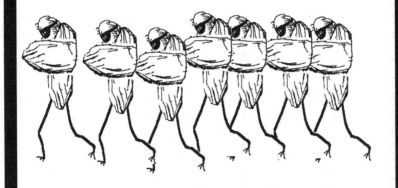

The subject of human life span cannot be presented without taking into account chronic disorders that accelerate the aging process and cause untimely death. It is curious that this subject is rarely, if ever, addressed by life span researchers. Perhaps that is so because that thorny problem throws a monkey wrench into their grand designs for extending the human life span to 115 to 120 years.

In matters of health, our legacy to the new millennium is a growing menagerie of mystery maladies. It includes epidemics of chronic fatigue syndrome, fibromyalgia, multiple chemical sensitivity syndrome, Gulf War syndrome, hyperactivity and attention deficit disorders, learning disabilities, chronic Epstein-Barr syndrome, "candidiasis" syndrome, and other related enigmatic chronic syndromes. None of those syndromes can be understood according to the prevailing systems of disease classification. Nor can any of those syndromes be treated successfully with any of the known drugs.

Beyond the matter of mysterious maladies, there is an equally distressing subject of the increasing incidence of common chronic disorders—such as cancer, coronary heart disease, asthma, viral infections, and others—for which there are neither any explanations for the cause according to the prevailing disease classifications nor any satisfactory treatment. The hype of drug companies and media notwithstanding, in this chapter I show a picture that does not bode well for aging-gene researchers.

How can I paint a negative picture of research in aging counter to the near-universal wave of optimism?, some readers might ask. How can I do so in the face of increasing longevity? On the surface, those are compelling questions. But first we must ask what the reasons are for extension of life span that we have witnessed during the last two hundred years. We owe our longer lives *primarily* to advances in sanitation, the technology of agriculture, and vaccination. In comparison, improved surgical techniques and drugs have made rather modest contributions. This view may also be questioned by some. I cite one example. From the mid-nineteenth century to the early 1900s in England, mortality from measles fell by over 90% *before* the advent of antibiotics *and* mass vaccination of children against measles. I have addressed that problem previously. In the endnotes of this chapter, I include some important citations to support my point of view.

DRUGS FOR DISCIPLINE

Our children are being drugged for discipline (considered behavioral problems by some) on an alarming scale. One of every nine children in some school systems is on Ritalin, Dexedrine, Adderall or other mind-altering drugs. The production of Ritalin has increased more than sevenfold during the last ten years, and 90% of its is consumed in the U.S.[1] The school psychologists consider hyperactivity, attention deficit disorder (ADD), learning disability, obsessive-compulsive disorder, autism, and Tourette's syndrome "mystery" maladies. They know their psychological theories do not hold water anymore. Mothers of such children know that the symptoms of such disorders are minimal on some days and very intense on others. They search for an explanation and discover that sugar, food reactions, mold allergy, and exposure to certain chemicals increase their children's symptoms. When such mothers keep their children from the suspected triggers, the symptoms are markedly reduced. When told of such associations, most pediatricians simply dismiss such clues. The abuse of mind-altering drugs for such reactions persists.

The relationship between the intensity of symptoms of hyperactivity and ecologic bowel imbalance is unmistakable. The same is true of some nutrients and metabolic factors and the spreading epidemic of attention deficit disorders. I observe a similar relationship among learning disabilities and events taking place in the liver, including food sensitivities and mold allergy. To some, such considerations may seem irrelevant to a discussion of the aging process. I see the relevance clearly.

ANTIDEPRESSANTS FOR FATIGUE

From New York to Nairobi, Bangkok to Beijing, Lahore to Istanbul, I have seen the spreading epidemic of chronic fatigue in children. And wherever I ask the doctors about what they think is behind those epidemics, they shrug. The Chinese physicians expressed the most exasperation. They were simply astounded by the mystery maladies. Their medical texts, ancient as well as modern, contained no references to such disorders. Can children with lives severely diminished by chronic fatigue be expected to grow into healthy 115-year-old men and women? I never hear aging-gene researchers address that question.

Our teenagers and adults suffer from persistent fatigue on an equally large scale. They are prescribed antidepressants, antianxiety drugs, and antibiotics with increasing frequency. Many pediatricians dismiss such fatigue as a part of "the teenage scene." In some areas, up to 21% of persons reported chronic fatigue as a dominant symptom.[2] In prevailing drug medicine, there is neither agreement on the cause of chronic fatigue nor is there any effective treatment. In the context of the present question, can young persons disabled with chronic fatigue be expected to grow into healthy 115-year-old persons? Would they even want to?

DRILLING SKULLS FOR FIBROMYALGIA

Fibromyalgia is rapidly climbing the list of disorders for which the government declares people physically disabled. It is also considered a medical mystery. Internists often think it is an imaginary problem. Rheumatologists treat it with steroids and strong painkillers. Neurologists present complex theories and then put such patients on heavy doses of neuroactive drugs. Psychiatrists think muscle pain and fatigue are psychogenic in origin and should be treated with antidepressants. Psychologists think what is really needed is some talk therapy. Neurosurgeons have the most perverted notions about fibromyalgia. Consider the following quote from *The Wall Street Journal* of November 11, 1999:

> **Jozan Plaza, a 45-year-old Alabama woman, visited Chicago recently to have a part of the back of her skull drilled off. Was this a good idea? Ms. Plaza is among the roughly eight million Americans diagnosed with a condition called fibromyalgia syndrome, which involves widespread muscle pain, sleeplessness, fatigue, and depression....For about $30,000 a case, they are**

**drilling and snipping away bone from the backs of
people's skull and spines to "decompress" their
brains, spinal cords and central nervous systems.**

In the 1860s, Baker Brown, a London surgeon, used genital
mutilation to treat headaches and menstrual syndrome in young
women. He performed clitoridectomies.[3] Thank God those days of
barbaric surgery are behind us, I remember saying when I first read
about Brown. But barbaric surgery still flourishes in the United
States. For $30,000 the poor patient not only gets a big hole in his
skull but also a big hole in the bank balance, if any is left.

While one of the nation's major newspapers reported skull
surgery for fibromyalgia, consider the following quote from another
major newspaper (*USA Today*, January 13, 2000) on the same
subject:

Real life with a 'phantom disease'

**Experts in the field say that many people,
including doctors, write off people like Hedrick [a
victim of fatigue/fibromyalgia syndrome],
attributing their symptoms to "phantom disease."**

One group of doctors drill holes in skulls for fatigue. The
other calls it a phantom disease! Such is the travesty of our Star Wars
medicine. Both groups of doctors demonstrate the worst type of
medical self-righteousness.

Fibromyalgia is *unmistakably* an oxidative-dysoxygenative
disorder[4] that cannot be reversed with drugs or surgery. The full range
of fibromyalgia symptoms can only be understood if we understand
dysfunctional oxygen metabolism. When oxygen metabolism is

restored in such persons, they regain their health.[5] I devote the companion volume, *Canary Two: Oxygen and Fibromyalgia,* to that subject.

The point of interest here is this: Can anyone expect millions of Americans to have holes drilled in their skulls and then go on to live to be 115-year-old men and women?

ALZHEIMER'S DISEASE:
Oxygen, Toxins, and Dead Brain Cells

The Centers of Disease Control and Prevention, the U.S. agency that keeps tabs on incidences of diseases, has forecast an epidemic of Alzheimer's disease. More than 35 years ago, when I first performed autopsies on persons who had suffered from Alzheimer's disease, I found dead and dying nerve cells caught up in a tangle of scar tissue—neurofibrillary tangles, in pathology terminology. I was then told the cause of Alzheimer's disease was not known, just as is the case of *all* other degeneratory disorders of the brain. Years later in 1995, in *RDA: Rats, Drugs and Assumptions,* I predicted that brain cell decay and death will prove to be due to oxidative damage to brain cells caused by accumulated toxins.[6] Within a year, *Nature* published an article validating my hypothesis. Many early cases of Alzheimer's disease responded well when my colleagues and I administered oxygenative therapies (such as intravenous hydrogen peroxide) and large doses (up to 30,000 mcg) of vitamin B_{12} along with other injectable nutrients. That provided us with some validation of our ideas that that disorder has something to do with insufficient oxygen and accumulated toxins. I revisit this subject in the chapter entitles, "How many Will Live Demented Lives."

Now there is much interest in developing a vaccine for Alzheimer's disease on the grounds that it is an inflammatory disorder. Of course, all inflammatory processes are triggered by oxygen-driven oxidative stresses. Neurologists are busy conducting drug trials for the disease. But will drugs (chemicals) bring dead brain cells back? I do not think so. Again, the important question is the same: Can anyone developing Alzheimer's disease in his sixties or seventies be expected to live to be 115-year-old?

EPIDEMIC OF BREAST AND PROSTATE CANCER —A LOST WAR

In 1971, Richard Nixon declared war on cancer and predicted victory. With hubris about medical matters that is not uncommon among politicians, he declared victory within a decade. Now thirty years later, where do we stand?

In 1958, in my medical school in Pakistan, I was taught that about one in fifty women will develop breast cancer in her lifetime. In 1965 in England, I learned that one in twenty women will develop breast cancer. In 1972 in the United States, I was told one in twelve women were expected to develop breast cancer. In the next twenty-five years, I saw that number change from one-in-eleven to one-in-ten to one-in-nine to one-in-eight to one-in-seven in some parts of Long Island and New Jersey. The incidence of cancer of the prostate in men has increased in a similar fashion so that one in five men are expected to develop prostate cancer. Would I be surprised if the incidence of breast cancer rises to one-in-six or even one-in-five in another thirty years? Similarly, would I be surprised if the incidence of prostate cancer rises to one-in-four in another thirty years? The folks at the American Cancer Society have no clues as to what is driving those cancer epidemics. In 1995, in *RDA: Rats, Drugs and Assumptions*, I presented my oxidative theory of cancer and published my view that the breast and prostate cancer epidemics were directly related to synthetic hormones and pesticides with hormone-like effects. In this volume, readers will learn that *a cancer cell hates oxygen, loves acidity, and thrives on dead and dying organic matter.*

How will those cancer epidemics affect longevity? What kind of progress have we made in curing cancer? Consider the following two quotes from reports analyzing cancer survival statistics published in *The New England Journal of Medicine*:

> **We are losing the war on cancer....The main conclusion we draw is that some 35 years of intense efforts focused largely on improving treatment must be judged a qualified failure.**
> 1986;314:1226.

> **In 1986, we concluded that "some 35 years of intense efforts focused largely on improving treatment must be judged a qualified failure." Now, with 12 more years of data and experience, we see little reason to change that conclusion.**
> 1997; 336:1569.

I point out here that the two reports cited above concern cancer survival statistics for the entire United States, not just one hospital, county, or state.

THE OTHER SIDE OF THE STAR WARS
MEDICAL TECHNOLOGY

During the last fifty years, we have witnessed one miracle of medical technology after another. The frequent and gross dramatization and distortion of TV notwithstanding, many medical inventions are breathtaking. We rarely blink at the sight of a heart being pulled out of one chest and put into another. Our surgeons demonstrate amazing dexterity. Medical procedures are routinely performed in our trauma units that could only be dreams a decade ago. Newer drugs for asthma control, acute coronary heart syndromes, and many other disorders are effective to degrees that were not imagined a few decades ago. A sheep named Dolly ushered in the era of cloning only a few years ago. We no doubt can expect many advances coming from such knowledge. Gene therapies will undoubtedly help some patients with genetic enzyme defects, though so far the results have been dismal.

But there is another face to that story that seems invisible to most people. Below, I cite a few examples.

THE OTHER SIDE OF THE ASTHMA STORY

Hardly a week goes by that some doctor on TV does not tell us about a new miracle drug for asthma. We see images of Star Wars technology with ventilators and gas machines controlled by flashing computers in intensive care units. We are told about saved lives. But there is another side to this story as well. Consider the following two quotes from *Nature* and the *Journal of the American Medical Association:*

> **[A]s we approach the millennium almost half the population of the West demonstrates sensitization to one or more environmental *allergens*. In countries such as Britain or Australia, this translates to 1 in 4 children under the age of 14 years having *asthma* and 1 in 5 having *eczema*. *Added to this* is the occurrence of serious allergic disorders caused by new allergens such as nuts, soya, and latex.**
>
> *Nature* 1999; 402/supp. 82.

How well are we treating such children? Consider the second quote:

> **From 1982 to 1992, the prevalence of asthma increased by 42% and the average annual death rate by 40%.**
>
> *JAMA* 1997;277:1503.

More asthma. More deaths from asthma. And that despite all the claims of miracle drugs and Star Wars medical technology! Again, the important question here is the same as for chronic fatigue, fibromyalgia, Alzheimer's disease, and cancer: Can children who develop asthma be expected to live for 115 years?

THE OTHER SIDE OF THE
CORONARY BYPASS STORY

A New Jersey hospital advertisement claims a 98% success rate for the coronary bypass operations performed there. *That is simply a sad and deliberate deception.* The real question is how they define the surgical success rate. The truth about bypass surgery and coronary stents is shown by the following recent reports of the *New England Journal of Medicine* (for exact quotes, see corresponding endnotes).

Elderly patients in the United States underwent coronary bypass surgery 7.8 times as often as similar patients in Canada. Despite these differences, the one-year death rates in the two countries were identical. The *Journal* blamed the fee-for-service system for ineffective operations.[7]

In an editorial titled, "Coronary-Artery Stents—Gauging, Gorging, and Gouging," the *Journal* reported a near five-fold increase in the number of coronary stents inserted in the United States and wrote,

Cardiologists have mistakenly believed that stents reduce the rates of heart attack and death.[8]

Indeed, *excess number of deaths* was seen among persons receiving stents.

In a series of more than 6,400 bypass and angiography procedures, the *The New England Journal of Medicine* reported that with "remarkable clarity and consistency," such procedures had offered no benefit over standard medical treatment.[9]

In 1997, my colleague, Omar Ali, and I described our oxidative theory of coronary heart disease and introduced the term oxidative coagulopathy for microclot and microplaque formation in the circulating blood.[10] We conclusively demonstrated that coronary artery heart disease is, first and foremost, caused by oxygen-driven oxidative stresses in the circulating blood. We also marshalled extensive evidence to support our view that natural cholesterol, an antioxidant, *cannot* cause coronary artery disease.

Returning to the subject of oxygen and aging, the essential question is the same: Can coronary bypass operations and stents that do not work help people with heart disease live to be 115 years old?

THE OTHER SIDE OF THE STORY OF CHOLESTEROL

Drugs for lowering blood levels of cholesterol bring the most money for drug companies. Predictably, doctors in university hospitals get the most grant money for writing cholesterol papers. So it is that at least every month one or more prestigious medical journals carry cholesterol papers extolling the virtues of cholesterol drugs. (How else would the doctors get the future grant dollars?) Amazingly, the current advice is that people should be taking cholesterol-lowering drugs even when the cholesterol level is within the so-called normal range. Such drugs have a clear risk of causing cancer, liver disease, fatigue, and other problems, but that does not seem to temper the infatuation with drugs.

There are two *real* issues in the cholesterol story which the enthusiasts of cholesterol-lowering drugs do not like to address. Those issues are:

Natural, unrancid cholesterol is an antioxidant. Blaming coronary heart disease on healthy cholesterol is like blaming pure water for illness. Rancid cholesterol, like polluted water, can cause disease. So, the focus must be on rancidity of cholesterol rather than on its blood level.

The second issue is how the results of cholesterol studies are deliberately distorted to support the use of drugs. In a survey of 22 large controlled studies, the *British Medical Journal* (1992;305:15) concluded:

Lowering serum cholesterol does not reduce mortality...Methods subject to bias, such as open trials or the use of drugs with characteristic side effects, or stratification instead of random allocation of participants, probably explain the overall 0.32% reduction recorded in non-fatal coronary heart disease.

An important issue here is that cholesterol papers always report *risk reduction rates* and never *actual rate reductions.* Rate, we all know, is a real mathematical number, while risk reduction is a contrived number. (Risk reduction rate has no denominator, hence has no mathematical validity.) For *13 lines of evidence* against blaming natural, unrancid cholesterol for coronary artery disease, I refer the advanced and professional readers to an article which my colleague, Omar Ali, and I published in *The Journal of Integrative Medicine*.[10]

Note how the *real* cholesterol story supports the *real* coronary bypass and stenting story. Neither approach is theoretically valid. And neither works in life.The relevant question here is the same as for the bypass/stenting story: Can cholesterol-lowering drugs help people live to 115 years when healthy cholesterol, an antioxidant, is not the culprit?

THE OTHER SIDE OF THE STORY OF SYNTHETIC HORMONES

The makers of synthetic hormones are as successful in persuading doctors to go on TV and advise women to take synthetic hormones as are the makers of cholesterol drugs. What is the *real* story there? Earlier in this chapter, I wrote about epidemics of breast and prostate cancer. I believe that those epidemics are directly related to permeation of our environment by synthetic hormones and xenoestrogens (synthetic chemicals with estrogen-like effects). An important question that is seldom, if ever, raised in discussions of synthetic hormone replacement therapy is: What happens to synthetic hormones passed in urine by millions of American women who take them? Such hormones—unchanged, as well as metabolites with potent hormonal effects—are passed into the urine, put into the large bodies of water, enter the food chain, and gain entry into the bodies of our babies, boys and girls.

The strongest evidence for my view is an analysis of the relationship between the introduction of synthetic hormones and epidemics of breast and prostate cancer in different countries during the last sixty years. Both types of cancers were quite uncommon among people in China, Japan, and other countries in the Far East, who lived on diets rich in soy (with a large content of natural estrogens). Both types are now occurring in epidemic numbers in big cities and other parts of those countries where synthetic hormone replacement was introduced American-style 20 to 30 years ago.

All over the world, wherever synthetic estrogens were introduced, the epidemics of breast and prostate cancer followed.

How do synthetic estrogens fare in the United States? There is a direct relationship between the use of synthetic hormones and death from breast cancer. Consider the following quote from a recent issue of *The New England Journal of Medicine*.[11]

[There was] a 43 percent increase in death due to breast cancer [among hormone users].

Another report published in the *Journal of the American Medical Association* reported an 80% increase in risk of breast cancer among hormone users.[12] The basic question here is the same: Can the life span of women and men be prolonged by giving them powerful carcinogenic hormones?

THE OTHER SIDE OF THE STORY
OF CHRONIC DISEASE

It does not seem necessary to continue this effort to lay bare the folly of claims of drug enthusiasts in the face of an ever-enlarging menagerie of maladies for which the Star Wars technology has no visible answers. I close this matter with an important quote from the *Journal of the American Medical Association:*[13]

The first National Health Survey conducted in 1935 found that 22% of the population had a chronic illness....[W]ith 100 million Americans [40% in 1995] with one or more chronic conditions, nearly every family is affected....[C]hronic conditions will increase to 148 million [estimated 50%] by 2030.

One of every two Americans will suffer some chronic disease in another thiry years! That certainly does not give us much confidence in the rosy pictures painted by the CNN futurists, does it? Nor does it increase our confidence in aging-gene enthusiasts.

SUMMARY

In earlier chapters, I presented my case that dysfunctional oxygen metabolism is at the root of not only the so-called mystery maladies but also the major chronic diseases of the present time. In this chapter, I have summarized a large body of data to demonstrate that the prevailing drug therapies and surgical procedures have yielded limited benefits for most of those disorders. To shed some light on why we have had such limited success with drugs and surgery, I make the following essential points:

1. Nutritional deficiencies, environmental sensitivities, chemical toxicities, and lifestyle stressors markedly increase oxidative stress on the human microecologic cellular and macroecologic tissue-organ ecosystems.

2. Excessive oxidative stress leads to dysfunctional oxygen metabolism.

3. Dysfunctional oxygen metabolism leads to a state of absence of health (dis-ease) and sets the stage for acute and chronic diseases.

4. Dis-ease and diseases speed up the aging process. Research in genes involved with aging will bring *limited* benefit to a small number of people, but will be of no value to the majority of people unless the larger issues that threaten oxygen metabolism are addressed.

In the United States we have failed to preserve health and promote healthful aging in spite of spending an estimated $1.5 trillion on health care. The reason for that is simple: We have ignored the fundamental issues of oxygenation, oxidation, and dysfunctional oxygen metabolism. Unless those matters are fully addressed, the promise of drugs and genes for longer life span is a false promise.

References
1. Gibbs N. The Age of Ritalin. Time Magazine, pp 85-96, November 30, 1998.
2. Kroenke K, Wood DO, Mangeldsroff AD, et al. Chronic fatigue in primary care: Prevalence, patient characteristics, and outcome. JAMA

1988;260:929-934.

3.   Journal of Obstretics and Gynecology of the Bristish Empire
      1867;67:1017-1034.

4.   Ali M. Ali O. Fibromyalgia: an oxidative-dysoxygenative disorder (ODD)
      J Integrative Medicine 1999;1:17-37.

5.   Ali M. Juco J, Fayemi AO, et al. Efficacy of ecologic-integrative
      management protocols for reversal of fibromyalgia: An open prospective
      study of 150 patients. J Integrative Medicine 1999;1:48-63.

6.   Ali M. Oxidative Theories of Diabetes and Alzheimer's Disease. RDA:
      Rats, Drugs and Assumptions. 1995, pages 199-304. Life Span Press,
      Denville, New Jersey.

7.   Krumholz HM. Cardiac procedures, outcomes, and accountability. N Eng
      J Med 1997;336:1522-3.

8.   Topol EJ. Coronary-artery stents -gauging, gorging, and gouging. N Eng
      J Med 1998;339:1702-3.

9.   remarkable Consistancy article N Eng J Med

10.   Ali M, Ali O. AA oxidopathy: the core pathogenetic mechanism of
      ischemic heart disease. J Integrative Medicine 1997;1:1-112.

11.   Grodstein F, Stampfer MJ, Colditz GA, et al. Postmenopausal hormone
      therapy and mortality. N Eng J Med 1997;336:1769-75.

12.   Okie S. Studies raise new concerns about hormone treatment. Washington
      Post News Service. 1999.

13.   Hoffman C, Rice D, Sung HY. Persons with chronic conditions. Their
      prevalence and costs. JAMA 1996;276:1473-9.

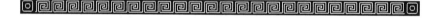

I see problems of health arise primarily in two locations: one in the head and the other in the bowel. In the head reside the problems of spiritual void, confused demands for love, and anger, in the bowel are the ecologic disruptions caused by sugar overload, antibiotics abuse, pesticides, food preservatives, and other toxins that weaken the bowel wall. Both types lead to dysfunctional oxygen metabolism and, in my view, both require focus not only on what caused those problems but also all relevant oxygenative therapies.

Chapter 11
What is Health?

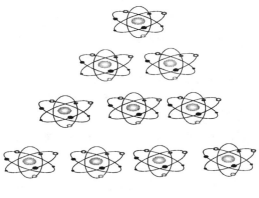

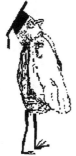
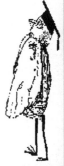

Health is usually—and quite superficially—defined as physical, emotional, and mental well-being. But what are the physical attributes of health? How may we define emotional well being? What is mental wholesomeness? I never reflected on those questions in more than 25 years when I worked as a surgeon and pathologist. I faced this problem only when my interest shifted from study and treatment of disease to deliberations of matters of health and healthful aging. Here is how I define health:

Health is rising in the morning with a sense of the spiritual —without any need to analyze what the spiritual might be. It is *knowing* that spirituality is a language without words.

Health is freedom from anger.

Health is waking up in the morning with a deep sense of gratitude—gratitude not for any accomplishment of the day before or for accumulations of yesteryears, but for simply being. An ENT surgeon from Greece once attended my lecture at the meeting of the American Academy of Otolaryngic Allergy and expressed a common frustration: "But this is utterly new to my Greek thought!" Well, if the concept of gratitude for simply being is foreign to us, we need to learn about it.

Health is waking up with a sense of energy, going through a day's work with that same sense of energy, and returning to bed at night with it.

Health is as much energy before meals as it is after them.

Health is the ability to treasure personal time in silence—with family, friends, or alone.

Health is a vigorous oxygen metabolism.

Health is two or three effortless, odorless bowel movements a day—without mucus and cramps.

Health comprises living, dynamic and vigorous bowel, blood and liver ecosystems—and of all cellular ecosystems elsewhere in the body.

Health is an intact and functioning gateway of life—cell membranes that mark the boundaries between life within the cell and that which exists outside. The cell membrane separates internal order of a cell from external disorder. It is a living, breathing, spongy and porous sheet that regulates the two-way energetic-molecular traffic between cells and the soup of life that bathes them.

The elements in the preceding paragraph of my definition of health may seem tedious to some readers. I discuss this essential subject in the companion volume, *RDA: Rats, Drugs and Assumptions*. In that volume I propose a conceptual model of what I call energetic-molecular (EM) medicine.

The essence of EM medicine is to seek a genuine understanding of the energetic-molecular dynamics of cells *before* the cells are injured, and not on our notions of cellular injury as seen through a microscope *after* the injury has occurred. All nondrug, restorative therapies used to reverse chronic diseases are based on EM dynamics of health. This model of clinical medicine promotes health with natural therapies that revive injured bowel, blood and cellular ecosystems.

It is not uncommon for me to see mainstream doctors criticize holistic physicians for their "unscientific" methods. The truth is that it is far more scientific to base restorative therapies for chronic disease on a genuine understanding of oxygen, oxidosis, and dysfunctional oxygen metabolism than on mere symptom suppression with drugs that block normal physiological processes. It is far more scientific to look at the bowel, blood and other organ ecosystems than on mere disease names that tell us nothing about the cause of suffering. Drug therapies for chronic disease—as necessary as they might be for symptom suppression—do not constitute a true solution to problems caused by damaged body ecosystems.

WHAT HEALTH IS NOT

And now, I define what health is not. Health is not the mere absence of disease. Health has nothing to do with the frivolous notions of RDAs (Recommended Daily Allowances) in the early 1940s by the Nutrition Board to prevent a handful of nutrient deficiency syndromes. Nor is it about the frivolous notions of balanced diets of doctors who practice drug medicine and consider nutritional medicine quackery.

Health is not high-fat or low-fat diet. Nor is it infatuation with this vitamin or that mineral.

Health is not the euphoria of eating nor is it the denial of dieting. Health is not preoccupation with recycling past miseries, nor is it precycling feared, future misery.

Health is not living with regrets, nor is it obsession with control in life.

Doctors who limit their work to drugs or scalpels shun the subject of health. Why? The answer is really quite simple: None of the essential aspects of health I define in this chapter can be addressed with drugs or with surgical scalpels. There are no drugs that make us spiritual, nor can they bring us gratitude and freedom from anger. There are no drugs for teaching us the limbic language of silence, nor for putting out the oxidative fires of stress. Drugs cannot revive injured energy enzymes, nor can they repair damaged detoxification enzymes. There are no synthetic chemicals that can upregulate energy and fat-burning enzymes. Drugs cannot restore a damaged bowel ecosystem, nor can they strengthen a weakened blood ecosystem. Drugs cannot normalize disrupted energetic-molecular dynamics at the cell membranes.

Injured tissues heal with nutrients—not with drugs. Blocker drugs—beta blockers, calcium channel blockers, proton pump inhibitors, and others—as necessary as they are for managing acute illness, cannot restore dysfunctional oxygen metabolism. Indeed, the tools of the Star Wars medicine are singularly ineffective for coping with most of the stressors that cause oxidosis and dysoxygenosis.

***

Good health is not about martyrdom before eating or guilt after it. It is not about low-carb, high-fat, no-yeast, or other silly notions of diets. Nor is it about calorie counting or clever schemes of losing weight.

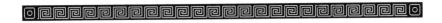

One can know only as much
divinity as exists within oneself

From *What Do Lions Know About Stress*

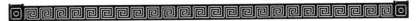

Chapter 12

The Pyramid

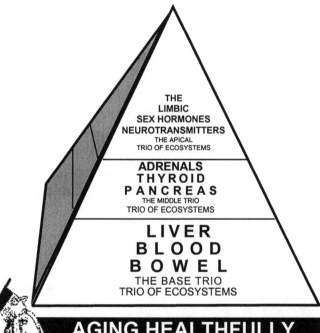

THE
LIMBIC
SEX HORMONES
NEUROTRANSMITTERS
THE APICAL
TRIO OF ECOSYSTEMS

ADRENALS
THYROID
PANCREAS
THE MIDDLE TRIO
TRIO OF ECOSYSTEMS

LIVER
BLOOD
BOWEL
THE BASE TRIO
TRIO OF ECOSYSTEMS

AGING HEALTHFULLY

Within the oxygen order of human biology, the bowel is where battles of health and disease are fought—and won or lost. The bowel is the guardian angel of the blood. The blood is guardian angel of the liver. The liver is the guardian angel of the rest of the body. To some, those may seem glib and trivial statements. For me, those are some of the most important lessons my patients have taught me during the last 42 years. Those simple statements cannot be understood except through ecologic thinking.

My own ecologic thinking, as I recall it, began one day in 1969. As a pathology resident, I received a large basin brimming with a messy inflamed and distended colon with copious bloody fecal matter spilling out of some tears in its wall. It was not much fun to clean that bowel and take tissue samples for preparing microscopic slides. The next day I examined the slides and observed the expected microscopic features of ulcerative colitis: acute and chronic inflammation, dead and dying immune and other types of cells, ulceration of the lining mucosa, disruption of the general architecture of the colon wall, and pockets of pus. After finishing my study, I took the case to one of my professors. He examined the slides and agreed that it was a case of ulcerative colitis.

The next day, something unexpected happened. Without purpose, I picked another slide of that colon, looked at it, and chanced upon a cluster of large, pale cells forming a discrete round structure. Such a formation is called a *granuloma* and is considered diagnostic of Crohn's colitis. "Look at that!" I said to myself in surprise. "Now, that granuloma makes it Crohn's colitis, doesn't it? Yesterday it was ulcerative colitis. Today it seems to be Crohn's colitis. Interesting!" I marked the microscopic field with ink and took the slides to a second professor, since the first one was out of the department. He looked at the case and readily diagnosed Crohn's colitis.

The next day as I prepared to carry the slides to one of the secretaries for filing, I picked another slide from the same case and started gazing at an area that showed discrete layers of tissue debris covering small patches of the inner surface of the bowel wall. Those are the features of another common type of colitis called pseudomembranous colitis. "Aha! Another diagnosis!" I exclaimed. "Let's see if I can get someone also to agree with me." That time I purposefully looked for a third professor and decided not to tell him about the diagnoses made by the other two. I pointed out to him the membrane-like structures and he agreed that we had a case of pseudomembranous colitis. I returned to my desk triumphantly. I knew I had a story to tell. Sometime after that Choua said, "Can you make more slides from that colon and see if you can get another professor to diagnose yet another type of colitis from the *same* colon?" he challenged. I smiled. Worth a try, I murmured to myself.

I went back to that colon and took many more sections of tissues. A technician looked at me, a little annoyed because she had to prepare the slides from all those sections. The next day she brought me several trays of slides and I went to work. In one of the slides, I found areas that showed well-preserved bowel architecture, congested blood vessels, pooled and disintegrating red blood cells in the tissue, and small surface erosions. Bingo! I knew those were the features of another type of colitis called ischemic colitis. I continued my search. I was not disappointed. I found some microscopic fields that showed diagnostic features of a type of colitis called collagenous colitis. "Ah! Another diagnosis!" I congratulated myself and continued study of the case with yet other slides. There were many fields which could only be diagnosed as nonspecific colitis. With some more persistence I found other areas qualifying for other forms of colitis. Getting my teachers to agree to those various diagnoses with different slides of the *same* colon did not prove to be difficult either. I spoke to Talat, my wife, about my accomplishment, but decided not to tell my professors about it. I did not know how some of them might take it.

Next I turned my attention to my pathology textbooks for a *critical* study of the causes of those various types of colitis. That turned out to be a yet more fruitful search. I made the second and equally important discovery: *The cause of none of those types of colitis was known.* It was not that dozens of pages of those texts were not filled with discussion of the etiology (cause) of all those types of colitis. For every type of colitis, some immune disorder, infectious agent, or vascular event was suspected or proposed, but in every case the final conclusion was always the same: *The cause is not fully understood.*

That search led me to a third important discovery: There is such a large overlap in the clinical symptomatology, microscopic appearances, and suspected causes that there was hardly any point in slavishly adhering to the system of classification of colitis which I was being taught as "science."

The young pathologist in me was jolted by his three discoveries. An image of several blind men surrounding an elephant arose in my mind's eye. During the weeks and months that followed, some vague, ill-defined notion of altered states of bowel ecology began to evolve. It took me several years before I could muster courage to begin writing about what I thought were my awkward notions of bowel pathology, which I thought would be heartily laughed at.

The Bowel Ecosystem

In my view, the most remarkable phenomenon in the entire field of human biology is this: A vast number of clinical problems that are seemingly unrelated to the bowel spontaneously resolve when the focus of clinical management turns to all the issues in bowel ecology. How often do symptoms of persistent debilitating fatigue in young men and women clear up when an altered state of bowel ecology is restored to normal? How often do troublesome mood swings subside when therapies focus on the bowel? How often does arthralgia (pain and stiffness in joints with or without joint swelling) resolve when all the bowel issues are addressed? How often do we successfully prevent chronic headache and anxiety; lightheadedness and palpitations; menstrual irregularities and incapacitating PMS; recurrent attacks of vaginitis and cystitis; recurrent sore throats and asthma; and eczema and related skin lesions by correcting the abnormalities in the internal environment of the bowel? The answers to these questions will vary widely among physicians.

THE GUT IS A MISUNDERSTOOD ORGAN

Physicians who regularly neglect the bowel (and those who never understood the issues of bowel ecology in the first place) will dismiss these questions with scorn. None of this has been proven with double-blind cross-over studies, they will strenuously protest. Other physicians who have learned to respect the bowel—as the ancients did—and care for their patients with a sharp focus on bowel issues will readily and unequivocally validate my personal (and fairly extensive) clinical experience.

LIFE IN THE BOWEL ECOSYSTEM

The bowel ecosystem teems with life. Shrouded in metabolic mists, it is as rich in biologic diversity and as broad in biochemical interrelationships as any other ecosystem on this planet Earth. The ancients seemed to have an intuitive sense about it. Death begins in the bowel, they pronounced in more than one way. Anton van Leeuwenhoek (1632-1723) studied fecal bacteria during his work with the microscope and thus was the first man to study life in the bowel ecosystem with modern scientific methods. Metchnikoff, the Russian biologist, who single-handedly developed the concept of the cellular arm of the immune system, became intensely interested in the aging process in his later years when he moved to Paris, where he served as the head of the Pasteur Institute. He studied the longevity of Bulgarians and provided strong evidence that certain bowel microbes played important roles in preserving health and promoting longevity among them. He named the microbe he thought was most prominent in this field as *Lactobacillus bulgaricus*. Metchnikoff's work opened the floodgates of basic research on the bowel flora.

WINDOWS ON THE WORLD

A cell looks at the world around it through its cell membrane. It is this membrane that separates the cell's internal order from external order. Although molecular host defense mechanisms of both immune and nonimmune types have progressed from simple single-cell forms to multicellular forms to highly developed complex organisms such as humans, the fundamental pattern of host defenses has remained the same: The cell membrane or its counterpart carries the primary responsibility for preserving the biologic integrity of the organisms. For the professional reader, I discuss at length the energy and biochemical events which occur at the cell membrane in health and disease in two monographs entitled, *Leaky Cell Membrane Dysfunction*[1] and *The Agony and the Death of a Cell*.[2]

For humans, the gut mucosa is the true counterpart of the cell membrane of unicellular organisms.

From an evolutionary perspective, the gut mucosa would be expected to be the primary host defense organ. In a biologic sense, man's gut lining is his window to the world around him. What do we ever get through our skin but a little vitamin D when we get a chance to bask in the sunshine? What do we get through our lungs? All our ancestors ever received through their lungs was oxygen. Now we receive— unwillingly and under severe protest—a heavy load of environmental pollutants. Everything else that enters our biologic systems enters through the gut lining. It is important to recognize that the mucosal linings of the mouth, esophagus and stomach essentially are extensions of the gut lining. The states of health and absence of health are expressions of the dynamics of foods within the gut ecosystem—the effects of foods on the digestive-absorptive processes, as well as the various life forms in the gut.

HUMAN DEFENSES AGAINST DISEASE EXIST AS PLANTS IN THE SOIL OF THE BOWEL CONTENTS

The ancients seemed to have known this intuitively. We seem to have taken a very circuitous route to grasp this most fundamental of all aspects of the immune system. I remember that the hakim (folk-doctor) in my village always prescribed laxatives for a headache. He prescribed remedies that seemed to work on the bowel for problems of the skin, joints, liver and other organs. Of course, I, then a medical school student, found it very amusing. It never occurred to me then why these folk-doctors would prescribe year after year remedies that couldn't work. More important, from my present perspective, I never wondered why people accepted those remedies year after year if they afforded no relief. I was into the science of medicine then. I wasn't into finding out what worked and what didn't. Nor did I ever doubt the science of my professors, who doled out prescriptions for drugs by the dozens for sheer symptom suppression. That was then. And that was poor Pakistan. Now I question the science of an average American family practitioner when he prescribes drugs for chronic bowel symptoms. How scientific is his use of antacids for symptoms of burning or pain in the pit of the stomach? How scientific is his use of antispasmodic drugs for abdominal cramps? How scientific is his use of antidiarrheal drugs for diarrhea? How scientific is his use of steroids for inflammatory bowel disorders? Steroids suppress the immune system. How scientific is it to further suppress the immune system for problems caused by an errant immune system in the first place? How scientific is the use of anti-inflammatory agents, anxiolytic drugs, antidepressants, antispasmodic agents, antihistamines, and, of course, broad-spectrum antibiotics for treating various types of bowel disorders that we—by our own admission—do not understand the causes of?

LAPs AND TAPs:
The Good and Bad Guys of the Bowel

LAPs and TAPs are my abreviations for lactic acid-producing and toxic agent-producing microbes in the bowel. LAPs preserve the normal bowel ecosystem; TAPs disrupt it.

In the companion volume, *The Canary and Chronic Fatigue*, I discuss many elements that increase oxidative stress on energy and detoxification enzymes. It turns out that almost all these elements also suppress LAPs and—both directly by inhibiting LAPs and indirectly by other mechanisms—promote the growth of TAPs. This subject is of enormous significance in the normal aging process, as well as in the accelerated aging process associated with chronic disease states.

LAPs confer many important host defenses upon the bowel, discussed later in this section. TAPs are equally versatile in their functions and produce a very large number of noxious substances in the bowel. Among these are ammonia; phenols; tryptophan metabolites; vasoconstrictive amines such as histamine, tyramine, agmatine and cadaverine; certain steroid metabolites; and many toxins — most notably mycotoxins derived from fungi (yeasts). This area has received rather limited investigative attention, and it is almost certain that future research will uncover a host of as yet undetected bacterial and fungal toxins and metabolic villains. Finally, the bowel flora both produce and potentiate some carcinogenic substances.

Not unexpectedly, LAPs-TAPs dynamics are profoundly influenced by food choices. American and British individuals show overgrowth of some TAPs, such as bacteroides and some types of clostridia, with much higher frequency than is seen in Japanese, Indians and Ugandans. It appears likely that these differences are due to excess use of antibiotics and an abundance of fats in the former populations' diet.

BACTERIA: THE MASTER CHEMISTS

Bacteria are living beings capable of executing an enormous number of biochemical reactions. Farmers used bacteria and fungi to turn compost into fertilizer long before biologists understood the metabolism of these single-celled bodies. A partial list of such reactions brought about by the normal bowel flora includes production of ammonia, conversion of amino acids into amines and phenols, inactivation of digestive enzymes such as trypsin and chymotrypsin and other enzymes located on the surface of cells lining the gut, deconjugation of hormones such as estrogen and bile acids, denaturation of bile steroids, breakdown of food flavonoids, hydrogenation of polyunsaturated fatty acids in food, utilization of certain amino acids such as B_{12}, conversion of some compounds into carcinogens, and many other enzymatic reactions.

I list below the three genera of LAPs and several genera of TAPs that most frequently populate the bowel ecosystem:

LAPs	TAPs
Bifidobacterium	*Proteus, Pseudomonas, Salmonella, Escherichia*
Lactobacillus	*Bacteroides, Clostridium, Peptococcus, Peptostreptococcus*
Streptococcus	*Streptococcus, Staphylococcus*

About 30 species of LAP microbes have been identified. Some important members of these three groups (*L, Lactobacillus; B, Bifidobacterium; S, Streptococcus*) include the following:

L. acidophilus	*B. bifidum*
L. bulgaricus	*B. adolescentis*
L. lactis	*B. infantis*
L. casei	*B. breve*
L. helveticus	*B. longus*
	S. faecium
	S. thermophilus

Most byproducts of modern technology threaten LAP microbes. In addition, alcohol, nicotine, various pharmacologic agents, and highly processed and "preserved" foods adversely affect LAPs.

LAPs: THE GUARDIAN ANGELS
OF HUMAN CANARIES

The LAP angels promote healthful aging in many ways.

First and foremost, LAPs keep TAPs under check. It appears that this essential role is played through different mechanisms that include simple physical crowding out of the potential pathogens as well as production of antimicrobial substances. *L. acidophilus* produces acidophilin, acidolin and bacterlocin; *L. plantartium* produces lactolin; *L. bulgaricus* produces bulgarican; and *L. brevis* secretes lactobacillin.

Second, LAPs produce many lifespan molecules. Notable among them are members of the vitamin B complex, especially folic acid and biotin, and vitamin K. Lactobacillic acid is an important fatty acid that is produced by some lactic-acid producers and is then converted into essential fatty acids. Another notable molecule in this context is tryptophan—this is likely to be one of the mechanisms by which yogurt has been reported to be beneficial in cases of fibromyalgia, chronic fatigue, and related conditions.

Third, LAPs play a pivotal role in digestion. Lactose intolerance is a very common clinical problem. It is often not fully appreciated that a major portion of lactose ingested in dairy products is actually broken down to simpler sugars by lactase enzymes produced by lactic acid producers. Lactic acid and lactase producers also play important roles in protein digestion. This is one of the primary reasons protein intolerance is so common among individuals with altered states of bowel ecology.

Fourth, LAPs actively break down some toxins produced during metabolism such as ammonia, free phenols and polypeptides.

Fifth, LAPs normalize bowel transit time and are effective in controlling infant and adult diarrhea.

Sixth, the antiviral and antifungal roles played by LAPs, having long been empirically suspected by nutritionists and holistic physicians, have recently been documented with research studies.

Seventh, the cholesterol-lowering effects of fermented milk have been attributed, among other mechanisms, to orotic acid, which facilitates fat metabolism in the liver.

Eighth, some LAP microbes suppress tumor cells in rats. This factor is not of direct relevance to human canaries — at least not yet, though in time oxidosis and dysoxygenosis is likely to increase the threat of cancer in persons with OD (oxidative-dysoxygenative) states.

It is noteworthy that all eight elements mentioned above increase, directly or indirectly, the fury of oxidosis, acidosis, and dyxoxygenosis.

In the late 1970s and early 1980s, for the professional readers I discussed many of the above issues in a series of articles published in the syllabi of instruction courses of The American Academy of Environmental Medicine.[3,4] In 1987, after examining an estimated 7,000 bowel and 1,500 stomach biopsies, I published a monograph entitled *Altered States of Bowel Ecology* to present a broad integrated ecologic view of the happenings in the bowel ecosystem.[5] For the general reader, I especially recommend a chapter entitled, "Battered Bowel Ecology and Chronic Fatigue," in *The Canary and Chronic Fatigue.*[6] For advanced and professional readers, I again recommend the following two articles published in *The Journal of Integrative Medicine*: (1) "AA oxidopathy"[7]; and (2) "Oxidative Regression to Primordial Cellular Ecology."[8]

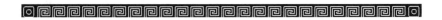

To cure chronic illness, England's Dr. Thomas Syndren prescribed trips on trotting horses. "I began to ride 2 or 3 hours every day," Thomas Jefferson wrote to a friend.

"While President...it was some time before the effects was sensible, because it takes time to strengthen the bowels, but in about a year I was completely cured, and am now perfectly well. 'Go thou and do likewise.'"

U.S. News & World Report, May 1, 2000

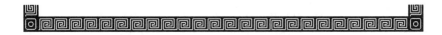

The Blood Ecosystem

The blood is also a dynamic, diverse, and delicate ecosystem. It is far from a sterile conveyer belt for transport of nutrients and wastes from one body organ to another.

The bowel dumps into the bloodstream much good stuff (nutrients) and much bad stuff (microbes and metabolic as well as external toxins). In the bloodstream, hunter immune cells swallow and kill microbes. The blood from the bowel is directed to the liver via a separate system of veins called the portal system, where it is cleared of most toxins. Thus, the circulating blood represents an ecosystem sandwiched between the two other major ecosystems of the body. When the bowel ecology is badly battered by sugar overload, antibiotic abuse, pesticides, and other insults, it causes adverse effects which my colleague, Omar Ali, and I designated "oxidative coagulopathy"[7] and which I discussed in the chapter entitled, "Oxygen: The Great Communicator." A similar set of conditions develop when the ability of the liver to detoxify toxins is exceeded and toxins back up in the blood.

THE BLOOD IS AN OPEN ECOSYSTEM

In 1995, in *RDA: Rats, Drugs and Assumptions*, I introduced the concept that the blood ecosystem is an open ecosystem.[9] This seemed necessary in light of my recognition that the circulating blood is not a closed and sterile stream. Rather, it is in a dynamic interface with the bowel ecosystem on one side and the liver ecosystem (along with other body ecologies) on the other. It is pertinent in this discussion to recognize that the bowel is estimated to harbor 50 to 100 trillion microbes at any time, a number similar to that of the total number of cells in the body. The author's microscopic studies suggest that the number of microbes that cross the bowel-blood barrier every day runs in tens of millions, perhaps in hundreds of millions. Indeed, in severe cases, as discussed in earlier chapters, I observed PLFs in the blood to outnumber red blood cells.

I discussed my reasons for assigning the circulating blood a place in the base trio of the Pyramid in the chapter, "Oxygen: The Great Communicator." For advanced and professional readers, I again recommend the article entitled, "Oxidative Regression to Primordial Cellular Ecology"[8] for detailed biochemical and microscopic evidence for my view that the blood ecosystem not only provides the essential link between the bowel and liver ecosystems, but also a field of PLF kept in check by oxygen and tracked down by hunter immune cells when they grow. In OD states, the blood ecosystem also teems with PLFs and spreads the adverse effects of oxidosis and dysoxygenosis to every microecologic cellular and macroecologic tissue-organ ecosystem of the body.

The Liver Ecosystem

Nature is generous. Nature is stingy. Nature creates ample reserves. Nature is a hard taskmaster. Nature is forgiving. Nature is unforgiving. Those are all aspects of nature's grand plan of economy. In matters of human health, next to the bowel, the liver is the most glorious mirror of nature's sense of economy.

The liver weighs two and one-half to three pounds in weight, yet it is the primary detox and metabolic organ of the body. It not only nourishes 50-100 trillion cells in the body, it is also responsible for keeping them clean and healthy. Thus, it comes as no surprise that the liver is the most frequently stressed organ of the body. It is one of the many wonders of nature that it has given this organ an enormous functional reserve. When 90% of the liver mass is removed in dog experiments, the dogs stay healthy. In my biopsy work I was more impressed by the regenerating capacity of liver cells than that in any other organ.

The ancient Greeks obviously understood some things about the liver's ability to regenerate. To punish the titan Prometheus for his transgression, the supergod Zeus had him chained to a mountain and sent an eagle to lunch at the prisoner's liver. Prometheus did not do too badly, however, as far as his liver was concerned. The liver grew back every day by the time the eagle returned.

Mother Nature has designed the liver in a most extraordinarily loving way. It has bestowed upon it a rare distinction: the liver gets its oxygen and nourishment from two sources. One face of *each* liver cell fronts oxygen-rich blood from the heart, while the other is covered with nutrient-rich blood from the bowel. To fully appreciate nature's benevolence, one needs to recognize that arterial blood from the heart brings 40 to 50% of the required oxygen, while that from the bowel delivers 50 to 60% of the liver's oxygen supply. That remarkable fact explains why pathologists rarely see liver infarction (large areas of cell death). The liver cell has yet another face that fronts ultramicroscopic bile passages. What mysteries abound in the innards of a liver cell, where hormones are built and broken down? A cell where some proteins are put together, while others are torn apart? A cell where the metabolic *soul* of a human being resides?

WHY IS THE LIVER ECOSYSTEM INCLUDED IN THE BASE TRIO OF THE PYRAMID?

The dual blood supply to the liver is a master stroke of nature's infatuation with Dr. Jekyll/Mr. Hyde architectural designs. The blood from the bowel not only brings nutrients and oxygen, but also a payload of natural and synthetic toxins, chemicals, and toxic metals. It is the responsibility of the liver to rid the blood entering it of all the toxic organic acids and other toxins before the blood can spread the toxins throughout the body. A fibro patient once remarked,

"Dr. Ali, for me it's bowel to the brain."

The sick have a way of crystallizing the truth about sickness. I cannot think of a more succinct and elegant way of stating the *essential* protective role of the liver. Medical students are taught the same thing in many convoluted ways. (Perhaps that's why they cannot seem to retain it when they leave medical schools.) In the medical jargon, when the liver fails and toxins cannot be cleared and reach the brain, the brain fog and problems of mood, memory, and mentation are designated as hepatic encephalopathy. *It is one of the profound ironies that we physicians so often laugh at the concept of early stages of liver toxicity and only too readily label the patients hypochondriacs.*

If the liver were not to filter the blood of its toxins and the blood from the bowel were to hit the brain directly, everyone would be brain-fogged at all times.

Human canaries who suffer from chronic fatigue syndrome, fibromyalgia, and severe bowel dysfunctions often suffer brain fog that clears when their battered bowel, blood, and liver ecosystems are restored.

Every young pathologist is intrigued by the liver. Nearly all give up on the liver, except the few who choose liver pathology as their subspecialty. Even that small group limits its work to the study of liver biopsies and classification of liver diseases caused by viruses, alcohol, chemicals, immune injury, and metabolic disorders. Treatment of most liver diseases in the hands of liver specialists is confined to the use of immune-suppressive therapies, such as steroids, chemotherapy drugs, large doses of agents such as interferon, or liver transplants. Otherwise, medical texts recommend "supportive treatment," which is a euphemism for symptom suppression with drugs.

There is simply no concept of liver detox among liver specialists. In most patients with nutritional, ecologic, immune, and heavy metal toxicity disorders, liver blood tests are often considered "within normal limits" and no attempt is made to prescribe nutritional, herbal, and natural detox therapies.

Every young naturopath is also intrigued by the liver. Nearly all develop an abiding lifelong interest in this organ. That is so because the use of liver-friendly nutrients and herbs and liver detox is emphasized as *the* core strategy in their schools. They recognize the clinical benefits of liver detox therapies, not only in patients with known liver diseases but also with chronic immune, nutritional, and ecologic disorders. Many of them are awkward in describing their concepts of the structure and function of the liver. And yet, their clinical results are superior to those obtained with drug therapies, except in cases of late stages of liver failure.

The above comments may seem to be glib simplification to some readers, but my view is based on the study of nearly 2,500 liver biopsies in hospitalized patients. During those years, I estimate I was also consulted by my associate pathologist for over 3,500 such biopsies. My work as an integrative physician with nearly 6,000 patients has been with generally advanced stages of nutritional, ecologic, immune, and degenerative disorders. The clinical results are far better when I focus on the issues of restoring the overburdened liver ecology with oxygenative therapies, including the liver detox. Such extensive study of the liver should have unraveled the secrets of this organ. In reality, the opposite has happened. My awe at the mystery of the liver continues to deepen. Indeed, I now think just as no one can ever fully know the healing energy of God, no one can ever fully know the liver. It is such a marvel of nature that it humbles everyone who ever reflects on its innards and its bioenergetic functions.

The above facts of the architecture and function of the liver explain why I include this organ in the base trio of The Pyramid of Trios of the Human Ecosystem. In summary, the liver is:

1.   The master detox organ;
2.   The master metabolic organ;
3.   The master nutrition organ;
4.   The master protein producer;
5.   The master fat metabolizer;
6.   The master sugar handler;
7.   The master vitamin producer and processor organ;
8.   The master mineral regulator organ;
9.   The master hormone modulator;
10.   The aging-gene organ; and, next to the bowel,
11.   The master lifespan organ.

The Pyramid

In 1997, I brought my concepts of the bowel-blood-liver and the thyroid-adrenals-pancreas trios together into a pyramid completed by adding the top trio of sex hormones, neurotransmitters, and the limbic brain. In the preceding paragraphs of this chapter, I have presented evidence that *all* mechanims of injury in the base and middle trios are oxidative in nature and lead to dysoxygenosis. The evidence for my view that the apical trio of neurotransmitters, sex hormones, and the limbic system is also damaged in oxidosis and dysoxygenosis is discussed elsewhere.[10]

In previous chapters, I have demonstrated that the core importance of the oxygen order of human biology to the aging process can be understood only through *ecologic thinking*. That also holds for my guidelines for healthful aging and reversing disease. Below, I include a schema of the previously published Pyramid of Trios of Human Ecosystems that shows:

1.   My sense of the *core* relationships among the major tissue-organ ecosystems of the body.
2.   My clinical priorities in proposing my guidelines for healthful aging as well as for reversing oxidosis, acidosis, and dysoxygenosis in illness.

I locate the trio of the bowel, blood, and liver ecosystems at the base of the pyramid because health is preserved or lost in these ecosystems. Accidents and some acute infections by highly virulent microbes are considered exceptions.

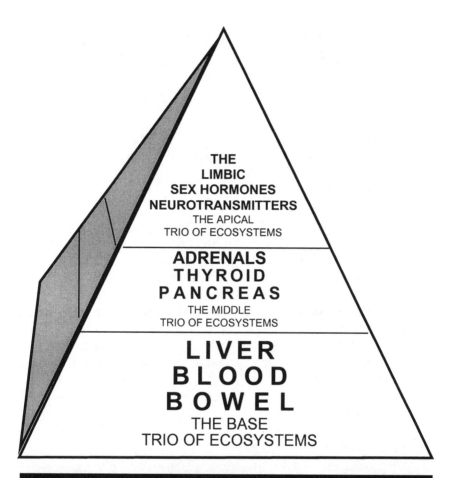

WHY ARE THE HEART, KIDNEYS, AND LUNGS EXCLUDED FROM THE PYRAMID?

Why have the heart, lungs, kidneys, spleen, skeletal muscle, and other body organs been left out in the Pyramid of Trios? The simple answer is that oxidative damage to such organs can be directly traced to the oxidative-dysoxygenative events taking place in the base trio of the Pyramid.

The heart is a pump. An air filter works well as long as the air it pumps is clean. A water pump functions well as long as the water it pumps if clean. The heart (a blood pump) beats well as long as the blood it pumps is clean. That, in simple words, is the story of coronary heart disease. As long as it pumps blood devoid of microclots and microplaques generated by oxidative coagulopathy and AA oxidopathy, there is no reason for its arteries to be clogged with plaques. Nor is there any reason for the heart muscle cells or the nerve cells in the conducting system of the heart to become damaged. The uncommon cases of viral and microbial damage to the nerve cells, of course, are exceptions. I discussed this subject at length in a recent publication.[11] Similarly, in the context of oxidosis and dysoxygenosis, the oxidatively triggered chronic lung lesions can be traced to macroecologic damages sustained by the bowel, blood and liver ecosystems. Again, infectious diseases and chemical toxicity caused by environmental pollutants are exceptions.

The kidneys are blood filters. They have a limited capacity for ridding the blood of its waste and toxins. I began this chapter by relating how I became disillusioned with classification of various types of colitis. Now I state that all thoughtful physicians find classification of kidney diseases equally disappointing. With the exception of some uncommon congenital and metabolic diseases, kidney failure is thought to be due to immune injury and/or oxygen-deficiency. The treatment, according to the kidney specialists, is either dialysis or transplant. At this point, readers will readily see the importance of keeping the blood free of microclots and microplaques in persons with diminished kidney function. Regrettably, the central roles of the bowel-blood-liver trio in causing and perpetuating kidney failure is not fully appreciated by most doctors. Indeed, my colleagues have successfully reversed early stages of kidney failure by a program of oxygenative therapies, including EDTA chelation.[12]

The same considerations also hold for disorders of muscle, soft tissues, and nonmetabolic brain disorders. For example, the myalgic patches and myofascial trigger points in fibromyalgia, CFS, and chemical sensitivity are also secondary to damage caused by oxidative coagulopathy and oxidative lymphopathy. From the standpoint of treatment, all such disorders require a broad, ecologic approach that addresses all issues of the Pyramid, and most importantly, of the base trio of the bowel, blood and liver ecosystems.

SUMMARY

The previously described Pyramid of Trios of the Human Body Ecosystems is presented in the context of the oxygen theory of aging. This model of relationships among the microecologic cellular and macroecologic tissue-organ ecosystems requires:

First, that oxidosis and dysoxygenosis be recognized as the core molecular mechanisms of accelerated aging process and the beginning of all chronic diseases.

Second, the prevailing one-disease/one-diagnosis/one-drug model of medical thinking must be replaced by an ecologic model. Furthermore, the base trio of the bowel, blood, and liver ecosystems must be given the most attention for healthful aging as well as reversal of chronic disease.

Third, all oxidants—metabolic, microbial, ecologic, industrial, and lifestyle stress-related—add to the cumulative burden of oxidosis and dysoxygenosis, and must be accepted as the cornerstone of all plans for controlling disease states and for healthful aging.

References

1. Ali M. Leaky Cell Membrane Dysfunction. Monograph. 1983. Teaneck, New Jersey.
2. Ali M. The Agony and Death of A Cell. 1987. Teaneck, New Jersey.
3. Ali M. Spontaneity of oxidation and molecular basis of environnmental illness. Syllabus of the 1991 Instruction Course of the American Academy of Environmental Medicine. Denver, Colorado.
4. Ali M. Molecular basis of cell membrane injury. Syllabus of the 1990 Instruction Course of the American Academy of Environmental Medicine. Denver, Colorado.AAEM bowel
5. Ali M. The Altered States of Bowel Ecology and Health Preservation, Monograph, 1993, Life Span, Denville, New Jersey.
6. Ali M. The Canary and Chronic Fatigue, Second Edition, 1994, Life Span, Denville, New Jersey.
7. Ali M, Ali O. AA oxidopathy: the core pathogenetic mechanism of ischemic heart disease. J Integrative Medicine 1997;1:1-112.
8. Ali M. Oxidative regression to primordial cellular ecology (ORPEC): evidence for the hypothesis and its clinical significance. J Integrative Medicine 1988;2:4-55.
9. Ali M. Blood: an open ecosystem. Rats, Drugs and Assumptions, 1995, pp. 424-442. Life Span, Denville, New Jersey.
10. Ali M. Ali O. Fibromyalgia: an oxidative-dysoxygenative disorder (ODD) J Integrative Medicine 1999;1:17-37.

Chapter 13

How Long
Will We Live?
How Many Will
Be Demented?

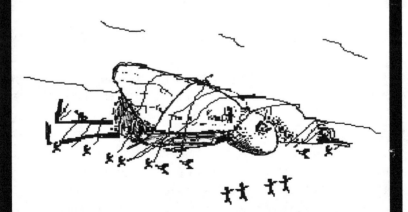

How long will we live? That question excites researchers in the field of aging most. For me, a more important question is: How many will live demented?

There is an epidemic of disorders of memory and mentation in the United States today. Three to four percent of Americans over 65 years of age suffer from Alzheimer's disease. Another five% suffer from other forms of dementia. During the early 1990s, one of every two Americans over the age of 84 was found to suffer from Alzheimer's disease.[1] Even the unflappable American Psychiatric Association (APA) has sounded alarm against "age-related cognitive decline" in people over the age of 50.

Age of 50! For decades, a debate raged among brain researchers whether age-related brain dysfunction (senile dementia and related disorders) should be considered as a "disease" or as a part of the *normal* aging process. But everyone understood senile dementia was a *senile* problem, something that one expects in the very elderly, say among those in their eighties, nineties or over. Now we are told that problems of memory and mentation should be of concern to Americans in their fifties!

I see even darker clouds on the horizon. *The Wall Street Journal* recently reported that eight million Americans, mostly young women and men, suffer from fibromyalgia, a condition of unremitting pain in muscles that progresses to cause brain fog and serious memory difficulties in most cases.[2] A second epidemic among the young, chronic fatigue syndrome, also causes serious, often disabling, problems of mood, memory, and mentation.[3] Multiple chemical sensitivity syndrome, long denied by most doctors, is now accepted as a real entity.[4] It is also spreading rapidly and claiming the cognitive functions of its victims. The brain researchers do not seem interested in such cognitive dysfunctions. As I wrote in earlier chapters, my colleagues and I observe evidence of OD (oxidative-dysoxygenative) dysfunction in all such cases. In the blood smears, I see deformed or dying cells and areas of congealed plasma and microclot formation. In the urine, I find increased amounts of organic acids (lactic acid, pyruvic acid, glyceric acid, and others) that indicate impaired oxygen metabolism. Can anyone say that teenagers and adults who cannot think well now will do so in decades to come?

The U.S. Department of Defense tells us that up to 100,000 Gulf War veterans are fully or partially disabled.[5] The non-government veteran organizations put the number close to 140,000. They were *all previously healthy* people, otherwise they would not have been sent to war. Most such persons report cognitive dysfunctions. Their case is also rejected by brain researchers, even though their SPECT and PET scans show clear evidence of diminished circulation and decreased metabolism in the brain. Does anyone really believe that the brain function of those Gulf War veterans will be intact fifty or sixty years from now?

Drugs for discipline in schools are being prescribed with increasing frequency. In some schools, one out of every ten children is on Ritalin or related drugs for hyperactivity, ADD, and learning disabilities. Does anyone seriously think that such use of mind-altering drugs for decades will not alter the brain function of those children in the future?

BRAIN DYSFUNCTION BY ANY NAME
IS BRAIN DYSFUNCTION

Just as the sleep specialists have been ingenious in inventing new names for sleep problems, psychologists and neurologists have been busy coining new terms for the problems of mood, memory, and mentation. Some of the names include mild cognitive impairment, primary degenerative dementia, early organic brain syndrome, senile dementia, frontotemporal dementia, multi-infarct dementia, cerebral ischemia, and TIA (transient ischemic attack). But to date neither group has shown serious interest in the events that occur below the neck and cause dysfunction above it. Specifically, they seldom, if ever, express concerns about the happenings in the bowel, blood, and liver ecosystems that lead to oxidative coagulopathy, oxidative lymphopathy, oxidosis and dysoxgenosis. They seem uninterested in how OD states so created cause oxidative injury to brain cell membranes, oxidative dysfunction of brain cell receptors, and oxidative damage to proteins, fats, sugars, enzymes, and DNA in the brain.

PLAQUES AND TANGLES OF ALZHEIMER'S
DISEASE

In the Iran-Contra affair, Ronald Reagan could not recall what his aids told him to forget. Since then, his health problems have made Alzheimer's disease a household name. When U.S. presidents come down with an ailment, research funding for that malady usually flows freely. That is a happy ending, though through an unhappy medium. But even before Reagan's personal battle, much progress was being made in understanding his disease.

In 1907, Alois Alzheimer laid the foundation for modern study of degenerative diseases of the brain. He described the microscopic appearance of plaques and tangles in the brain of patients who were thought to have senile dementia. Today we honor him by calling that condition Alzheimer's disease. There is accumulation of an abnormal protein called amyloid (also called beta amyloid) in the plaques and tangles. Many researchers believe amyloid to be a potent neurotoxin. However, at autopsy examination, amyloid deposits are seen in the brains of many persons who did not suffer from Alzheimer's disease. So the presence of amyloid protein cannot be accepted as a sure sign of Alzheimer's disease. However, much larger amounts of amyloid are seen in the brains of the victims of the disease.

The officials at CDC also use the word epidemic when they talk about the rising incidence of Alzheimer's disease. (CDC, the Centers for Disease Control and Prevention, is the U.S. agency that keeps tabs on disease patterns.) They consider Alzheimer's disease an enigma. I do not. In my view there is sufficient evidence that Alzheimer's disease is caused by states of oxidosis and dysoxygenosis created by:

1. Poor circulation.
2. Heavy metal toxicity.
3. Chemical pollutants—especially the fat soluble pesticides and other synthetics that get literally fixed to the brain tissue.
4. Immunologic stressors.
5. Chronic lack of mental activity.

As for the last item, there is some evidence that Alzheimer's disease occurs more frequently in persons with chronic lack of mental activity, such as problem solving, writing, and others. However, such lack of activity may indeed be the *consequence* rather than the cause of OD stress on the brain caused by the first four factors.

To understand denatured proteins in Alzheimer's disease, such as amyloid, we need to understand how proteins perform under stress in health and disease.

CHAPERONS AND CHAPERON NANNIES

Protein molecules are long strings made up of amino acids. The functions of proteins depend on how those strings are folded in specific three-dimensional forms.[6] Just as the twists in a rope are determined by the twists in its fibers, the folds in a given protein are determined by the amino acids in its structure.

It has been known for several years that proteins fold and unfold to respond to changes in their environment. Some proteins have a special function of guarding other proteins against excessive stress, bending, and damage. Such proteins are called molecular chaperons. Without such chaperons, proteins under oxidative stress get deformed, irregularly folded, and scrambled—literally as incompatible with the life of a cell as a scrambled egg might be in a hen's nest. There is yet another family of proteins called "chaperonins" that binds with newly formed proteins—hold hands, so to speak—until the baby proteins can grow up, fold properly into their "adult" structure, and act responsibly. But there is a limit to how much chaperon proteins and nanny chaperons can do. When oxidative stress exceeds their limits, proteins get tangled—aggregate and insolubilize, in scientific terms—and are deposited as amyloid material.

TOXIC METALS AND BRAIN DYSFUNCTION

The clinical and biochemical patterns of acute and chronic brain dysfunctions caused by acute ronic heavy metal toxicities are well established. The problem of sidious and cumulative toxicity of such metals in persons with bowel is an altogether differnt matter, and is rarely addressed by mainstream doctors. That is so because they seldom, if ever, order measurement of levels of toxic metals in post-chelation 24-hour urine samples. Without such testing, heavy me

Chronic heavy metal toxicity in chronically ill persons poses some vexing questions. How does one tell whether toxic metal overload is adding to the total toxic burden of an individual person? And how much? Notwithstanding the difficulty, some clinical aspects of such patients are revealing. My colleagues and I have seen patients in which acute brain dysfunctions were clearly triggered by rapid mercury chelation with intravenous administration of DMPS, a potent mercury chelator. Less frequently, we have seen limited symptoms of confusion and memory lapses that developed after oral DMSA, a less potent mercury chelator, therapy. For those reasons, we do not prescribe mercury chelation in persons with documented mercury overload until we have stabilized their bowel, blood, and liver ecosystems.

SYNTHETIC CHEMICALS AND BRAIN DYSFUNCTION

As in the case of heavy metal toxicity, the clinical and biochemical patterns of acute and chronic brain dysfunctions caused by acute and chronic exposures to many synthetic compounds are well established. Many pesticides and related chemicals love fats —are lipophilic, in chemistry lingo—and have a special affinity for fatty tissues, including those in the brain. Thus, such chemicals easily get stuck to the brain tissue and do not come off it easily. That explains why problems of mood, memory, and mentation caused by such compounds— designated neuropsychiatric symptom-complexes by some—are among the earliest and most common symptoms seen in chemical-induced disorders. It is important to recognize that such symptoms may be dose dependent (and be considered chemical toxicity) or dose independent (and be regarded as chemical sensitivity). I addressed some aspects of this subject in the chapter titled, "Guidelines for Healthful Aging."

OXIDOSIS-INJURED CHAPERONS AND CHAPERON NANNIES

It should be apparent from the brief preceding comments about protein folding and misfolding that amyloid protein formation results from oxidative injury. Indeed, formation of plaques and tangles in Alzheimer's disease fits *elegantly* in the OD (oxidosis-dysoxygenosis) model I present in this book. For me, the story of Alzheimer's disease was utterly predictable—and I did predict it in *RDA: Rats, Drugs and Assumptions*—on the basis of the OD model long before actual experiments proved the oxidative nature of the disease.[7] Even though the focus in Alzheimer's disease research in the past has been on amyloid proteins, I am confident future research will also show clear evidence of injury caused by oxidatively modified fats, sugars, enzymes, and DNA.

Since the publication of my monograph, *Spontaneity of Oxidation in Nature and Aging* in 1983,[8] I have presented extensive evidence of the oxidative nature of many specific disorders.[9-14] In 1994, in *RDA: Rats, Drugs and Assumptions,* I presented my view that plaques and tangles seen in Alzheimer's disease are formed when proteins and fats in the brain are oxidatively damaged. Specifically, amyloid protein is an abnormal protein that is formed when excessive oxidative injury is too much for the chaperon proteins and chaperon nannies to cope with. The result is damaged and tangled proteins. In outlining my oxidative theory of Alzheimer's disease in *RDA*, I wrote the following (page 279):

Is the beta amyloid protein found in plaques of Alzheimer's disease a product of oxidative damage to natural proteins present in the brain? Objective evidence for that has not been published. So it remains speculative on my part at this time. However, I have absolutely no doubt that such evidence will be forthcoming with future research in this area.[7]

Now it is established that the basic mechanism of injury involved in plaque and tangle formation in Alzheimer's disease is oxidative injury. *Now, of course, I believe oxidative injury leads to dysoxygenosis, and together those two mechanisms continue to damage brain cells and cause memory loss and diffuse brain dysfunction of Alzheimer's disease.*

VACCINE FOR MICE AND MEN

In July 1999, a paper published in *Nature* caused much excitement in the world of Alzheimer's disease.[15] Researchers at Elan Pharmaceutical claimed they could arrest, and even reverse in some cases, lesions of Alzheimer's disease in mice with a vaccine. Again, I have serious reservations that any vaccine against Alzheimer's disease will prevent the disease in any significant way, nor do I think that brain dysfunction will be restored by such vaccine in any significant number of people. That is not because I do not recognize the enormous value of vaccination in controlling many dangerous infectious diseases. Nor because I fail to foresee miraculous technologic breakthroughs in the coming decades. But I do see a *real* difference between vaccination for an infectious process and that for a degenerative process. Vaccines prevent infections by enhancing the body's own immune defenses against microbial invaders. The case in Alzheimer's disease is fundamentally different. It is an oxidative-dysoxygenative disorder. To date, there has never been an effective vaccine against a degenerative process caused by an oxidative disorder. Free radicals not only cause disease but are also *essential* for life. Thus, in my view, one cannot hope to prepare a vaccine against free radicals and hope to promote healthful aging.

If that is true, why did the vaccine work in mice?, readers might ask. One needs to look deeper for an answer to why a vaccine for Alzheimer's disease might work in mice but not in men. Experimental Alzheimer's disease in mice is produced by causing acute injury to the brain, thus provoking an acute and subacute inflammatory response. An immune response triggered by a vaccine under such conditions can bring excess blood and nutrients, and so initiate a healing response. The case of slow plaque and tangle formation in humans over decades is quite different. As I outline above, Alzheimer plaques and tangles are caused by slowly choking off the blood, oxygen, and nutrient supply to the brain tissue. Cumulative loads of toxic metals and synthetic chemicals add to brain injury. One cannot hope to bring back dead brain cells by triggering an immune response against them. Some limited benefits with Alzheimer's disease vaccine, indeed, may be realized in humans at some future time. However, such vaccination will not have long-term effects unless the oxygen metabolism can be preserved.

DENATURED FATS, SUGARS, ENZYMES, AND REDOX-RESTORATIVE SUBSTANCES

The subject of amyloid proteins in Alzheimer's disease has drawn the most attention recently, largely because amyloid research raised the specter of quick cure with drugs or vaccine that might block amyloid formation. It seems safe to predict that continued research will also show that oxidative-dysoxygenative injury to fats, sugars, enzymes, and redox-restorative substances in the brain also play important roles in the genesis of plaques and tangles. That is another important reason why I believe vaccines directed against amyloid protein will not be effective against Alzheimer's disease in the long run.

I reiterate here a point I have made repeatedly in this chapter: Alzheimer's disease is an oxidative-dysoxygenative disorder, and its control will require broad-based therapies that address *all* the relevant issues of the bowel, blood, and liver ecosystems.

OXIDATIVE-DYSOXYGENATIVE (OD) BRAIN DYSFUNCTIONS

What do Alzheimer's disease and other brain disorders associated with memory loss have in common? The answer: oxidosis, acidosis, and dysoxygenosis. To my knowledge, those three furies were found at work in all studies of brain dysfunctions, including Alzheimer's disease, in which the focus was on uncovering the molecular basis of the problems of the mind. I predicted that in 1983 in my monograph *Spontaneity of Oxidation in Nature and Aging*, in which I concluded that spontaneity of oxidation was the core driving mechanism in *all* types of molecular and cellular injury. The different diagnostic labels we use for them do not in any way indicate that there are any differences in the underlying pathophysiologic processes. In nearly two decades of my own work and review of that of others, I have not seen any evidence to the contrary.

The enormous importance of the OD model of brain dysfunctions is this: Regardless of the clinical picture of the patient and the diagnostic category we use, *the basic game plan for arresting the disease process is the same.* I can safely predict that the degree to which future drugs, vaccines, or gene therapies will work for those disorders will depend on how safely and effectively those measures will control the two basic problems of oxidosis and dysoxygenosis.

Now consider the following quote from an Alzheimer researcher from Johns Hopkins University:

Postmortem examination remains the gold standard for the diagnosis of Alzheimer's disease....The problem is the need to decide the cause of dementia during a patient's life.[16]

During my years of pathology residency I saw plaques and tangles, that are considered diagnostic of Alzheimer's disease, in persons who had died without any evidence of Alzheimer's disease. None of my professors then could answer why I should accept those plaques and tangles as microscopic proof of Alzheimer's disease in one person and not in another. Nor can anyone explain why that is so even now.

TESTS, BUT NO TREATMENT

In recent years, several important advances have been made in the diagnosis of brain dysfunction syndromes. Functional diagnostic tests for Alzheimer's disease and related disorders have been improvised. A gene test for Alzheimer's disease (apolipoprotein E4 allele) is now available for young persons to predict the risk of subsequent development of the disease. It is now possible to study the utilization of oxygen in the brain (by measuring sugar metabolism) with PET brain scans. With such scans, one can document the presence of dysoxygenosis not only in Alzheimer's disease, but also in *all* related brain dysfunction disorders, including patients with fibromyalgia and chronic fatigue syndrome.

However, not much progress has been made in treatment (which is the only important thing for the afflicted person). It is regrettable that oxy therapies have been, and continue to be, ignored by most doctors. Unaware of the value of such therapies, they continue to express hopelessness in the area of treatment. Consider the following two quotes:

> **"We have no treatment for the disease," he notes. "What good does it do for someone to find out at age 45 that they have a chance of developing the disease?"**

> An Alzheimer's disease researcher expressing his disillusionment with diagnostic tests. Quoted in *Science News* 1996; 149:312.

Four years later:

> **The twentieth century has witnessed a dramatic prolongation of lifespan, but little progress in preventing age-related cognitive decline. The anticipated further prolongation of human life in the twenty-first century will be a hollow victory unless cognitive function can also be preserved.**

> *Nature* 2000;404:125.

A Century of Cognitive Decline is the title of the millennium essay by a Harvard professor from which the above quote is taken. The subtitle of the essay asked: If we live long enough, will we all become demented?[17]

OXY THERAPIES FOR BRAIN DYSFUNCTIONS

From the preceding discussion, the readers will expect oxy therapies to be of substantial benefit for persons with brain dysfunction disorders, such as mild cognitive impairment, Alzheimer's disease, senile dementia, and TIA. That, indeed, is true. Oxy therapies in the form of intravenous ozone infusions and hyperbaric oxygen for managing strokes and pre-strokes have been extensively used in Europe and, to a lesser extent, in the United States. A large number of reports attest to the clinical benefits of such therapy.

At the Institute, my colleagues and I have had extensive experience with nasal oxygen, intravenous infusions of hydrogen peroxide and ozone, and EDTA chelation. In the preceding chapter, I cite several outcome studies documenting the clinical efficacy of such therapies. Our group has not yet published any systematic clinical outcome study of our true-to-life experience with oxy therapies. Below, I include two case histories to make two important points: (1) how the refusal of insurance carriers to reimburse for nutritional and other natural therapies leads to interruptions in care; and (2) how sometimes the benefits of such therapies are more apparent when therapies are withdrawn.

A woman asked me to see her husband, who was diagnosed with Alzheimer's disease two years earlier. He was unable to attend to his basic needs at home. Six weeks after weekly infusions of EDTA and hydrogen peroxide plus multivitamins on alternating basis, she reported a "substantial improvement" in his doing household chores. Several weeks later, she sadly told me of her decision to discontinue treatment because her insurance company had refused to reimburse her.

A man asked me to see his aunt who had serious difficulties of confusion and memory loss. Several weeks later, her home-care practitioner reported "some improvement" in those functions. No further progress was reported during the next several weeks. That led to a shared decision by all involved to discontinue treatment, largely because the benefits observed were deemed not worth the effort necessary to proceed with the therapy. About four months later, the lady returned for additional treatment. Her nephew and the home-care provider had not noticed appreciable improvement while receiving the treatment, but had observed "disturbing" deterioration of the status of her mentation, mood, and memory after treatment had ceased.

Strokes and TIAs (pre-strokes or transient ischemic attacks) are also caused by oxidative injury. As is the case with coronary heart disease, those disorders also begin with oxidative coagulopathy. It follows that a rational approach to those disorders must also be directed to arresting oxidative coagulopathy and reversing its adverse effects on the brain tissue.

I REMAIN OPTIMISTIC

I end this chapter with the same words with which I began this book:

This book is about a simple idea: Oxygen is *the* organizing influence of human biology and governs the aging process. From that idea I develop two other dominant themes of this book. First, *dysfunctional oxygen metabolism* is the *primary* cellular mechanism of aging and will be the single most important threat to the human life span in the coming decades. Second, a growing understanding of relationships among man's internal and external environments will govern *all* our plans for preserving health and reversing disease.

Until now, the medical profession has largely ignored the above three issues, to the great detriment of the sick. Hundreds of billions of dollars were spent on Star Wars medicine, largely committed to dealing with late stages of diseases and with predictably limited results. Hundreds of billions of dollars were also spent on mapping out the human genome. Those dollars also have had limited, if any, benefits in clinical medicine. I am an optimist. I believe eventually there will be general acceptance of the three central ideas of this book outlined above. I am also confident that in the future, substantial public funding will be allocated to research how dysoxygenosis affects the human microecologic cellular and macroecologic tissue-organ ecosystems. Then we will see *real*

progress in   disease prevention and healthful aging. I remain
optimistic.

References

1.   Hebert LI, Scherr PA, Beckett LA, et al. Age-specific incidence of
     Alzheimer's disease in a community population. JAMA 1995;273:1354-9.
2.   Surgery on the skull for chronic fatigue? Doctors are trying it. The Wall
     Street Journal, November 11, 1999. pp, A1 and A8.
3.   Buchwald D, Sullivan JL, Karmaroff A. Frequency of chronic active
     Epstein-Barr virus infection in general medical practice. JAMA
     1987;257:2303.
4.   Sparks PJ, Daniell W. Black DW, et al. Multiple chemical sensitivity
     syndrome: clinical perspective. J Occupational Medicine 1994;36:718-
     737.
5.   Hurley D. Fighting to explain Gulf War syndrome. Healthstate.
     1998;16:27-31.
6.   Taubes G. Misfolding the way to disease. Science 1996;271:1493-5.
7.   Ali M. Oxidative theory of Alzheimer's disease and diabetes. In: RDA:
     Rats, Drugs and Asssumptions, Life Span Press, 1995 Denville, New
     Jersey, pp. 279-81.
8.   Ali M. Spontaneity of Oxidation in Nature and Aging. Monograph.
     Teaneck, New Jersey, 1983.
9.   Ali M. The agony and death of a cell. Syllabus of the Instruction Course
     of the American Academy of Environmental Medicine, Denver, Colorado,
     1985.
10. Ali M. Molecular basis of cell membrane injury. In: Syllabus of the
     Instruction Course of the American Academy of Environmental Medicine.
     Denver, Colorado, 1990.
11. Ali M, Ali O. AA oxidopathy: the core pathogenetic mechanism of
     ischemic heart disease. J Integrative Medicine 1997;1:1-112.
12. Ali M. Oxidative regression to primordial cellular ecology (ORPEC):
     evidence for the hypothesis and its clinical significance. J Integrative
     Medicine 1988;2:4-55.
13. Ali M. Fibromyalgia: an oxidative-dysoxygenative disorder (ODD). J
     Integrative Medicine 1999;3:17-37.
14. Ali M. Darwin, oxidosis, dysoxygenosis, and integration. J Integrative
     Medicine 1999;1:11-16.
15. Schenk D, Barbour R, Dunn W, et al. Immunization with amyloid *b*
     attenuates Alzheimer's disease-like pathology in the PDAPP mouse.
     Nature 1999;400:173-7.
16. Check W. Puzzling out a role for Alzheimer's tests. CAP Today
     1998;12:1.
17. Yankner BA. A century of cognitive decline. Nature 2000;404:125.

Chapter 14
Guidelines to Aging Healthfully

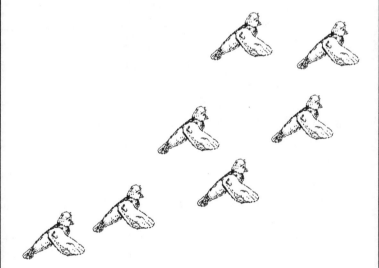

In this chapter, I include my guidelines for healthful aging that include meditation and spiritual awareness; proper hydration and optimal food choices in the kitchen; nutrient supplementation; herbs for restoring the bowel, blood, and liver ecosystems; and detox procedures, such as liver flush, EDTA chelation, short-term vegetable juice fasting, and others. My guidelines are based on the following:

1. My studies of elderly persons who are aging healthfully.
2. My experience with long-term effects of autoregulation, meditation, and spiritual awareness on health (both personal as well as that related to me by my patients who agreed to do serious work with me in those areas).
3. My evaluation of the clinical benefits of limbic (non-competitive, non-goal-oriented) exercise.
4. My advice to healthy persons concerning the use of foods, nutrient supplementation, herbs, and other substances which normalize or optimize oxygen metabolism.
5. My prescriptions of foods, nutrient and herbal therapies, and other oxygenative therapies for my patients to restore damaged bowel, blood, and liver ecosystems.
6. My review of the relevant and *valid* literature concerning the physiological and pathological aging processes.
7. My observations, experimental as well as clinical, of oxidosis and dysoxygenosis in health and disease.

I have tried to stay away from what I consider are misleading or fraudulent claims of the merchants of the "anti-aging" industry. Specifically, I have dismissed:

1. Studies done by feeding this or that nutrient to mice or medical students for weeks or months, which are then cited to support absurd claims of lifespan benefits.

2.   Recommendations of nutrient or herbal recipes with claims of longevity advantages stated by some obscure tribal healers.

3.   Use of the so-called anti-aging hormones or prehormones.

The deceptions of the hormone promoters, in my view, are of the worst kind. Hormones are pieces that play many a changing role in the web of life. If we change one hormone in one way, we change *all* hormones in some way. Hormone chemistry is far too complex to allow prudent practitioners to assign lifespan advantages to a given hormone or prehormone. One must consider integrity of the cell receptors for a given hormone, functions of response elements, workings of genes, and the variability in their products. In short, no single hormone must ever be used to extend lifespan.

The anti-aging movement has rapidly grown into a robust industry. Earlier I indicated that the term anti-aging is a poor choice. It is intellectually dishonest, since no one has ever "anti-aged" or "un-aged." Notwithstanding its commercial success, its claims are misleading or brazenly deceptive. The gurus of the industry do not conduct any studies of their own. Rather, their expertise is in distorting data of other people's studies to promote their favorite products.

TWO AILMENTS

Sometimes I think there are really only two basic ailments that afflict humankind; the first begins above the head and the second in the bowel ecosystem. The ailment taking shape above the head involves issues of the spiritual void, confused demands for love, and anger. The one beginning in the bowel stems from disharmony among elements outside the body and those within the bowel ecosystem. Both ailments create symptoms through dysfunctional oxygen metabolism. Accidents of birth (genetic defects) and of life (injuries) are exceptions to the ailments. However, how well a person copes with consequences of accidents also depends on whether or not oxygen can be preserved. This simplified view of human afflictions is not only of theoretical interest from the standpoint of causation of human suffering, but also of central importance for healthful aging.

THREE CORE MOLECULAR ISSUES

Three *core* issues in *all* considerations of health and healthful aging are: (1) oxidosis; (2) dysoxygenosis; and (3) the man-microbe disharmony. The nature and importance of that trio should be clear from the preceding chapters. I support my dysoxygenosis theory of aging with a large number of clinical and experimental observations.

As a hospital pathologist, I examined over 100,000 biopsies and other pathology specimens. As a laboratory director, I directed a facility that performed over one hundred million tests over a period of 25 years and headed an active team of researchers. As an integrative clinician, I studied with high-resolution microscopy and chemically analyzed the blood samples of nearly 6,000 patients with nutritional, ecologic, metabolic, immune, and malignant disorders. During that period of clinical research I continued my experimental work to shed light on my clinical observations. Above all, I stayed focused on the state between health and disease—what I have called a state of absence of health in my past writing.[1,2] Based on those observations, I concluded that *the trio of oxidosis, acidosis, and dysoxygenosis mostly begins with spiritual issues and with damage to the bowel, blood, and liver ecosystems.* However, the trio can also be triggered by any of the stressors listed below.

1. Unresolved anger.
2. Confused demands of love.
3. Spiritual void.
4. Lack of physical fitness.
5. Sleep difficulties.
6. Chronic dehydration.
7. Poor choices in the kitchen.
8. Constipation and slow bowel transit time.
9. Rapid sugar-insulin-adrenaline shifts, and metabolic roller coasters.
10. Food allergies and incompatibilities.
11. Mold (yeast) allergy.
12. Environmental (chemical) sensitivity.
13. Functional nutritional deficiencies.
14. Hormonal dysregulations.
15. Toxic metal overload.
16. Cumulative synthetic chemical overload.
17. The battered bowel ecosystem.
18. The polluted blood ecosystem.
19. The overburdened liver ecosystem.

The central issue in this discussion is the *cumulative total body burden* of all oxidants. In essence:

We age healthfully or unhealthfully depending on whether or not the body's self-cleansing mechanisms can cope with the *total* body burden of metabolic and environmental toxins that lead to oxidosis, acidosis, and dysoxygenosis.

In the following pages, I include brief comments about each of the above elements. For readers interested in additional information about those subjects, I also suggest some chapters from the companion volumes of this series.

1. UNRESOLVED ANGER

My patients have taught me two lessons about anger. First, angry persons do not heal well. Second, the answer to the problem of anger is spirituality, not psychology.

Psychologists and psychiatrists recognize anger as the root of many disorders. That has also been my observation. They think the solution to the problem of anger is in verbal unleashing of the hidden rage. They prescribe therapies for empowerment and control. I have not seen those approaches work well in the long run.

ANGER IS OXIDIZING

Neither the chemistry nor the energetics of anger have been worked out. Yet, based on my work with many angry patients, I believe anger is a powerful oxidizer. And I am certain future research will clearly establish that. On a basic level, acute anger causes muscles to tighten up, and that produces local excess of free radicals, lactic acid, and other toxic organic acids (such as pyruvic, glyceric, and 2-hydroxybutyric acids). Chronic anger is worse and causes chronically tightened muscles, producing chronic oxidosis and acidosis, both of which lead to local as well as systemic oxidosis and dysfunctional oxygen metabolism.

The discomfort and pain of acute and chronic conditions characterized by muscle spasms are caused by hypersensitivity of nerve fibers due to *local* oxidosis, acidosis, and dysoxygenosis. I have put local in italics because this matter is rarely appreciated by most doctors. More than one pulmonologist has criticized my use of nasal oxygen to treat severe pain of fibromyalgia. Their reason for rejecting my therapy was that their blood oxygen studies showed what they consider a normal level of blood oxygenation. The fact that my oxygen therapy had clearly helped those patients was dismissed by them as a placebo effect. I return to this essential issue in the chapter, "Oxy Therapies for Healing." However, some enlightened physicians have recognized the central role of lack of oxygen in the causation of pain in acute and chronic backache, neck pain, and other related syndromes. One such physician is John E. Sarno, M.D., who has authored two highly acclaimed books, *Mind Over Back Pain* and *Healing Back Pain.* I consider those books must-reads for anyone with painful muscle disorders of the back.

Anger is a child of the thinking mind—the cortical monkey, in autoregulation language. That monkey cannot be banished with mere words. Indeed, he thrives on clever schemes and convoluted theories. The mind forever recycles past misery and, when that is not enough, precycles feared future misery.

Healing is not an intellectual function. No clever mind can order healing in injured tissues. The cortical monkey decorates doubt. It embellishes fear. Clever thinking is of little value in coaxing rebellious tissues to behave. The pain of muscle spasm in the back or neck is not relieved by mere talking. Nor does the deep anguish of depression abate with so-called positive thinking. What is needed is *true* spiritual surrender. I return to that subject later in this chapter.

2. CONFUSED DEMANDS OF LOVE

My patients have also taught me another important lesson: *Love, like water, flows only one way.* It may be offered, but cannot be demanded.

Sending love sustains one,
demanding love depletes one.

Of course, demands for love also demean one. I once saw an athletic young man who was paralyzed by an accident. Some months later his blood tested positive for HIV infection. Some more months later he developed chronic fatigue syndrome. He was wheeled in by his girlfriend. His parents followed. I was struck by how serene he seemed. Maybe the next visit will reveal something else, I told myself. But he showed no signs of anger during the next visit and the one that followed. Then I probed him about stress in life.

"What stresses you most?," I asked.
"Do you really want to know?," he asked with a grin.
"Yes."
"My parents."
"Your parents?," I asked, incredulous, recalling how anguished his parents had looked.
"Yes, my parents. We live upstairs," he replied, glancing at his girlfriend, then added, "My parents live downstairs. There is no end to their demands on me. I can't move out. If I could, I would have moved out long ago." He finished with a sadness that he couldn't hide anymore.

Facilitating the healing process in others by offering love is a powerfully healing influence for the sufferer himself. The ancients recognized that and counseled the sick to try to find ways to serve others. In my native Urdu language, the word for that is *saadhaqa (saa-dhaa-kaa)*. To my knowledge, all religions and all earlier cultures emphasize that. Even the sacrificial rituals of the ancients, in my view, were in recognition of the same phenomena. (Though, it seems to me, that the *spirits* they thought were mad and needed to be appeased by their sacrifices were really not mad.)

In the companion volume, *What Do Lions Know About Stress?*, I suggest several ways to reach out and serve others, including helping an elderly person in ordinary chores, befriending a sick child, or being kind to an animal. This path to healing is especially needed by those who have been chronically sick. To paraphrase John Ruskin,

The true reward for one's service to others is not what one receives for it, but what one becomes by it.

The core aspect of this path to resolving anger for healthful aging is the matter of simply being present with the sick or the needy. Telling a severely depressed person to cheer up is a cruel joke. The same holds for common utterly frivolous platitudes used by people when speaking with the sick or grieved.

A true gift of service is the gift of presence, and the essence of that presence is listening to what goes unspoken.

Another practical aspect of compassion through silence is that it is usually difficult for the visitor to divine what troubles those who are suffering and who need comforting most. What such persons need most is to be with someone. Of course, when that person is ready to say anything, she knows she is free to speak up. Thus, the easiest thing for the visitor is to simply *be*.

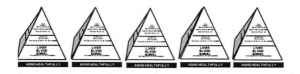

3. SPIRITUAL VOID

The third important lesson taught me by my patients is this: Spirituality is a language without words. As long as one continues to struggle to define what spirituality is, one is out of it. That is the fundamental limit of humankind.

The wisdom of the ancient notion of mind-body-spirit trio is this: Whatever can be sensed with physical senses or perceived by the mind cannot be spiritual. For the spiritual to be discrete from the body and the mind, it must be beyond the reach of either. One cannot reach the spiritual either by seeing, smelling or hearing clearly—nor by superior thinking. Indeed, if that were true, there would be no need for the trio; the mind-body duo would have sufficed. How does one go about searching for the spiritual? One doesn't!

The spiritual has something to do with surrendering in silence to the larger *Presence* that permeates each of us. Why is silence essential? Because sights, smells and other sensory perceptions are aspects of the physical body—and language is the mind's turf. None of that constitutes the core of the spiritual. Clever thinking, after all, is just that: thinking. And thinking, by definition, is not spiritual. A thinking mind cannot *know* the spiritual.

In *What Do Lions Know About Stress?* I suggest some simple ways for escaping the tyranny of the thinking mind—the relentless clutter of the cortical monkey. What that monkey cannot cope with is the silent energy of the spiritual. Specifically, I make two suggestions that I have found to be clinically useful: meditation with the silence of a candle flame in winter, and with the silence of stone during summer. In essence, we can only hope that through a candle flame or a stone we will enter that domain and experience some of our essential link with the larger Presence. These two simple approaches are usually far more rewarding—and revealing—than any elaborate ritual created by shrewd schemes.

GRATITUDE, NOT HAPPINESS

Happiness is an illusion. That is one reason why no two people ever agree on what constitutes happiness. No matter which way one chooses to define happiness, it is an empty notion—now you have it, now you don't.

Few things make people more unhappy than the search for happiness.

The best reason for practicing gratitude I know is that it makes getting out of the bed in the morning less demanding. For others, it makes the morning hours a profoundly spiritual time.

Gratitude, of course, cannot be gained with clever rituals or by traveling to exotic places either. It can be practiced anywhere, at any time. It requires neither any outside support nor any special inner capacity. I have seen patients who lived with profound gratitude even when they suffered progressive paralysis of body muscles by disorders such as multiple sclerosis and Lou Gehrig's disease (amyotrophic lateral sclerosis). I know of many young people who are incarcerated in their homes with incapacitating fibromyalgia, chronic fatigue state, and other chronic disorders. And yet, they are grateful for simply being alive.

I know many chronically ill patients and angry persons for whom the word gratitude is a cruel joke. Then there are those who live in rage but do not quite understand why they are consumed by it. Both groups need a lot of work with the wordless language of spiritual awareness. Those who persist *always* succeed. Then they learn what is known to *all* who choose that path.

Gratitude is a river that flows endlessly, neither revealing its true origin nor its destiny.

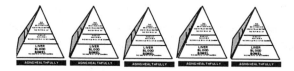

4. LACK OF PHYSICAL FITNESS

Limbic exercise is my term for slow, sustained, noncompetitive and non-goal-oriented exercise. Such exercise done every morning, in my view, is essential for healthful aging. The core philosophy of such exercise is to integrate physical activity with a deep spiritual awareness.

> How does an African tribal messenger run on his wilderness trail? What state of energy is he in? How does an American executive run on his sidewalk? What does his cluttered head demand from his tired and hurt tissues? How do hurt tissues rebel? Can physical exercise provide a deeply personal, treasured retreat from the relentless chatter of the thinking mind?

I wrote those words in the companion volume *The Ghoraa and Limbic Exercise.* Below, I include some more text from that volume.

> Roosters flutter their wings to announce their morning. Canaries flap their feathers before they fly off their nests. Dogs stretch before they take their first steps. So do cats. We humans wake up to our coffee and begin to recycle the misery of our yesterdays and map out the feared future suffering of our tomorrows.

Is limbic exercise right for everyone? Extensive clinical experience has convinced me that it is not only possible, it is essential for long-term good health. A physically more demanding plan of evening workout is also desirable when feasible. Of course, athletic persons must include a structured, vigorous exercise program suitable for their particular sport.

This volume has become much larger than I envisioned it originally. A satisfactory account of my recommendations for limbic exercise is outside the scope of this book. For interested readers, I suggest *The Ghoraa and Limbic Exercise.* Or the reader may obtain a copy of my video entitled, "Limbic Exercise." Limbic exercise is:

> **...a state of body awareness in which the right stroke or the right movement happens by itself, effortlessly, without any interference of the conscious will....The game plays the game; the poem writes the poem; we can't tell the dancer from the dance....the doer has wholeheartedly vanished into the deed....It happens when we trust the intelligence of the universe in the same way that an athlete or a dancer trusts the superior intelligence of the body.**

> Lao Tzu in Tao Te Ching
> Translated by Steven Mitchell

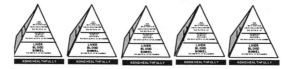

5. SLEEP DIFFICULTIES

As is the day, so is the night. That, in simple words, is the *full* story of sleep disorders.

I know the above statements will draw some chuckles from

sleep specialists, who will consider them amusingly simple-minded. I have good reasons to support my view.

There is an ever-growing list of sleep disorders in the United States today. Consider the following quote from *Science News*:

Much controversy surrounds the definition of sleep disorders....Many sleep specialists criticize DSM (*Diagnostic and Statistical Manual of Mental Disorders*) for ignoring physical ailments linked to sleep problems, and some prefer an alternative classification that lists nearly 70 sleep disorders.

Nearly 70 sleep disorders! But how relevant is such a classification to those who do not sleep restfully?

Kirto is my ancestral village in Pakistan. During my boyhood there, people slept soundly, on the bare cots under an open sky, on the ground under the trees, and in the fields. I don't remember anyone complaining about chronic sleep problems then. No one there ever took sleeping pills. There were no sleep specialists there. There were no sleep disorders there. No one ever complained of morning fatigue. No one was ever tired, except after hard manual labor. Darkness after sunset brought them all the sleeping aids they ever needed. The light of the eastern sky provided all the pick-me-uppers. It was a different time. I wonder how things might be there now. The villagers now have TV, and they probably stay up late watching American reruns. TV probably has also taught them a hundred ways to stay awake when they finally reach their beds. They now probably suffer from sleep difficulties. They probably *do* know about sleep disorders. Many of them probably have self-diagnosed various sleep disorders. Our sleep specialists probably will face no difficulties diagnosing and categorizing many different types of sleep disorders according to the numbers spewed by the sleep machines of Star Wars medical technology.

How common is sleep difficulty in the United States? Consider the following quote from *The New England Journal of Medicine* (328:1230; 1993):

> **The estimated prevalence of sleep-disordered breathing, defined as an apnea-hypopnea score of 5 or higher, was 9 percent for women and 24 percent for men....Undiagnosed sleep-disordered breathing is associated with daytime hypersomnolence.**

Twenty-four percent of young men! The authors of the article studied a random sample of 602 young corporate employees. The important question here is: Why does one of every four young men in corporate America not sleep well? Or, to be more blunt, what is it that corporate America does to its young men to create such frequency of sleep disorders? On a larger scale, what keeps people everywhere restless during sleep? Why is sleep not deep and sound for so many people? Why do so many people wake up tired and stale?

When one sleeps, one is not dead. The state of sleep must be accepted as a continuation of the conscious state. How do adverse food reactions interrupt sleep? How do bowel problems interfere with sound sleep? What are the effects of muscle and joint pain on the depth of sleep? How does chronic anger change the quality of sleep? How do lifestyle and work stressors influence the sleep patterns? Those are the important questions. I rarely see sleep specialists make any *real* efforts to address those issues. Consider another quote from the *Journal* article cited above:

Evaluation by current standards includes full-night polysomnography, at a cost per procedure of approximately $1,100. Sleep-disordered breathing can usually be eliminated by the nightly use of a nasal device that delivers continuous positive pressure to the upper airway. Since patients must continue to receive this therapy throughout their lives, it is often viewed as a hardship.

The authors did not address any of the real issues concerning the causes of poor sleep I raise above. What they seem to advocate is that the use of sleep machines should not be viewed as a hardship. How can anyone sleep with his face covered with a mask and not find that a nuisance? Or, have a tube stuck up his nose for several hours and not consider that a hardship?

There is a growing tendency among sleep specialists to attribute various patterns of ill health to sleep disorders, including chronic fatigue syndrome, fibromyalgia, anxiety states, panic attacks, restless leg syndrome, and related disorders. Next, they prescribe sleep machines. *I strongly disagree with that.* The sleep "disorders" in such patients are caused by the same mechanisms that cause their other symptoms. As a matter of fact, my colleagues and I have managed nearly 5,000 persons with chronic fatigue syndrome and/or fibromyalgia—successfully, in most cases—with natural restorative therapies.[3,4] When their damaged bowel, blood, and liver ecosystems are restored, they get better and their sleep disorders disappear. Most of such patients do need specific measures to restore sleep—such as meditation, music therapies, melatonin, St. John's wort, SAMe, tryptophan, and sleeping pills—until their general health is restored. Indeed, in most such patients the natural therapies listed above are necessary for long periods of time.

In certain cases of advanced sleep apnea—such as those associated with severe obesity, extreme cases of restless leg syndrome, and intense anxiety—the temporary use of a sleep machine may become necessary. But that does not in any way support the position of sleep specialists that the sleep disorders are the cause of their other ailments.

I have been blessed with deep sleep. On rare occasions when I have experienced sleep difficulties, I found the answer in what happened during the day. Recently, I developed a prolapsed lumbar disc that interfered with sleep, necessitating the use of a Halcion (a sleeping pill) for four days. That followed another period of six days when I could not fall asleep without the continued use of the Halcion. I lay awake until 4 am every night until I took a double dose of Halcion. I spent long hours thinking about the *process* of falling asleep. I had never wondered why the moment of passing into the sleep state is called falling asleep. "How do we *fall* into that state?," I could not stop wondering. "If only I could *know* that, I could *make* myself fall into it," I told myself repeatedly during those interminable hours. "Throw myself into that pit, so to speak, and put myself out of that misery," What also irked me greatly was that during that period I felt well enough to carry my usual heavy schedule at the Institute without pain. Then I made the decision to change something in my day to get back to my normal nights. "Isn't sleep the continuation of wakefulness?" I asked myself. "After all, one is not dead when one is asleep," I responded to my own question. I did extra limbic breathing (a method of meditation[5]) during the evening and reduced my reading and writing work during the late evening hours. That night I had much less difficulty in *falling into* sleep, though I still needed melatonin, the natural compound made by the pineal gland that makes us fall asleep. The next night, I slept soundly without any sleeping aid. I began to fall asleep without wondering what the mystery of such falling process might be, just as I had for years. I have good reason to disagree with sleep specialists.

The practical suggestion here is to search for the answer to the puzzle of poor sleep in the events of the day. Except in extreme cases, one need not worry about the precise *diagnosis* of one's sleep disorder and rush to a sleep disorder center. Meditation, limbic breathing, music therapy, and natural remedies—such as melatonin—are usually adequate. In chronic illness associated with chronic sleep deprivation, use of other remedies—such as melatonin, St. John's wort, tryptophan, SAMe, kava kava, valerian, and sleep medication under supervision of a physician—become necessary.

I also advise my patients to try different combinations of the natural sleep-promoting remedies listed above until they can find two effective combinations, and not always depend on just one remedy. Furthermore, I suggest that they initially begin with smaller doses—melatonin, 1.5 mg; St. John's wort, 150 mg; tryptophan, 500 mg; SAME, 200 mg; kava kava, 75 mg; and valerian, 150 mg. After establishing the safety of small doses, they can increase the dose by two- or three-fold. Of course, I strongly recommend that persons with chronic illness stay under professional supervision. In extreme conditions, short-term use of sleep machines may not be avoidable.

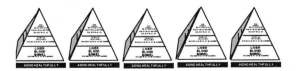

6. CHRONIC DEHYDRATION

Next to spiritual silence, my first and best prescription for oxidosis is water. The same is true for acidosis. Next to spiritual silence, my first and best prescription for dysoxygenosis is also water.

Chronic dehydration is a pervasive problem in the United States. Physicians generally diagnose dehydration by testing for dryness of tongue and skin. That, of course, works only in advanced stages of dehydration in ill persons and is wholly inadequate for determining whether or not a person is optimally hydrated. That statement can be easily validated by doing the following test:

An experienced clinician first helps the person to achieve optimal hydration for two weeks. That person is then asked to describe his overall sense of well-being. The next step in the test is to ask that person to limit his water intake to the pretest level for two weeks and again describe the general state of well-being or lack of it.

I have conducted the above test many times. The chronically dehydrated person can almost always see the benefits of optimal hydration with the above simple test.

I prescribe water *therapy* for every patient for many reasons. I discuss water therapy and the state of hydration during almost *every* visit with each patient. The most basic reason for water therapy is the dilution effect of drinking additional water. It simply carries the excess oxidizing substances as well as toxic acids into the urine.

Water is equally important to the integrity of all three major ecosystems of the body. In the bowel, water is the *single* most important laxative. In the blood, water is the single most important *functional* antioxidant. Without water none of the antioxidant enzyme systems of the blood can function well. The same is true for the liver ecosystem.

One of the fundamental differences between the cells in the body of a seven-year-old and a 70-year-old is that the cells in the older person are dehydrated, dried out, and shrunken. *All* cells need to be optimally hydrated to carry out their functions. None of the cell membrane channels, receptors, enzymes, and organelles can function well without optimal hydration. For example, neurotransmitters in the brain literally are like buds that do not bloom well without water.

My patients living stressful lives frequently complain that they need to drink large quantities of fluids to take their prescribed nutrients and herbs. I tell them that is good news. Nutrient protocols force them to increase their water intake. So much the better! The simplest and most effective practical measure for reducing excessive acidotic and oxidative stress on biology in acute and chronic disorders—including cancer, heart disease, respiratory disorders, fibromyalgia, chronic fatigue syndrome, and other disorders is to dilute the toxins and eliminate them with increased fluid intake. Parenthetically, one of the fundamental changes of the general aging process is cellular aging. Aged cells are shrunken and dehydrated. Chronic fatigue is clearly a state of accelerated molecular and cellular aging. A state of overhydration is not only desirable, but necessary.

One-third of kidney diseases in the United States are considered to be iatrogenic — caused by prescription drugs. Three major culprits are nonsteroidal anti-inflammatory painkillers, antibiotics such as aminoglycosides, and contrast media used for X-ray and scan studies. The simplest safeguard against such kidney damage when taking drugs is optimal hydration.

A LESSON FROM AN ALOE LEAF

Next to spiritual silence, water is the *best* antioxidant. That probably will surprise most, if not all, readers. I myself did not understand the profound significance of that statement until recently. I was peeling an aloe vera leaf for preparing fresh pulp for personal use. Looking at the spines of the leaf, my mind drifted to the intensely hot and dry summer days of my boyhood in Lahore, Pakistan. I recalled the blazing sun baking everything on the roadside. Most plants died, and the few that survived were browned out and withered. The aloe plants were different. They stood defiant. When a leaf was cut by a passerby, the pulp looked like freshly made Jell-O. At that time oxygen was not a part of my world, which was populated by clay toys I had molded myself and dreams of one day owning my own bicycle.

A blazing sun burns everything that is green by oxidation. Water prevents that. That is why one sees green oases around water springs in deserts. And that is why we water our lawns in summer months more often. But why didn't the oxidizing fires of the scorching sun also burn the roadside aloe plants of my boyhood? There was no extra water for them there. Those aloe plants shared the same soil and survived, while the powerful oxidizing sunlight destroyed all other plants in their vicinity. That must be accepted as a proof that this plant contains something magical.

More than fifty years later, looking at the fresh opalescent aloe pulp, I suddenly saw the miracle of the aloe leaf and recognized why this plant made the list of top ten medicinal plants of herbologists wherever it grew. A patient recently showed me the picture of the national symbol of Aruba, which includes aloe as the symbol of health in its first quadrant. A large number of recent research studies have documented the various clinical benefits of this plant.

"What is an optimal state of hydration?," many patients ask me. Depending on the size of the patient, I recommend from three to five quarts of water a day. I advise them that organic vegetable juices and prescribed herbal teas may be considered part of that volume of water. Coffee, cocoa, caffeinated sodas, and black tea and alcohol are not to be included. In reality, under many circumstances such beverages are dehydrating.

I drink fifty to fifty-five ounces of water with nutrient supplements in the morning. This amount of fluid includes my breakfast, in which I put one and one-half heaping tablespoons of soy or rice protein powder in eight ounces of organic vegetable juice and then add another eight ounces of water to it. Such fluid intake assures me a state of overhydration and obviates any need for coffee or tea. A few trips to the bathroom are a small price to pay for the overall benefits of such a state of overhydration during the morning hours. How can I take so much fluid on an empty stomach?, some readers may ask. I take the stated quantity of water in portions of eight to ten ounces during twenty to thirty minutes of my limbic exercise. Readers may wish to add a piece of fruit to their protein drink for additional support or add small amounts of fruit juices to change the taste of the protein drink.

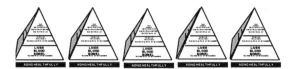

7. POOR CHOICES IN THE KITCHEN

In the preface, I expressed my doubts about the wisdom of the gurus of the dieting industry, as well as of other high-fat/low-carb and low-fat/high-carb diet experts. The nearly equal life expectancies in Japan (with low-fat diet) and Switzerland (with high-fat diet) clearly demonstrate the fallacies of those experts. In their passion, they ignore both sound empiricism and good science. I recognize that acute and chronic illnesses require that prudent clinicians must take into account the specific needs of the individual patient. For example, persons with battered bowel ecosystems do not tolerate sugars and starches well. Those foods further feed the PLF populations in their bowel ecosystems and fan the fires of oxidative coagulopathy in their blood ecosystem and oxidative lymphopathy in their lymphatic ecosystem. Those changes markedly increase the detox burden in the liver ecosytem and lead to progressive oxidosis and dysoxygenosis. Thus, specific dietary measures taken to reverse various disease processes cannot be blindly recommended as optimal choices for healthful aging.

Good health is neither the denial of dieting nor the euphoria of eating.

I wrote the above words in *The Butterfly and Life Span Nutrition.* I recommend that volume for an in-depth discussion of the relevant issues of choices in the kitchen for aging healthfully.

Good nutrition for healthful aging is common sense and the making of food choices that have stood the test of time. Modern science, in my view, helps us *understand* the mechanisms underlying the empirical observations of hundreds of generations that have gone before us. No studies conducted in mice or medical students for weeks or months must be allowed to negate the empirical experience of astute observers of the past centuries.

Martyrdom in the kitchen does not work. I cannot overstate the case for a sound philosophy of nutrition. One cannot eat well for a full life span except through a deep visceral-intuitive sense about how various foods affect his general level of energy and well-being. This cannot come from cortical obsessions about studying food charts and calorie tables. It requires a *learn-experiment-observe-learn* approach for adopting a *food philosophy.*

Specific plans for choices in the kitchen may be selected for addressing specific disorders, or even for different patterns of absence of health. For example, patients with damaged bowel ecology generally do better with food plans that comprise high-protein, high-fat (with emphasis on unoxidized fat) and low-carb food choices. Such plans prevent sugar roller coasters and insulin dysmetabolism. For those reasons, that diet plan is usually also effective for *short-term* programs for weight loss. I emphasize short-term here because, in my view, a high-fat, high-protein, no-starch diet probably carries more risk for more diseases than any other commonly used diet plan. Thus, from the standpoint of healthful aging, I do not recommend *long-term* use of high-fat, high-protein, no-carb diets.

Below, I include some text from *The Butterfly and Life Span Nutrition* to provide some general guidelines to the readers.

1. Seek steady-state energy metabolism.
   - Avoid starving-gorging-starving cycles.
   - Avoid sugar-insulin-adrenaline roller coasters.
2. Maintain an optimal state of hydration.
   - Drink 50 to 70 ounces of high-compatibility fluids every day.
   - Drink fluids even when you are not thirsty.
3. Know your food reactivities.
   - Avoid foods that cause allergic reactions.
   - Avoid foods that deplete energy.
   - Avoid foods that cause abnormal bowel responses.
4. Focus on what you can eat.
   - De-focus foods that should be avoided.
   - Try new foods, observe their effects.
   - Think high-compatibility foods when food shopping.
5. Never miss breakfast.
   - Body tissues need to be energized in the morning.
   - Missing breakfast is fasting for 15 to 18 hours and sets us up for nutritional roller coasters.
   - Missing breakfast increases the need for undesirable stimulants such as coffee and tea.
6. Get the most out of vegetables.
   - Develop a taste for uncooked vegetables. (Taste is changeable.)
   - Develop a taste for steamed or stir-fried vegetables.
   - Reduce acidotic stress on metabolism. (Vegetables are alkaline-ash foods.)
7. Cut back on fruits.
   - Avoid allergenic fruits such as oranges.
   - Avoid very sweet fruits.
   - Avoid overripe fruits.
8. Increase proteins in food choices.

●Proteins are time-release energy sources.

●Proteins are building blocks for tissues and for energy and detoxification enzymes.

●Minimize meat intake; increase lentils and beans.

9. Favor alkaline-ash foods.

●Favor vegetables. (All biologic stressors increase acidotic stress. SAD [standard American diet] increases the body acid burden significantly.)

10. Minimize acid-ash foods.

●Reduce intake of all meats.

●Grains are, in general, acid-ash foods, but are needed to balance the alkalinity of vegetables and fruits.

11. Understand food cravings.

●Food craving is the same thing as food addiction.

●Reduce salt intake.

●Reduce sugar intake.

●Eliminate or reduce intake of artificial sweeteners. (Salt, sugar and sweeteners increase sugar cravings.)

12. Have free access to healthful snacks.

●The ideal snacks: uncooked or steamed vegetables.

●Eat low-fructose fruits—those that are not very sweet.

●Soynuts, pumpkin, sunflower and other seeds are also recommended.

●Avoid walnuts and other tree nuts. (Tree nuts are among the most allergenic foods.)

13. Rotate foods.

●High-compatibility foods may be eaten on three or less days a week.

●Low-compatibility foods should not be eaten more often than once a week.

14. Ensure a healthy gut ecosystem.

●Seed the bowel with healthful lactic acid-producing

microbes.
- Feed the lactic acid producers with nutrients such as pantothenic acid, vitamin B_{12}, fructose oligosaccharides and others.
- Weed out the toxin-producing microbes such as yeasts, bacteria and parasites.

15. Eat limbically.
- Follow visceral-intuitive impulses in making food choices. That, of course, is usually very difficult for those in the throes of sugar-insulin-adrenaline roller coasters. However, patience and persistence with these guidelines pays.
- Dieting plans are cortical traps.

(Reading food labels becomes unnecessary after some time.)

16. Do not omit nutrient supplements.
- Take morning supplements with breakfast.
- Take evening supplements with dinner.
- Split daily supplements into three, four or more portions if problems of tolerance exist.
- Pollutants in the air can only be neutralized by nutrients.
- Contaminants in food can only be neutralized by nutrients.
- Toxins in water can only be neutralized by nutrients.

17. Don't be a skunk in someone's garden party.
- It is not necessary.
- It is not desirable.
- Enzyme detoxification systems can cope with an occasional lapse—but only occasionally.

18. Bring some spiritual dimensions to your day.
- From extensive clinical work, I know that is the *single most* important matter in developing a long-term *livable* food philosophy. To reiterate what I wrote earlier, martyrdom doesn't work in nutrition. Good nutrition is neither the denial of dieting nor the euphoria of eating.

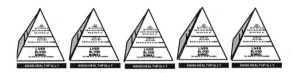

8. CONSTIPATION AND SLOW BOWEL TRANSIT TIME

In the chapter, "What Is Health?," I consider two to three effortless, odorless bowel movements every day an important criterion for health. Under physiological conditions, many changes occur throughout the gastrointestinal tract—including the mouth and the esophagus—that increase bowel motility and lead to evacuation. Thus, it is common for people in tribal cultures to have a bowel movement almost after every meal. Of course, there are no real lifestyle-related impediments to bowel evacuation in their lives. Many teachers consider that frequency of elimination simply impractical. Their teaching schedules make it difficult for them to respond immediately to their bowel signals with such frequency. I advise them to find two hours when they have free access to restrooms and overhydrate themselves in the beginning of that period.

I try not to complete an office visit with any of my patients without ensuring that their bowel habit is regular and effective, or without taking some measures to achieve that. Of course, many of my patients report chronic constipation for years—some, in their words, all their lives. Years of neglect make the bowel very sluggish. Several of them were told, sometimes by their doctors, that it is normal for some people to have a bowel movement once every two or three days. Such statements amaze me. I wonder if engineers ever make similar statements about the exhaust systems of their machines.

In the chapters, "The Pyramid" and "Oxygen and Primordial Life Forms," I present evidence for regarding the bowel as a dynamic, diverse, and delicate ecosystem. Dehydration and constipation are among two of the most important threats to the integrity of the bowel system. The bowel must not simply be seen as a dark, gurgling tube. It teems with life that can either preserve health or put it in jeopardy.

Most of the recommendations in the sections for optimal hydration and healthful choices in the kitchen restore bowel motility and prevent constipation. Uncooked vegetables are especially beneficial. Such measures are usually enough to relieve constipation and restore normal bowel motility in persons with occasional episodes of constipation. In general, certain vegetables—such as turnips, daikon, squashes, burdock, red radish, and green leafy vegetables—are very beneficial for preserving bowel health. Many people experience specific effects on the bowel transit time with specific uncooked vegetables and fruits. To learn about such food-bowel relationships, one needs to be aware of his bowel health and then observe. As I write this, I recall one patient who reported excellent bowel results with peaches and poor results, including staining of stools with blood, with mangoes.

What is food to one, is to others bitter poison.
Lucretius.

The above primarily food-based approach may not be enough for persons with chronic and persistent constipation. Such individuals often have additional problems of adverse food reactions and unsuspected mold allergy that further diminish bowel motility. They require an integrated approach incorporating therapies including: (1) ample doses of magnesium, potassium, and taurine supplementation (doses used at the Institute are included later in this chapter); (2) natural substances, such as turkey rhubarb, triphala, cascara, and senna; (3) healthful microbes, such as *L. acidophilus* and *Bifidobacterium bifidus*; (4) judicious use of water, coffee, or sodium phosphate enemas; and (5) bowel detox protocols, such as colonic irrigations in selected cases. I make additional recommendations for restoring bowel ecology in the section dealing with that subject.

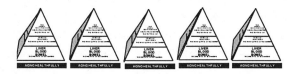

9. RAPID SUGAR-INSULIN-ADRENALINE SHIFTS AND OTHER METABOLIC ROLLER COASTERS

Many people live lives in metabolic roller coasters without ever realizing the cause. Some live with sugar-insulin-adrenaline roller coasters, while others suffer adrenaline-cholinergic roller coasters. Many women live with PMS, wild mood swings and hot flushes caused by estrogen-progesterone-adrenaline roller coasters. Yet others are tormented by neurotransmitter roller coasters. In my clinical work, I consider elimination of such roller coasters as one of my primary goals.

Dysregulation of blood glucose level is a widespread problem in the United States. Below, I reproduce some text from *The Butterfly and Life Span Nutrition* to show how sugar roller coasters are produced.

An eight-year-old child has a blood sugar level of 100 mg/dl (or 1,000 mg in one liter of blood). Since he has a total circulating blood volume of about 5 liters, the total quantity of glucose in his circulating blood is 5,000 mg or 5 grams. A teaspoonful of sugar holds 4 grams of sugar. Now this boy drinks a can of soda that contains 8 to 10 teaspoonfuls of sugar. This means that by drinking a can of soda, that child pours six to eight times as much sugar into his blood as exists at any time. Such a massive overload of sugar throws him into a sugar roller coaster, followed by an insulin roller coaster, which in turn triggers an adrenaline roller coaster. Similar molecular roller coasters are caused when he drinks a 12-ounce glass of commercial orange juice. How is the sugar molecular roller coaster initiated? With sugar overload. How is the sugar molecular roller coaster perpetuated? By withdrawal symptoms. "Highs" in the blood sugar levels are followed by the "lows" that create biologic demands for yet more sugar. Sugar craving is another name for sugar addiction. An American child at the turn of the century consumed between 5 and 10 pounds of sugar per year. His counterpart today ingests 150-175 pounds. How many thousands of molecular roller coasters does that come to? The numbers add up. This is the essence of the hypoglycemia problem. How does our sugar industry respond to all this? They keep physicians on their payroll to publish absurd studies showing that our children are not hurt by sugar. This is the simple truth behind the hypoglycemia controversy.

In *What Do Lions Know About Stress?* I devote a large chapter to a discussion of sugar and insulin roller coasters. The best way to preserve the integrity of carbohydrate metabolism is to protect it from large and sudden sugar overloads. For this purpose, I strongly recommend breakfast comprised of suitable protein drinks containing eighty or higher percent calories in proteins and amino acids.

I protect the carbohydrate metabolism of my patients during afternoon and evening hours with prescriptions for supplemental cold-pressed essential oils to be taken cold. Specifically, I recommend that they take one to three tablespoons of one of the recommended oils an hour or so before dinner. The oil may be taken with steamed (and cooled) vegetables, salads, goat or sheep cheese, a small amount of grapefruit juice, or be simply taken as oil. My list of recommended oils includes extra virgin olive oil, flaxseed oil, sesame oil, avocado oil, grapeseed oil, pumpkin oil, safflower oil, almond oil and canola oil.

Ample but judicious prescriptions for vitamin and mineral supplements are needed for controlling metabolic roller coasters. I give my recommendations for this purpose later in this chapter.

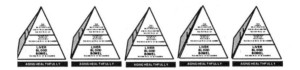

10. FOOD ALLERGIES AND INCOMPATIBILITIES

Food reactions are widely misunderstood. There are three important issues in understanding food allergy and sensitivity reactions: (1) allergy-causing genes; (2) frequency of consuming the food in question; and (3) the temperature of the *oxidative plate* of the body.[6,7] In my clinical work, I find the last element to be most significant.

I introduced the concept of the oxidative plate in *The Canary and Chronic Fatigue* to emphasize the impact of the oxidative-dysoxygenative state in the body. I used the analogy of the hot plate in a popcorn machine. When the plate is cool, the corn put on it does not pop. When it is heated partially, some kernels will pop while others will not. When the plate is fully heated, nearly all kernels pop. I see the same phenomenon in my patients with fibromyalgia, chronic fatigue syndrome, and many chronic immune disorders. This phenomenon is sometimes called *spreading phenomenon.*

In general, the sicker the person, the more frequent and troublesome the food reactions in food-sensitive individuals.

I see the reverse of that phenomenon when the general health of such patients improves with restorative oxygenative therapies. Their food reactions become fewer and less intense. When some of such patients relapse due to infections or chemical exposures, their food reactions become more frequent and intense. For advanced and professional readers, I have discussed this oxidative-dysoxygenative (OD) perspective of allergy elsewhere.[7]

A source of confusion about food allergy and sensitivity reactions arises from failure to differentiate between *fixed* food allergy and *variable* food sensitivity reactions. The former is caused by a specific type of antibody called IgE antibodies and triggered by ingestion of a food against which such antibodies exist in the body. This type of reaction is fixed in the sense that every exposure to that food provokes a reaction. Such fixed food allergy can be reliably diagnosed by appropriate diagnostic skin test or micro-ELISA blood tests. The variable food reactions are more dependent on the state of the oxidative plate, i.e., the level of OD stress.

> **The practical advice for the readers here is to learn to be *sensitive* to what is eaten and how that affects the state of their health. That may be possible by following the guidelines for eating and the tables giving lifespan and aging-oxidant food choices in the Appendix. For persons with chronic illnesses in which food reactions constitute significant clinical problems, it becomes necessary to work with a clinician experienced with food allergy and sensitivities.**

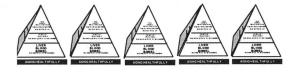

11. MOLD (YEAST) ALLERGY

From the material presented in the chapters entitled, "Oxygen and Primordial Life Forms" and "Oxygen Settles the Great Pasteur-Bechamp Debate," it will be evident to the reader that I think the "mold issue" is one of the most significant in my guidelines for healthful aging.

The mold issue—including the so-called yeast problem—has four faces: (1) IgE-mediated mold allergy; (2) overgrowth of PLFs in the bowel and blood; (3) mold toxins (mycotoxins); and (4) mold (yeast) infections.[8,9]

Mold allergy and toxicity are among the most important causes of chronic illness. It is noteworthy that in true desert communities, serious chronic immune disorders such as multiple sclerosis, rheumatoid arthritis, lupus, scleroderma and vasculitis are virtually unknown. In my view, this is largely due to the fact that molds require closed, humid and dark places to flourish and such places are rare in deserts. Reduction of exposure to molds—also called yeasts—is of central importance in successful management of inhalant allergy. Pollens are in the air for limited periods of time; mold spores are in the air throughout the year in most instances. It is not possible to eliminate mold exposure altogether. I reproduce here some text from my monograph, "Allergy: Diagnosis and management," to provide some guidelines for reducing exposure to molds[10]:

1. Humidity levels at home should be kept low—in summer below 35% if possible with the air conditioner or dehumidifier. Minimize the use of humidifiers in the winter.
2. Exhaust fans should be used in the bathroom and above the stove when cooking.
3. Visible mildew and other molds in the home should be removed with nontoxic solutions. A solution of two tablespoons of baking soda in one cup of vinegar and one pint of water may be used to remove visible deposits of mold. An alternative cleansing solution is to use equal parts of household bleach and water for this purpose.
4. Heavy leather items should not be kept in the bedroom.
5. The number of mold-breeding indoor plants should be kept low. Molds grow well in indoor planters.

6. Some long-term measures include substituting paints for wallpaper. Heavy drapes should be avoided, and heavy garments and sleeping bags should not be piled on the floor of closets.
7. Prolonged periods of time in dark and humid (moldy) areas should be avoided, such as basements, attics, barns, and areas with decomposing grass and compost.
8. Discretion should be used during extended hiking in woods or working on lawns in the height of pollen season if you suffer from pollen allergy. (Pollen exposure will increase mold sensitivity in this setting.)
9. Discretion should be exercised in visiting antique shops, old book shops and other such areas where molds flourish.

Foods that may trigger allergic reactions in mold-sensitive persons are: fermented foods (especially beer and wine), vinegar and salad dressings, aged cheeses, malt and foods containing malt, dried fruits, mushrooms, peanuts and peanut butter, and pickles and pickled foods. Another issue is that of mycotoxins—toxins produced by molds. In general, the longer the time yeasts have to grow in foods, the greater the risk of toxicity with mold toxins. Thus yeast in baked bread does not have the same risk as yeast in fermented foods.

The practical advice for the readers here is to learn to be *aware* of relevant mold exposures and how such exposures affect their state of health. For persons with chronic illnesses in which mold allergy reactions constitute significant clinical problems, it becomes necessary to work with a clinician experienced with mold allergy and sensitivities.

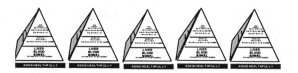

12. ENVIRONMENTAL (CHEMICAL) SENSITIVITY

Chemical sensitivity is dose independent, while chemical toxicity is dose related. The failure to appreciate this critical difference between chemical sensitivity and chemical toxicity leads confusion among many doctors as well as patients.

During the last twenty-five years, there have been great advances in understanding allergic reactions. And yet, *certain basic questions about such reactions remain unanswered.* For example, skin allergy conditions, such as eczema lesions, flare more in some weeks than in others in the same person. Lifestyle stressors cause more wheezing on some days than on others in the same asthma sufferer. Abdominal cramps, bloating, and diarrhea in Crohn's colitis and ulcerative colitis ease off or intensify for no apparent reason in most persons with those conditions. Food sensitivity reactions vary over a broad range in the same individual. Nasal and sinus congestion become more intense on some days when pollen count is low and abate on days when pollen counts are high. This spreading phenomenon is increasingly recognized in chronic fatigue syndrome, fibromyalgia, and multiple chemical sensitivity syndrome. The molecular cause of none of the above can be understood on the basis of the classical knowledge of allergy. Those considerations led me to look beyond the matter of allergy caused by IgE antibodies and put forth an oxidative-dysoxygenative disorder as the molecular model for fibromyalgia.[11] It should be evident from the preceding chapters that *all* mediator responses of allergy would be greatly amplified by oxidative coagulopathy and its cellular consequences. *The clinical symptoms of allergy in conditions of increased oxidative-dysoxygenative stress must be seen as the visible tip of a much larger iceberg of foundational changes in the trio of the bowel, blood, and liver ecosystems.*

CHEMICAL SENSITIVITY SYNDROME

During the past few decades, a wide gulf developed between the views of university-based allergy researchers and clinical ecologists (physicians who focused on *clinically verifiable* patterns of hypersensitivity reactions that can be explained neither on the basis of IgE antibodies nor with any of the other recognized immunologic sensitivity mechanisms). The pioneers of clinical ecology included Theodore Randolph,[12] William Rea,[13] Francis Waickman,[14] and others. The core concepts of clinical ecology included the following: (1) total load, (2) sensitization; (3) maladaptation; and (4) deadaptation. In the author's own opinion, the classical view of atopy simply could not explain a broad spectrum of clinical manifestations of hypersensitivity responses. The academicians continued to focus on effects of injection therapy with single allergens, such as cat dander or ragweed. The ecologists, while recognizing the theoretical value of such work, found such observations of very limited value to the care of the ill, who invariably suffered multiple sensitivities. After decades of doubt and denial,[15,16] the existence of multiple chemical sensitivity syndrome was finally acknowledged and its relevance to the management of classical allergy understood.[17]

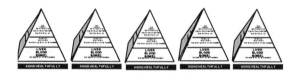

13. FUNCTIONAL NUTRITIONAL DEFICIENCIES

Nutritional status is impoverished in many Americans. My colleagues and I perform laboratory assessments of the body reserves of essential vitamins, minerals, and other natural redox-active nutrients in all patients with chronic disorders. It is uncommon for us to find persons who show levels of such nutrients within a healthy range. For example, a 24-hour urine mineral analysis which we conduct routinely on all patients nearly always reveals deficiencies of essential minerals as well as excesses of toxic metals. This is also true in most patients who consult us for disorders that are commonly *not* considered to be associated with nutrient deficiencies, including coronary artery disease, stroke, Alzheimer's disease, arthritis, vasculitis, and others.

A SINGLE ROBBER GOES DOWN WITH SIX COPS

Our nutrition is in jeopardy for many reasons. The prevalent use of highly processed foods, sugar overload, and regular exposure to preservatives and pesticide residues in food items creates many *functional* nutritional deficiencies. I often use the following analogy to explain why functional nutritional deficiencies are so common today. Suppose the people in a town are deeply troubled by a high rate of robberies in their houses and the frequent escape of robbers from the town prison. In their frustration, they establish a strict rule that whenever a cop catches a robber, the cop will also stay in the prison cell handcuffed to the robber. That may seem irrational, but that is exactly how the cops-and-robbers game is played in the human body. Robbers are the synthetic chemical poisons and toxic metabolic waste substances. Cops are the nutrients. The toxic molecules (robbers) are literally trapped by the nutrient molecules (cops) and both stay bound to each other.

Then I extend the analogy. The town people learn of a big tragedy. They are shocked to find out that the robbers again escaped the prison, but took along the cops handcuffed to them. A fight broke out among the cops and robbers and they shot and killed each other. Something very close to that happens in human detox pathways. Sometimes as many as six molecules of glutathione (an especially good detox cop) are bound to some pesticide (a particularly nasty robber) and are wasted by the kidney. *Six cops wasted for every robber gotten rid off!*

This nutrient-toxin relationship is not fully appreciated by many doctors who question the value of nutrient supplementation in integrative medicine. Such doctors often ask for proof that functional nutritional deficiencies indeed do exist. My colleagues and I see the proof of that every working day when patients report recovery from fibromyalgia and disabling fatigue after such therapies. Furthermore, on many occasions when our patients discontinue their nutrient supplementation, their symptoms recur. We also document the biochemical evidence of their value by appropriate laboratory tests.

In the table below, I furnish some general information about vitamins, minerals, and other redox-restorative substances which my colleagues and I prescribe for our patients.

Table 1. General Guidelines for Nutrient Supplementation for Healthful Aging for Persons With and Without Chronic Disorders

	Healthy Subjects	Persons With Chronic Illness
Vitamins	Vitamins: C, 1,000 to 2,000 mg; . E, 200 to 400 IU; A, 5,000 to 7,500 IU; D, 100 to 250 IU; B-complex, 25-50 mg; B12, 1,000 mcg weekly for four weeks.	Vitamins: C, 3,000 to 5,000 mg; E, 400 to 800 IU; A, 10,000 to 15,000 IU; D, 100 to 250 IU; B-complex, 30-50 mg; B12, 1,000 to 5,000 mcg weekly for four to six weeks .
Minerals	Magnesium, 1,000 to 1,500 mg; Calcium, 1,000 to 1,500 mg; Potassium, 200 to 400 mg; Chromium, 50-100 mcg; Selenium, 50-100 mcg; Molybdenum, 50-100 mcg.	Magnesium, 1,500 to 2,500 mg; Calcium, 1,000 to 1,500 mg; Potassium, 400 to 600 mg; Chromium, 200-400 mcg; Selenium, 200-400 mcg; Molybdenum, 200-400 mcg.
Redox-Restorative Substances	Glutathione, 200-300 mg; N-acetylcysteine, 200-300 mg; MSM (Methylsulfonylmethane) 200-500 mg; Lipoic acid, 100 to 200 mg; Taurine, 500 to 1,000 mg; Coenzyme Q10, 30 to 50 mg; Pycnogenol, 50 to 100 mg.	Glutathione, 600-800 mg; N-acetylcysteine, 600-800 mg; MSM, 500 to 1,500 mg; Lipoic acid, 100 to 500 mg; Taurine, 500 to 1,500 mg; Coenzyme Q10, 100-150 mg; Pycnogenol, 100 to 150 mg.

Seven G's For the older person with chronic illness

In my view, the following seven items stand out in their healthful benefits for older persons with chronic disease and require special focus under professional supervision.

1. Ginger   2. Garlic   3. Ginseng   4. Glutathione
5. Geranium   6. Ginkgo   7. Growth Hormone

14. HORMONAL DYSREGULATIONS

From the standpoint of oxygen and aging, the following are the important issues:

1. Hormones are molecular messengers.
2. Hormones play many and *varying* roles in the web of life.
3. When one hormone system is changed in one way, something is changed in every other hormone system. Hormones turn into each other according to the prevailing cellular ecologic conditions.
4. Hormones are essential to *every* cellular function, and not just the limited roles that are assigned to them in medical texts.
5. Disruptions of the base trio of the bowel, blood, and liver ecosystems are at the root of problems such as premenstrual syndrome (PMS), endometriosis, and menstrual irregularities (including loss of menstruation in young women with fibromyalgia, chronic fatigue syndrome, and chemical sensitivity syndrome).
6. The epidemics of breast and prostate cancers (two of the most common malignant tumors) are directly linked to the avalanche of synthetic hormones that children and adults are exposed to in their daily lives.
7. *All* hormone systems are essential for healthful aging; however, no single hormone or prehormone can be used for extending the lifespan.

In *RDA: Rats, Drugs and Assumptions*, I addressed the above subjects at length. I suggest that volume to the general as well as specialist readers.

Some readers are likely to raise their eyebrows on my assertion that menstrual disorders are related to battered bowel, blood, and liver ecosystems. My colleagues at the Institute and I published the evidence for that view in a clinical outcome study of young women with fibromyalgia and CFS who also reported oligomenorrhea (fewer or scanty periods) and amenorrhea (complete loss of menstruation). Their menstrual functions were completely or nearly completely restored by our integrative plans with focus on restorative and oxygenative therapies that *primarily* addressed issues of those ecosystems.[18]

Others might be surprised by my statement that epidemics of breast and prostate cancers are due to exposure to synthetic hormones. I state my case simply. Consider the incidence of those two cancers in different regions of the globe during the last century. You will note that widespread use of synthetic hormones and xenoestrogens (pesticides and related chemicals with estrogen-like effects) in all countries was followed by rising incidences of those two cancers. Both cancers were distinctly uncommon among the Japanese prior to World War II, and became increasingly common during the post-war decades as the population was increasingly exposed to synthetic hormones and pesticides. China today makes for an illuminating study of that phenomenon. In the wealthy big cities of eastern China (Beijing, Shanghai, Nanjing, and others), the incidence of both cancers is rising. In the rural and poor populations of western China, those cancers are still uncommon.

For preserving or restoring hormonal equilibrium for healthful aging, my colleagues and I focus heavily on all relevant issues of the bowel, blood, and liver ecosystems. Next, based on appropriate laboratory test results, we offer an integrated program employing natural substances that support hormone ecosystems, such as licorice, wild yam, dong quai, black and blue cohosh, false unicorn root, fennel and sarsaparilla. In persons with chronic illness, we also offer a "layered" approach that includes such substances as DHEA, pregnenolone, androstenedione, and others. In many cases of chronic illness, blood and urine tests often reveal significant abnormalities and it becomes necessary to prescribe hormones derived from soybean and other natural sources.

The practical advice for the reader here is to learn the importance of *all* hormone systems for healthful aging of *all* cellular and tissue-organ ecosystems of the body, and not merely for improving sexual function or controlling menopausal symptoms. I strongly recommend that readers resist the temptation of taking any hormone or prehormone for preserving health without the direct and *ongoing supervision* of an experienced clinician.

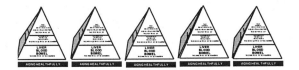

15. TOXIC METAL OVERLOAD

A California dentist consulted me for severe rheumatoid arthritis and debilitating fatigue, which forced her to stop work several months before I saw her. She had been a vigorous person who worked 50 to 60 hours a week and then had energy to live an active social life. She had no prior symptoms of joint or muscle pain. A doctor had performed a urine mercury test following a test dose of DMPS (a potent mercury chelator). The next day she did not feel well. Within a few days, she developed progressive generalized joint stiffness and pain and increasing fatigue. Within weeks she was totally disabled. Since that case, I have seen other similar examples of serious illness caused by acute mercury toxicity resulting from rapid mercury chelation with DMPS.

A young woman with multiple sclerosis suffered from progressive muscle stiffness and pain, numbness in limbs, urinary difficulties, and increasing fatigue. She responded well to our integrative program and within several months was completely symptom free. A urine mineral profile performed after an intravenous dose of 1.5 grams of EDTA (a very weak mercury chelator) revealed raised levels of mercury and some other toxic metals. She wanted to have mercury fillings in her teeth replaced with composite ones. I agreed with her, since she had been stable and free of any signs of the disease for several months. With additional nutrient support, we cautiously began the process and scheduled one removal session every two months. *After each such session she missed her next menstrual cycle.* Several months following the last session, at the age of 29, she conceived her first child.

Heavy metal overload and toxicity are widely misunderstood areas. Except for integrative physicians and clinical ecologists, doctors rarely, if ever, order tests for 24-hour urine or blood levels of toxic metals, such as mercury, lead, aluminum, cadmium, and arsenic. Hence, the problem, when it exists, remains undiagnosed and ignored. Pediatricians who diligently look for lead overload in children often find clear evidence for that. Integrative physicians who routinely order mineral analysis for their patients fully recognize how widespread heavy metal toxicity is in Americans.

The clinical pictures of acute heavy metal toxicities are well characterized and generally described at length in medical textbooks. What is rarely, if ever, addressed in those texts is the critical issue of *cumulative* toxic metal burden in persons compromised with chronic nutritional, immune and ecologic disorders. Of course, that further feeds the fires of dissent in this important area.

In the context of oxygen and aging, it is noteworthy that many toxic metals inflict heavy damage on antioxidant enzyme systems of the body. For example, mercury rips apart the sulfhydryl bonds in such redox-essential substances as glutathione.

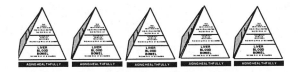

16. CUMULATIVE SYNTHETIC CHEMICAL OVERLOAD

Three things come to my mind as I begin this section. First, during summer months, we occasionally lost air conditioning in our hospital laboratory for several hours. At such times, the test results obtained with some equipment showed mild elevations in the enzyme activities in the blood samples of some patients. In the chemistry section, some staff members also experienced irritability, headaches, and related problems.

Second, one of my associate pathologists examined biopsies and surgical specimens sent to the laboratory in Formalin (formaldehyde) on Tuesdays and Fridays. Sometimes emergencies and conference and vacation schedules forced her to do such work on two consecutive days. She often developed a headache on the evening of the second day.

Third, formaldehyde is a very strong irritant, a common cause of chemical sensitivity, and a carcinogen in animals. The law required that we monitor exposure of our staff in the histology section (where they worked with formaldehyde all the time). So they carried formaldehyde sensors during work hours. We were all very sensitive to the issue and used multiple specially exhausted air filter systems there. While establishing the monitoring mechanism, on an impulse I asked the laboratory manager to get one control person in our personnel department to also wear the formaldehyde monitor for a comparative study of exposures. He smiled and accepted my challenge, humoring my eccentricity, I'm sure. He came to my office some weeks later, laughing and holding the survey reports. The results showed that the person in the personnel department had a greater exposure to formaldehyde than *any* of the laboratory staff! We realized that the air in the personnel department without special air filters actually contained more fomaldehyde than in the laboratory.

THREE ISSUES OF CHEMICAL OVERLOAD

There are three core issues in the matter of synthetic chemicals and healthful aging: (1) *cumulative* body burden of synthetic chemicals; (2) *cumulative* toxicity of chemicals; and (3) *cumulative* cellular functional and structural damage caused by chemicals.

Cumulative Burden of Synthetic Chemicals

As for cumulative chemical burden, it is estimated that Americans are exposed to nearly 65,000 synthetic chemicals in their daily lives. The liver, as indicated in the chapter entitled, "The Pyramid," is the first-line-of-defense organ for most such chemicals. Even though the liver has enormous functional reserves, it cannot eliminate or detoxify *all* such substances, so their accumulation begins. Many synthetic chemicals are fat soluble and have a greater affinity for brain tissue than many other tissues. Having gained entry into the brain, such chemicals are not in any hurry to leave. Indeed, they *accumulate* there for years. Those facts explain why chemical detox plans give delayed results.

Cumulative Toxicity of Synthetic Chemicals

My father, a judge, used to say that one and one in a court of law do not make two. Sometimes we get 11. That, it seems to me, happens more often to synthetic chemicals in the body than in the courts of law. Many chemicals not only add to the toxicity of other chemicals, they also *amplify* each other's toxic effects. Of special relevance to the present discussion are the oxidative-dysoxygenative *chain* reactions that are triggered by synthetic chemicals and involve fats, proteins, sugars, enzymes, cell receptors, and DNA in the body. Again, I emphasize the *cumulative* aspect of the above processes.

Cumulative Cellular Damage Caused by Chemicals

There is a wide gulf on this subject among academics and clinical ecologists. The academics rarely, if ever, assess the *functional* consequences of chemicals on the human body. Their studies are largely limited to effects of exposures of small animals to large doses of chemicals—they use terms like minimum lethal dose to characterize the toxicity of the chemical. Such an approach is *fundamentally* irrelevant to the subject of functional and structural cellular changes caused by chemicals.

Blood and urine tests for measuring chemical overload are routinely performed by many clinical ecologists. However, the state of the art seriously limits their efforts. Evidence for such toxicity is amply clear to clinicians who undertake slow and steady detox programs for their patients with ecologic and immune disorders.

I believe the *cumulative* threat posed by chemicals to human health is a very serious issue which is rarely, if ever, addressed by the main physician body in the United States.

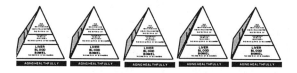

17. THE BATTERED BOWEL ECOSYSTEM

The bowel ecosystem *is* the foundation of the pyramid of human ecosystems. Readers by now should be familiar with the experimental and clinical evidence I present in this volume to support that view. It should not come as a surprise that I consider measures taken to preserve the integrity of the bowel ecosystem in health and its restoration in disease as *fundamental* to the goal of aging healthfully. Below, I adapt some text from my monograph, *Altered States of Bowel Ecology,* first published in 1987.[19]

The Seed, Feed, and Occasionally Weed Approach

An integrated *seed, feed, and occasionally weed* approach is the centerpiece of *all* my attempts for preserving the bowel ecology for healthful aging, as well as for restoring bowel ecosystems battered by antibiotic abuse and sugar overload.

Seeding is the repopulation of the bowel ecosystem with microbes that normally preserve it. I call such microbes guardian angels of human health. It is necessary because our bowel ecology is under unrelenting assault by antibiotics fed to our poultry and cattle, as well as those prescribed by doctors. Another important factor is sugar overload. Both factors lead to overgrowth of oxygen-hating, acid-loving primordial life forms (PLFs) in the bowel that literally crowd out the healthful microbes.

Feeding is the use of growth factors required by the healthful bowel microbes, such as *Bifidobacterium bifida* and *Lactobacilus acidophilus*. Those growth factors include vitamin B_{12}, pantothenic acid, biotin, and others. I do not think it is coincidental that both vitamin B_{12} and pantothenic acid are essential for the health of humans as well as their guardian-angel microbes.

Occasional weeding is accomplished by the use of several natural substances that suppress the overgrowth of PLFs, as well as viruses and disease-causing bacteria. The best known—and the most widely used worldwide—is plain yogurt. However, that may not be enough to prevent damage to the bowel ecology caused by antibiotics.

**Table 2. Therapies for Restoring
the Battered Bowel Ecosystem***

For Healthy Persons:
Water therapies
Organic vegetable juices
Bowel-friendly vegetables
Optimal choices in the kitchen
Freshly fileted aloe
Ginger/garlic
Magnesium, potassium, and taurine
Psyllium husk and apple pectin
For persons with history of bowel disorders:
Vitamin B_{12}
Pantothenic acid and pantotheine
Fennel seeds, fenugreek, licorice, and pau d' Arco
Echinacea, astragalus, goldenseal, and burdock root
Grape seed extract
Oral hydrogen peroxide
Coffee, water, and probiotic enemas
Hydrogen peroxide baths
Colon hydrotherapy
Diagnosis and management of food sensitivities and mold allergy

Table 3. Composition of Adjunctive Nutrient and Herbal Protocols for the Bowel
Bowel Ecology Protocol #1
One billion spores of *Lactobacillus acidophilus, Lactobacillus bulgaricus, Bifidobacterium* in a base of complex vegetable fiber, magnesium sulfate, vitamin B complex, l-histidine, l-arginine, pantethine, aloe vera.
Bowel Ecology Protocol #2
Alfalfa, 500 mg; pau d'Arco, 100 mg; allium, 100 mg; licorice root extract, 200 mg.
Bowel Ecology Protocol #3
Calcium caprylate, 50 mg; magnesium caprylate, 50 mg; grapefruit seed extract, 25 mg; aloe vera, 1 mg; spirulina, 10 mg.
Bowel Ecology Protocol #4
Grapefruit seed extract, 50 mg; allium, 50 mg; pau d'Arco, 500 mg.
Bowel Ecology Protocol #5
Par-quing, 150 mg; pau d'Arco 150 mg; beet root fiber, 200 mg; guar gum, 100 mg.
Bowel Ecology Protocol #6
Echinacea, 200 mg; goldenseal root, 150 mg; astragalus root, 150 mg; burdock root, 150 mg.

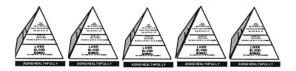

18. THE POLLUTED BLOOD ECOSYSTEM

From the chapters, "The Pyramid" and "Oxygen: The Great Communicator," it will be obvious to the reader why I consider the bloodstream as an ecosystem sandwiched between the other two great ecosystems of the body: the bowel and liver ecosystems. Next to the bowel, oxygenative therapies that address *all* issues of the blood ecology are the most effective treatments for acute and subacute disorders. Such therapies also rank high among my priorities for healthful aging. Furthermore, it will be obvious to the reader by now that, in my view, a drop of blood smeared on a slide provides us the *best windows to the world of human biology*, including the matters of healthful aging and disease.

Table 4. Therapies for Restoring the Polluted Blood Ecosystem
Nasal oxygen Oral hydrogen peroxide Hydrogen peroxide bath Intravenous hydrogen peroxide infusion Intravenous ozone infusion Intravenous EDTA infusion Intravenous nutrient infusions Intramuscular infusion Mercury and other toxic metal chelation

As is the case with nutrient therapies, doctors unfamiliar with the therapies listed in the above table frequently make derisive comments about treatment methods. For those who wish to directly assess the efficacy of such therapies, I suggest simple examination of blood smears of the patient before and after such therapies are administered. They will quickly recognize what my colleagues and I see every working day.

A drop of blood smeared on a slide and seen with a high-resolution microscope provides the *best windows* to the state of oxidation and oxygenation of the person.

The blood smears are much *cleaner* after such therapies. See the chapter entitled, "Oxygen: The Great Communicator," for detailed description of the observed changes.

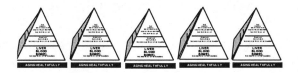

19. THE OVERBURDENED LIVER ECOSYSTEM

Next to the bowel, the liver is the most important guardian angel of oxygen metabolism. I support that view with several lines of evidence and my personal observations in the chapter entitled, "The Pyramid." Thus, I believe the liver, next to the bowel, must be the focus for all oxygenative and antioxidant therapies for reversing dysoxygenosis and preserving health. For emphasis, I again point out that all therapies that primarily address issues of the bowel and blood ecosystems also restore the liver ecosystem and health.

In Table 5, I list therapies that my colleagues and I prescribe for restoring the damaged liver ecosystem.

Table 5. Therapies for Restoring the Overburdened Liver Ecosystem
Therapies that normalize cellular oxygen metabolism by focusing on restoration of the bowel, blood, and liver ecosystems include the following: 1. Liver-protective foods, such as ginger, garlic, onions, black radish, turmeric, beets, turnips, burdock, dandelion, and others   2. Liver-friendly nutrients, such as inositol, choline, lecithin, methionine, glutathione, N-acetylcysteine, MSM, lipoic acid, and others   3. Liver-friendly herbs, such as aloe, milk thistle, catnip, goldenseal, red clover, fennel seeds, Jerusalem artichoke, and others   4. Liver and gall bladder flush   5. Liver castor oil packs   6. Kidney flush   7. All measures taken to prevent chemical overload on the liver   as well as all therapies designed to reduce total chemical overload

I refer the advanced and professional readers to *Integrative Medicine: The Principles and Practice* for detailed descriptions and discussion of the above therapies and procedures.

In Table 6, I include two protocols composed of liver-friendly nutrients and herbs that my colleagues and I prescribe for our patients with chronic disorders characterized by liver congestion and enlargement with or without elevated blood activities of enzymes (which indicate the presence of liver injury). We also employ those protocols for all patients with various types of viral hepatitis.

Table 6. Composition of Liver Protocols Composed of Liver-Friendly Nutrients and Herbs

Liver Ecology Protocol #1
Dandelion root, 100 mg; beet root fiber 50 mg; black radish 50 mg; goldenseal 50 mg; catnip 50 mg; methionine 400 mg; choline bitartrate 200 mg; inositol 20 mg.

Liver Ecology Protocol #2
Turmeric, 100 mg; milk thistle, 100 mg; red clover, 100 mg; ginger root, 100 mg; goldenseal, 100 mg; Jerusalem artichoke, 100 mg; fennel seed, 100 mg.

LIVER CASTOR OIL PACK AND LIVER FLUSH PROTOCOL

Two natural therapies that have stood the test of time for liver detoxification are liver castor oil pack and liver flush protocols. As for other specific therapies I include in this volume, I recommend that both liver pack and flush should be undertaken under professional supervision first. I myself prescribe castor oil liver packs to facilitate liver detox and reduce liver congestion as a part of our basic bowel-blood-liver detox program in most patients with chronic ailments. Both protocols are included in the Appendix of this volume.

The practical advice here is to undertake liver detoxification under the supervision of a clinician experienced in this area.

SUMMARY

In preparing my guidelines for healthful aging, I have been mindful both by the wisdom of the ancients and modern science. It is amazing how closely the latter has validated the former. Indeed, in many ways, my work may be seen as efforts to develop as well as marshal experimental and modern clinical evidence to support the ancient healing philosophies. *Moderation, they counseled, was the best strategy in eating.* That, in essence, is one of the messages of this chapter. *Know thyself,* they also advised. That is another important message. To me, *knowing oneself* means how one can move towards *one's own* spiritual surrender, *one's own* freedom from confused demands of love and anger, *one's own sense* of sancity of his environment, and *one's own sense* of right food choices. The ancients understood—intuitively, it seems to me—that diseases of the body are rooted in the bowel. I came to the same conclusion after the study of over 14,000 bowel and 5,000 stomach biopsies, and after caring for over 5,000 patients with nutritional, ecologic, immunologic, and degenerative disorders.

Earlier I expressed my disillusionment with the gurus of weight-loss industry. The issue is not whether some of those diets can help some people lose weight some of the time—or that weight loss is not desirable for many Americans. The real issue in the context of healthful aging is this: Weight loss that ruins metabolism cannot promote healthful aging.

Two lead articles in a recent issue of *The New England Journal of Medicine* told us that fiber and low fat diets (factors that promote health) do not reduce the incidence of colon polyps. *That is bad science* because it only indicates *bad study design* that fails to take into account the diversity, dynamics, and delicacy of the bowel ecosystem. There is no substitute for learning, trying, observing, and knowing.

References
1.   Ali M. "Absence of Disease Is Not Always Presence of Health." The Cortical Monkey and Healing. 9-11. The Institute of Preventive Medicine Press, Denville, New Jersey, 1990.
2.   Ali M. "Absence of Disease Is Not Always Presence of Health." RDA: Rats, Drugs and Assumptions, 175-197, Life Span Press, Denville, New Jersey, 1995.
3.   Ali M. Hypothesis: Chronic fatigue is a state of accelerated oxidative molecular injury. J Advancement Medicine 1993;6:83-96
4.   Ali M, Juco J, Fayemi O, et al. Efficacy of ecologic-intgrative managment protocols for reversal of fibromyalgia. J Integrative Medicine 1999;3:38-47.
5.   Ali M. The Ghoraa and Limbic Exercise. Life Span Press, Denville, New Jersey, 1993.
6.   Ali M. Oxidative Plate and Oxidative Board. The Canary and Chronic Fatigue, 293-298. Life Span Press, Denville, New Jersey, 1995.
7.   Ali M. Recent advances in integrative allergy. Current Opinion in Otolaryngology. Philadelphia. 2000 (in press).
8.   Ali M. In-Vitro Allergy: Diagnosis and Management. Textbook Otolaryngology and Head Neck Surg, pp 320-346. Elsevier, New York, 1989.
9.   Ali M, Ali A. Oxidative coagulopathy in fibromyalgia and chronic fatigue syndrome. Am J Clin Pathol 1999;112:566-567
10.   Ali M. Oxidative regression to primordial cellular ecology (ORPEC): Evidence for the hypothesis and its clinical significance. J Integrative Medicine 1998;2:4-55.
11   Ali M, Ali O. Fibromyalgia: an oxidative-dysoxygenative disorder (ODD). J Integrative Medicine 1999;3:17-37.

12.   Randolph TG. Human Ecology and Susceptibility to the Chemical
      Environment. Springfield, Illinois, Charles C. Thomas. 1962.
13.   Rea WJ. Chemical Sensitivity: Tools of Diagnosis and Methods of
      Treatment (Volume 4). Lewis Publishing, Dallas, Texas, 1997.
14.   Waickman FJ, Vojdani A. Putting chemical and environmental
      sensitivities in perspective.Otolaryngologic Clinics of North America,
      Vol 31, No. 1, Feb, 1998.
15.   Kahn E, Letz G. Clinical ecology: Environmental medicine or
      unsubstantiated theory? Ann Int Med 1989;111:104-6.
16.   Sparks PJ, Daniell W. Black DW, et al. Multiple chemical sensitivity
      syndrome: a clinical perspective. J Occupational Medicine 1994;36:718-
      737.
17.   Cullen   MR. The worker with multiple chemical sensitivities: an
      overview. State Art Rev Occup Med. 1987; 2:655-661.
18.   Ali M. Amenorrhea, oligomenorrhea, and polymenorrhea in CFS and
      fibromyalgia caused by oxidative menstrual dysfunction (OMD-I). J
      Integrative Medicine 1998:3;101-124
19.   Ali M. Monograph: Altered States of Bowel Ecology and Health
      Preservation. Life Span Inc. Denville, New Jersey, 1987,1993

Chapter 15

Oxy Therapies and Healing

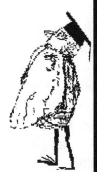

Two case histories given below underscore the main issue I address in this chapter: a pervasive and gross misunderstanding of oxygenative ("oxy") therapies in the general medical profession.

OXYGEN FOR A NEW YORK LAW PROFESSOR

A law professor in New York City was disabled with chronic fatigue syndrome. He showed only moderate improvement after several months. At that time I prescribed nasal oxygen for him in doses of 3 liters per minute for one hour three times a day. Some months later, he felt well enough to return to his teaching work on a part-time basis. One day I asked him which one of the many therapies we included in his treatment helped him the most. "Oxygen," he replied without hesitation. "My brain fog began to lift when you put me on oxygen. Even now I have to use oxygen when I prepare my lectures. Without that I just can't seem to put my material together."

This was one of the many conversations I have had with my patients with chronic fatigue syndrome, fibromyalgia, and other states characterized by ODD (oxidative-dysoxygenative dysfunction). I started evaluating the clinical benefits of intermittent nasal oxygen as a direct oxy therapy for such patients several years ago. It made much theoretical sense and was clearly safe and inexpensive. Positive experience with some early patients led to my work with a much larger number that validated the early impression. Now I generally prescribe nasal oxygen to be administered with a mask or a canula in doses similar to those given to the law professor. "Why don't all doctors treating similar patients prescribe this simple, inexpensive therapy?," some readers may ask. The answer is that no one with a strong commercial interest is promoting it. Thus, it is ignored in our medical schools and postgraduate medical conferences.

NO OXYGEN FOR A TORONTO DESIGNER

One of my Canadian patients, a designer in her forties, consulted me for severe, progressive and debilitating fatigue accompanied by brain fog and abdominal symptoms. One of her passions in the past had been landscape painting north of the Arctic circle that necessitated backpacking all her equipment and food for days on end. After developing the fatigue syndrome, on her worst days she could not "walk from one end of her living room to another." Almost two years later, she felt well enough to go north again for painting. I was inspired by the progress she had made and by her courage to consider such a trip, but was afraid that it would cause a return of her fatigue. So I had vigorously opposed her plans but to no avail. My fears came true and she suffered a severe relapse during the trip. However, the mere fact that she made that trip still amazes me.

Last week, I received an urgent request from her for a telephone visit. All her original symptoms had reappeared a few weeks after she bought a new car. She suspected carbon monoxide exposure, which was later confirmed by her car company.

That problem was not new to me. I outlined an integrated detox program for her bowel, blood, and liver ecosystems that focused on oxygenative therapies, including nasal oxygen, just as I had prescribed for the law professor. "I don't think I can get oxygen in Toronto," she sighed. "The last time you prescribed oxygen for me, the oxygen company would not deliver the tank without a prescription from a Canadian doctor, and my doctor here absolutely refused to write a prescription for that. He insisted that was quackery."

OXYGEN, THE CORE NUTRIENT

In my view, the *single most* important nutrient regularly ignored by doctors, even those practicing integrative medicine, is oxygen. The *most* effective antimicrobial treatments neglected by most doctors are oxy therapies.

In medical school, I was taught that oxygen is useful for patients with failing hearts, bleeding stomachs, lungs filling up with water, and other critically ill patients in intensive and coronary care units. No one ever spoke of oxygen for patients with chronic disorders. Things have not changed in that area during the last four decades. I sometimes wonder how and why did we physicians decide that oxygen was not helpful in *every* illness. Isn't oxygen the *primary nutrient?* Doesn't every injured cell heal with oxygen? Doesn't every cell need more oxygen when injured than when in health? *Oxy therapies that I include in this discussion are safe, efficacious, and inexpensive.* It is unfortunate that such therapies are neither part of the curriculum in most medical schools nor prescribed by the main body of physicians in the United States. I sometimes hear that there is no scientific proof of efficacy of such therapies. That is even more unfortunate, since it indicates the total ignorance of such persons of the *vast* body of literature attesting to the clinical value of oxygenative treatments, including papers published in *The New England Journal of Medicine* and other widely read journals.

Oxygen metabolism is in jeopardy in *all* acute and chronic disorders. Many physicians among the readers may look at that statement as too broad of a generalization to be theoretically valid or clinically useful. I ask them to consider the following:

During nearly thirty years of performing autopsies, I never saw a disease process in which the cells and body organs did not show the microscopic features of oxidosis, acidosis, and dysoxygenosis.

That should not surprise any professional reader. It is well known that lactic acid accumulates in the tissues and in blood rapidly when cellular oxygen metabolism is impaired. Other organic acids that accumulate in tissues and are passed in increased amounts in the urine in cellular dysoxygenosis include pyruvic acid, glyceric acid, and hydroxybutyric acid. So it is that whether a person died of cancer, heart attack, stroke, pneumonia, hepatitis, or AIDS, I *always* observed the OD changes at autopsy.

"But aren't those changes caused by the process of dying?," some readers may ask. "Shouldn't oxidosis and dysoxygenosis in that setting be considered the consequences and not the causes of the death?," some others might ask. The answer is that *all* disease processes that lead to autopsy actually *begin* with oxidosis and dysoxgenosis. Of course, that is also true of disease processes that are arrested before threatening or ending life. In the chapters, "The Spontaneity of Oxidation Theory of Aging" and "The History of Oxygen and Dysfunctional Oxygen Metabolism," I present several lines of evidence to support my view. Controlling those two mechanisms must be accepted as the primary goal in case management.

OXY (OXYGENATIVE) THERAPIES

I define an oxy (oxygenative) therapy as a treatment that, directly or indirectly, achieves one or both of the following objectives:

1.   Increased availability of oxygen to cells;
2.   Normalization of *dysfunctional cellular* oxygen metabolism.

A complete discussion of the clinical indications, procedural details, and efficacy of oxygenative therapies is clearly outside the scope of this book. However, I recognize that most readers at this stage would want some general information on those subjects. I also hope that the brief information included here will spark the interest of physician-readers and encourage them to learn more about oxygenative therapies.

In 1987, I published the details of intravenous and intramuscular therapies I used in my practice in a monograph entitled, "*Intravenous Nutrient Protocols in Molecular Medicine.*"[1] In that monograph, I also discussed issues which I thought would be important to physicians, nurses, and the IV teams interested in administering those therapies in their medical offices or outpatient clinics. In the subsequent editions of that monograph, I included clinical outcome data obtained with my own studies with oxygenative and antioxidant therapies.

During the last several years, my colleagues and I have published the results obtained with several clinical outcome studies conducted at the Institute.[2-6] For the advanced and professional readers, I include abstracts of some of those articles in the Appendix. In 1998, in an article published in *The Journal of Integrative Medicine*[7] and entitled, "Guidelines for intravenous therapies in integrative medicine," my colleagues and I presented a detailed description of technical procedures in use at the Institute. Finally, I devote a large part of my forthcoming book, *Integrative Medicine: The Principles and Practice*, to theoretical and clinical aspects of oxygenative therapies.

CONFUSION ABOUT OXYGENATIVE THERAPIES

In general, there is little, if any, understanding of the antimicrobial efficacy of oxygen among mainstream doctors. Indeed, they often make derogatory (and irresponsible) remarks about the clinical efficacy of oxgenative therapies. However, I see a big change on the horizon. In its January 20, 2000, issue, *The New England Journal of Medicine* reported dramatic reduction in the rate of serious infections with oxygen therapy.[8] Patients who received 80% oxygen with a nasal mask during colon surgery had half as many infections as those who received 30% oxygen for the same period. In an accompanying editorial, the *Journal* recommended the use of oxygen for reducing the frequency of infections in surgical patients.[9] It is noteworthy that there are no known drugs that have shown such a high level of efficacy in preventing serious abdominal infections as oxygen.

The study reported in the *Journal* did not surprise me—and others well versed with antimicrobial potency of oxygen—since it only reported what we have seen in our patients for decades. For emphasis, I ask the reader to recall my discussion of how oxygen arrests microbial growth (PLF overgrowth, as well as that of other types of microbes) in health and how such microbes rapidly multiply in states of dysoxygenosis. I devoted the chapter, "Oxygen Settles the Great Pasteur-Bechamp Debate," to this subject. My basic conclusion is the following:

Specific microbial species invading the body from the outside cause specific infections when oxygen metabolism is normal. However, when the cellular oxygen metabolism is dysfunctional, the primordial life forms from within the body multiply rapidly and become more troublesome sources of "infections." Thus, in chronic illness, oxy therapies are as important as in acute illnesses.

CLINICAL DISORDERS TREATED WITH OXY THERAPIES

In this volume, I present extensive evidence to support my ODD model of illness. Still, I recognize that all new models of illness must be vigorously tested and verified with true-to-life experience. In order to meet that requirement, my colleagues and I tested the validity of that model with extensive clinical outcome studies. We carefully designed such studies to employ integrative management plans that focus on *all* the relevant issues of oxidosis and dysoxygenosis.

Specifically, such outcome studies included patients with advanced coronary heart disease[2], chronic fatigue syndrome,[3] fibromyalgia,[4] young women with loss of menstrual function and other menstrual irregularities,[5] A third group was children with arrested growth following chemotherapy and steroid therapies.[6] The abstracts of those papers are included in the Appendix.

A full discussion of conditions that my colleagues at the Institute and I successfully manage with oxy therapies is outside the scope of this book. From the preceding chapters, the readers have probably suspected that I focus on such therapies for *all* of my patients. That, indeed, is true. For the general interest of the reader, I include in this section lists of acute and chronic disorders that are successfully managed with integrated protocols, including vigorous use of oxygenative therapies. Some brief comments about selected disorders follow.

Table 1. Acute Disorders Treated with Oxygenative Therapies

1. Acute coronary syndromes (including persistent angina and impending heart attacks) 2. Suspected or proven stroke, TIA (transient ischemic attack), and accidental brain injury 3. Acute viral, bacterial, yeast and other infections 4. Rapidly spreading cancers 5. Acute autoimmune disorders, including
     * Progressive multiple sclerosis and lupus
     * Crohn's colitis and ulcerative colitis
     * Rheumatoid, psoriatic, and other immune arthritides
     * Vasculitis with or without brain involvement
 6. Acute oxygen deprivation states (see "Air Travel Dysoxygenosis (ATD))" 7. Acute chemical toxicity syndromes 8. Acute pain syndromes 9. Acute asthma, pneumonia, and other respiratory disorders 10. Acute and widespread skin eruptions 11. Acute kidney failure

The above table does not include a complete list of acute clinical indications for which I prescribe oxy therapies. There are many other acute clinical states for which oxy therapies work well.

Table 2. Chronic Disorders Treated with Oxygenative Therapies
1. Malignant tumors
2. Chronic viral infections, such as hepatitis C and HIV
3. Chronic autoimmune disorders
4. Fibromyalgia and chronic fatigue syndrome
5. Chronic bowel disorders that do not respond to other therapies, such as Crohn's colitis and ulcerative colitis
6. Chronic pain syndromes
7. Multiple chemical sensitivity syndrome
8. Heavy metal toxicity, such as mercury overload
9. Chronic oxidative stresses (chronic oxidative coagulopathy)
10. Insidious cumulative chemical overload
11. Asthma and chronic lung disorders
12. Chronic kidney failure

As in the case of acute disorders, the above table does not include a complete list of chronic clinical indications for which I prescribe oxy therapies. There are many other chronic clinical states for which oxy therapies work well. Indeed, I consider oxy therapies as my top priorities in *all* chronic disorders.

OXY THERAPIES FOR CORONARY HEART DISEASE

Coronary heart disease is caused by oxidative injury. It begins as oxidative injury to blood plasma and cells (collectively designated as oxidative coagulopathy) and ends with dysoxygenosis of heart muscle and nerve cells. As described in the chapter, "Oxygen: The Great Communicator," oxidative coagulopathy results in microclot and microplaque formation in the *circulating* blood.[10,11] *All* known risk factors for coronary heart disease increase the degree of oxidative coagulopathy. Furthermore, all factors that are known to reduce such heart disease decrease the intensity of oxidative coagulopathy. In 1997, we marshaled extensive evidence for our view.[12] Specifically, we argued against the prevailing cholesterol theory of coronary heart disease. (Cholesterol is an antioxidant and cannot cause coronary disease. Rancid cholesterol is an oxidant and does contribute to that disease.)

In recent years, the evidence for the view that coronary artery disease is also caused by microbial species has rapidly accumulated. It is noteworthy in this context that *all* such infections inflict oxidative injury on blood elements and trigger changes of oxidative coagulopathy.

Oxidative coagulopathy not only *fully* explains how coronary heart disease is caused, it also provides a rational and logical approach to reversal of heart disease. In 1998, my colleagues and I published a clinical outcome study of 26 patients with advanced coronary heart disease (five with failed coronary bypass operations, six who had undergone one or more angioplasties, and fifteen who failed to respond to multiple drug therapies).[2] Sixty-one percent had complete relief of symptoms and all drugs were discontinued, while in 17% the relief of symptoms was more than 75%. The results were considered fair in 13% and poor in nine percent. The complete abstract of that paper is included in the Appendix.

OXY THERAPIES FOR ALZHEIMER'S DISEASE, OTHER MEMORY DISORDERS, AND STROKE

The subject of oxy therapies for acute and chronic brain dysfunctions is critically important and is discussed in a previous chapter entitled, "How Long Will We Live? How Many Will Live Demented?" It should be evident from the preceding comments about coronary artery disease that all therapies that improve cerebral circulation—increase oxygen and nutrient supply to the brain— should be of value to persons with acute and chronic memory disorders. That would include degenerative brain disorders—such as Alzheimer's disease and senile dementia—and other disorders that are not considered as brain problems but lead to poor circulation— such as fibromyalgia and chronic fatigue syndrome.

My colleagues and I have substantial positive experience with both direct and indirect oxy therapies. The former type includes nasal oxygen, intravenous hydrogen peroxide, intravenous ozone infusions, and EDTA chelation therapy. Some other therapies include oral hydrogen peroxide drops (3 to 10 drops with a glass of water before meals) and hydrogen peroxide baths. Injected (IM or IV) redox-restorative substances that we find especially helpful include large doses of vitamin B_{12} (up to 30,000 mcg), coenzyme Q10 (up to 200 mg), SAM-e (up to 1,200 mg), glutathione (up to 1,000 mg), MSM (up to 750 mg), and others.

Strokes and TIA (pre-strokes or transient ischemic attack) are also caused by oxidative injury. As is the case with coronary heart disease, those disorders also begin with oxidative coagulopathy. It follows that a rational approach to those disorders must also be directed to arresting oxidative coagulopathy and reversing its adverse effects on the brain tissue. Oxy therapies in the form of intravenous ozone infusions and hyperbaric oxygen for managing strokes and pre-strokes have been extensively used in Europe and, to a lesser extent, in the United States. A large number of reports attest to the clinical benefits of such therapy.

OXY THERAPIES FOR ACUTE AND CHRONIC INFECTIONS

Next to the disorders of the heart and the brain, treatment of acute and chronic infection is where oxy therapies offer the most clinical value and where the benefits of such therapies are most ignored. Such therapies are also very effective for *prevention* of infections in persons who suffer repeated infections due to a weakened immune system. Working six days a week, I generally write fewer than five prescriptions for antibiotics a week. Some weeks I write none. This is all the more noteworthy because many of my patients consult me for chronic immune disorders and recurrent episodes of infection that could not be controlled by multiple antibiotic therapies. Indeed, in my view such use of antibiotics had significantly contributed to their immune dysfunction.

My colleagues and I rely heavily on oxygenative therapies to minimize the use of antibiotics. It is often not fully appreciated that all of us have microbial populations in our bodies, which are kept under surveillance by oxygen in health. I explain this point repeatedly because it is very important. Acute and chronic viral infections, when not rapidly controlled, lead to secondary bacterial infections. The reverse also obtains. Uncontrolled bacterial infections lead to *viral activation syndromes.* Thus, antimicrobial oxy therapies are useful in *all* infections.

> **For acute and chronic viral infections, my colleagues and I have found a hydrogen peroxide drip followed by a vitamin drip to be the *single* most effective therapy. That includes serious viral infections, such as hepatitis B and C viruses, HIV, and certain cases of aggressive herpes and Epstein-Barr viruses.**

REDUCTION OF HEPATITIS C VIRAL LOAD

I include here a brief case history of a patient with hepatitis C and debilitating fatigue to make two important points: (1) oxy therapies significantly decrease the total viral load; and (2) antibiotic therapy, as important as it may be, often further weakens the immune cells in individuals with compromised immune defenses.

A 69-year-old man with hepatitis C presented with a viral count of over five million per milliliter of blood. His liver was enlarged. His other problems included severe fatigue for three years, high blood pressure, enlarged prostate, nasal allergy, constipation, impotence, and low blood immune cell count. His legs showed edema (water retention). With our integrative protocols and 14 intravenous hydrogen peroxide infusions on a weekly or alternate-week basis, he showed slow and steady improvement in symptoms of allergy, fatigue, and constipation over a period of twelve months.

Table 3 shows how his hepatitis C viral count dropped from over 5 million per ml to 489,230 per ml in about seven months of oxy and antioxidant therapies. During that time, his immune cell count rose from 2,900 to 3,600. Two months later, he developed upper abdominal pain and was given antibiotic therapy for *H. pylori* for three weeks by his gastroenterologist. When I saw him two months later, his viral count had climbed back to 1,879,000/ml and his immune cell count had fallen to 3,000.

Had he seen me for his *H. pylori* infection, I probably would not have prescribed antibiotics for him. He had had that infection previously and, in my experience, antibiotic therapy rarely eradicates recurrent *H. pylori* infections. Furthermore, I have had generally good results controlling *H. pylori* infections by herbs, changes in diet, oxy therapies, and bismuth.

The readers should especially take note how changes in the total viral count were associated with the changes in the immune (white blood) cell count. That association has been recognized for decades by physicians, who primarily prescribe drug therapies for chronic viral infections, as well as those who employ integrative therapies including oxy therapies.

Table 3. Hepatitis C Viral Counts During Integrative Oxy Therapies			
Date	**Viral Count***	**Immune Cells****	**Comments**
11/30/1998	over 5 million/ml	2,900	Treatment begun
3/13/1999	898,000/ml	3,100	14 IV hydrogen peroxide on alternate weeks
7/22/1999	489,230/ml	3,600	
11/15/1999	1,879,000/ml	3,000	Antibiotics received in September

*Viral counts performed with RNA PCR technology.
** Immune cell count represents white blood cells.

An interesting facet of the relationship between oxygen and hepatitis C viral count is presented later in the section dealing with air travel dysoxygenosis.

OXY THERAPIES FOR ARRESTED GROWTH IN CHILDREN

The problems of arrested growth in children are attributed either to hormonal dysregulations or malabsorption. My experience with several children with arrested growth has given me a different viewpoint. The first two girls who changed my entire thinking on this subject had been hospitalized for Crohn's colitis for progressive malnourishment and weight loss. One weighed 55 pounds at age 15 and the second 65 pounds at age 16. Both had not grown in height for about a year. Since all standard drug therapies had failed, I reluctantly prescribed intravenous therapies as a last resort. Growth in both girls was restored. I include here brief comments about the efficacy of oxy therapies in two cases, one of them being the 15-year-old girl with colitis. The full abstract of the paper published in *The Journal of Integrative Medicine*[6] appears in the Appendix.

A 15-year-old girl suffered from a severe form of Crohn's colitis. She had been hospitalized on several occasions and treated with steroids. *She weighed 55 pounds and measured 57 inches in height.* During an 18-month program, she gained four-and-one-half inches in height and 26 pounds in weight, and reported the appearance of her first menstrual cycle at age 16 1/2. The second patient, a 13-year-old, stopped growing after receiving chemotherapy for a highly malignant tumor of the jaw. *He weighed 51 pounds and measured 50 inches in height.* During a nine-month program, he gained two-and-one-half inches in height and 11 pounds in weight.

OXY THERAPIES FOR FIBROMYALGIA AND CHRONIC FATIGUE SYNDROME

Fibromyalgia and chronic fatigue are oxidative-dysoxygenative disorders. Indeed, my very notion of dysfunctional cellular oxygen metabolism emerged during my extensive work with those twin disorders. In 1994, I published my observations concerning the oxidosis in chronic fatigue syndrome in *The Canary and Chronic Fatigue.* I discuss at length my work with dysoxygenosis in the forthcoming book, *Canary Two: Oxygen and Fibromyalgia.*

Here, I include the summary data of a clinical outcome study my colleagues and I recently published.[4] The study included 150 consecutive patients with fibromyalgia who met the study criteria and followed our integrative plans for a minimum period of six months. The following are the outcome data: over 90% relief of symptoms in 65.4%; between 75% and 90% improvement in 19.3%, and less than 25% improvement in 10%. The full abstract of that article appears in the Appendix.

OXY THERAPIES FOR LOSS OF MENSTRUATION AND MENSTRUAL IRREGULARITIES

Very few, if any, gynecologists think of oxygen or liver function when their patients complain of menstrual irregularities, loss of menstruation, PMS, endometriosis, or menopausal symptoms. My insights into those relationships came to be by simple observation of my patients with those difficulties who were under my treatment for fibromyalgia, chronic fatigue syndrome, bowel disorders (such as Crohn's colitis and ulcerative colitis), and other serious autoimmune disorders. I was not focused on their menstrual difficulties. Almost all of them reported relief of PMS and normalization of menstrual cycles when their chronic disorders (which I was treating vigorously) came under control. Of course, that should have been entirely predictable from an oxidative-dysoxygenative standpoint.

It is common knowledge among doctors focusing on fibromyalgia and chronic fatigue syndrome that menstrual irregularities are very common in such patients. Furthermore, not uncommonly, young women with those disorders cease menstruation completely. However, most of those physicians seek to address those problems by prescribing synthetic hormones which, in my view, is a serious error. During my early years of work with such patients, I also recognized the relationship between liver detox therapies and menstrual health. I presented my view in two articles entitled, "Oxidative menopausal dysfunction (OMD-II): hormone replacement therapy (HRT) or receptor restoration therapy (RRT)?"[13] and "Amenorrhea, oligomenorrhea, and polymenorrhea in CFS and fibromyalgia are caused by oxidative menstrual dysfunction (OMD-I)."[5]

In the OMD-I article cited above, I published data of a clinical outcome study concerning 35 young women who had scanty periods or had ceased all menstrual function. The menstrual cycles were completely normalized in 12 of 14 women with total loss of menstruation (amenorrhea) of longer than six months duration and in 19 of 21 women with scant periods (oligomenorrhea).

NONDRUG CONTROL OF ASTHMA
An Example of Indirect Oxy Therapies

For instance, for a child with asthma I consider diagnosis and treatment of mold allergy an oxy therapy. That may seem to be a stretch to some. But the *primary* cause of asthma in almost all asthmatics is mold and food allergy. Viral infections often unmask asthma. A careful study of events that trigger bronchial spasm and wheezing —asthma by another name—reveals that all such events are oxidative-dysoxygenative in nature. I know for a fact that success in asthma control without drugs depends on addressing all issues—nutritional, ecologic, and others—that threaten normal oxygen metabolism. My experience with about 150 children and adults with asthma has convinced me that the ability to control asthma without drugs depends on how effective one can manage *all* the relevant issues in the bowel, blood, and liver ecosystem. The air hunger which a child experiences during an asthma attack is rooted in the bowel, blood, and liver ecosystems. Wheezing is simply the visible symptom of underlying OD events in those three ecologies. In a recent article concerning an outcome study of fifty asthma patients, my colleagues and I described our "integrative-ecologic management plan" in which *all* essential oxygenative issues are discussed.[14] In a previously published clinical outcome study of 44 consecutive patients with asthma that proved refractory to the standard bronchodilator therapies, regular use of drugs was discontinued in 77%, reduced by more than 50% in 12%, and by about 25% in another 11% of subjects. In the steroid dependent subgroup of 11 patients, steroids were discontinued in 4 patients (35%).[15]

OXY THERAPIES FOR KIDNEY FAILURE

At present, nephrologists offer their patients with kidney failure two choices: lifelong dialysis or a kidney transplant. It is a little-known fact that kidney failure in *most* early and intermediate stages can be reversed with oxygenative therapies. Kidney failure may be triggered by many causes but, in most cases, it is perpetuated and worsened by changes that severely interfere with blood supply to the kidneys. In 1981, my colleague, Professor Alfred Fayemi, and I presented extensive evidence for that view developed in our laboratory as well as in some others, in our book, *The Pathology of Maintenance Dialysis.*[16] Thus, it seems logical that oxy therapies that restore blood supply to the kidneys and address all issues, which caused the kidney damage in the first place, are likely to be of much clinical benefit. This, indeed, is the case.

In Figures 1 and 2, I demonstrate how EDTA chelation and other oxy therapies reversed kidney failure in two patients. The graphs show the falling values for blood creatinine levels, indicating improved function and reversal of kidney failure.

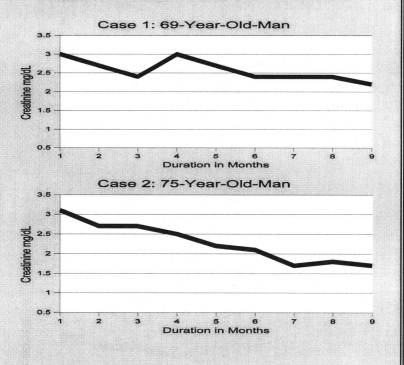

**IMPROVEMENT IN KIDNEY FUNCTION
IN TWO PATIENTS WITH KIDNEY FAILURE.**
(Oxygenative therapies included EDTA chelation.)

Dialysis was avoided in both patients.
Creatinine levels remained low during the three
follow-up years in case one and four years in case
two.

OXYGENATIVE THERAPIES FOR CANCER

A cancer cell hates oxygen and loves acid. That, in simple words, is the basis of my *metabolic* approach to control of cancer. In an earlier chapter, I described how dysfunctional oxygen metabolism leads to excess acid production. Thus, the problem of excess acidity in cancer cannot be addressed except through restoration of oxygen metabolism.

In caring for my patients with cancer, I rely heavily on oxy therapies, including intravenous hydrogen peroxide and ozone administration, nasal oxygen, hydrogen peroxide baths, and EDTA chelation infusions. And, of course, I diligently address all the bowel, blood, and liver issues that threaten oxygen metabolism. Again, the scope of this book does not permit full discussion of this issue. However, the following may interest many readers. Many cancers of the chest cause accumulation of fluid in the chest called pleural effusion. That occurs when cancer cells invade the pleural lining of lungs. It is an extremely serious condition for which oncologists have no effective therapy. In a paper published in *Explore* magazine (1999;9:43), Chinese doctors reported successful treatment of that condition in all 16 patients they treated. They aspirated the fluid and instilled oxygen instead. This report should not be a surprise to anyone, since oxygen kills cancer cells.

AIR TRAVEL DYSOXYGENOSIS (ATD)

I have recognized a pattern of illness related to prolonged air travel which I attribute to insufficient oxygen supply in the passenger cabins of the planes and which I designate "air travel dysoxygenosis (ATD)."[17] In ATD, persons with chronic illness experience marked worsening of their symptoms. Specifically, patients with fibromyalgia suffer more pain and their trigger points become more tender. Asthma sufferers suffer more wheezing attacks. Those with autoimmune disorders describe a greater intensity of joint pains and bowel symptoms. Sometimes, persons without previous neurologic symptoms develop an acute syndrome of brain dysfunction (encephalopathy). I see firm evidence for oxidative injury in their blood with microscopy, with other laboratory tests (such as increased urinary organic acids), and sometimes with positive signs at physical examination (such as skin rashes, sore throat, white coating of tongue, and bruises). A commonly seen evidence for dysoxygenosis is the sense of air or oxygen hunger.

I include below four brief case histories that dramatically illustrate those phenomena.

TOXIC ENCEPHALOPATHY CAUSED BY ATD

A 72-year-old physician-friend who practices environmental medicine went to Australia in good health to give a series of medical seminars. After his flight, he experienced mild nonspecific and temporary symptoms that cleared within a few days. His return trip to the United States was not so uneventful. He developed progressive confusion and memory difficulties soon after the flight. Within a week, his symptoms became disabling and he was forced to cancel all his patient appointments. Even though he had never experienced symptoms of poor circulation prior to that long flight, initially he suspected he might have suffered a mini-stroke or a TIA (transient ischemic attack). His doctor agreed with him. When his confusion persisted, he and his doctor began to think of other possibilities. Weeks later, he realized that he was suffering from chemical toxicity in some way related to his flight. It took him nearly three months to regain enough of his cerebral functions to resume his medical practice.

RELAPSE OF MULTIPLE SCLEROSIS

A 29-year-old woman saw me for multiple sclerosis (MS) in April 1997. She suffered from persistent muscle spasm, fatigue, balance and urine control difficulties, and numbness in her limbs. She made a dramatic recovery with a vigorous program that focused on treatment of her mold allergy, food sensitivities, restoration of her battered bowel, blood, and liver ecosystems, and improved cellular oxygen metabolism (control of oxidosis-dysoxygenosis). In the spring of 1999, she told me she felt as healthy as before the diagnosis of MS and that her "MS was behind her." In summer of that year, she went to Moscow, Paris, and some other European cities for about three weeks. The airplane trip to Europe made her very fatigued, but she recovered within days. The return trip also caused severe fatigue.

Rather than recover with rest that time, she rapidly developed all her original symptoms of multiple sclerosis.

We restarted our original plan of treatment in its entirety, including two intravenous hydrogen peroxide infusions followed by an infusion of one of our multivitamin protocols every week. That treatment, our clinical and experimental studies had shown, was a potent oxygenative therapy. Her recovery the second time was much more rapid than at the time of initial treatment and she felt her health was completely restored in about six weeks.

RISES IN PSA LEVELS IN A MAN WITH PROSTATIC CANCER

A 65-year-old man with prostate cancer traveled to Europe for a two-to-three-week vacation yearly from 1996 to 1999. After each trip, his PSA value rose. (PSA is a marker for prostate cancer.) After the first trip, the PSA value returned to the pre-travel number after two months with his nutrient and herbal protocols. A year later, he went to Europe again and had his PSA measured there. There was no change. When tested again on his return, his PSA value had nearly doubled. The value returned again to the pre-travel level with his regular program. Table 4 shows PSA values before and after each trip.

Table 4. PSA Values Changing With Air Travel			
Date	PSA Values Before Trips	PSA Values After Trips	Comments About Treatment*
1995	12.2	22	on phytohormones
1996	7.9	23.2	on phytohormones
1997	21.1	25.3	on Zoladex and Casadex
1998	23.5	32.2	on PC-SPES
1998	3.6	11.1	on PC-SPES
1999	2.5	3.1	on PC-SPES
1999	2.2	6.6	on PC-SPES
2000	1.1	3.3	* On antioxidant andHerbal protocols throughout

RISES IN HEPATITIS C VIRAL COUNT AFTER AIR TRAVEL

Earlier in this chapter, I illustrated the efficacy of hydrogen peroxide as an oxy therapy for reducing the hepatitis virus with a case history. The following values for hepatitis C viral counts in another man show how he initially responded well to oxy therapies. A trip to Europe caused fatigue and abdominal symptoms along with a dangerous rise in his viral load. Aggressive oxy therapies dramatically lowered the viral count and restored his health within months.

Dates	Hepatitis C Counts
10. 06. 96	203,000
03. 22. 97	1,078,000
06. 17. 97	1,731,000
10. 07. 97	414,000
02. 06. 98	367000
06. 19. 98	2,133,000*
08. 06. 98	926,000
08. 27. 98	497,000
10. 28. 98	118,308
03. 08. 00	199,000

* He traveled to Europe and developed abdominal discomfort and fatigue within a few days of the trip. He felt better while traveling in Europe by car. After the return flight, he became progressively fatigued and develped abdominal symptoms. A viral count showed a dangerous rise of viral count from 367,000 to over two million copies of the virus.

AIR IN AIRPLANES

I include below two quotes that have obvious relevance to our subject matter.

In the last two decades, in a highly competitive travel environment, airlines have been under pressure to increase their efficiency. That drive for lower costs has left passengers gasping for air—literally—as the levels of fresh air circulated to the average passenger have been cut.

New Science, July 1999

Of course you realize that as an airplane climbs in altitude the cabin pressure is allowed to decrease for airplane structural reasons. However, the cabin pressure is not allowed to drop below that value equivalent to an 8,000 foot altitude. For your information, the cabin pressure at 8,000 foot equivalent altitude is approximately 74 of sea level, but oxygen concentration remains at approximately 20.95% by volume....a change in airplane cabin equivalent altitude from sea level to 8,000 feet reduces the blood oxygen by only 6% for an unacclimatized individual.

Taken from a letter to my patient from the manager of Transport Airplane Directorate, U.S. Dept. of Transportation, January 5, 2000.

Now, the figure of 6% loss of oxygen saturation may not mean much to airlines, but it is evidently of great concern to the persons like those described in the above three case histories. There is yet another important issue here. The figure of 6% loss in oxygen creates a false sense of security. The airplane cabins carry a much greater load of chemicals, including carbon monoxide, than air in other areas. That creates a double jeopardy for many people.

Here is another common observation: Many people become lethargic within several minutes of entering the planes. And we cannot blame all that on the *uniquely bad* food served there!

The letter mentioned above also included a table giving the rates of approximate percentage of recirculation for various types of aircrafts, ranging from 0% to 53%. Of great interest to me was the fact that it was possible with known technology to keep the rate of recirculation for Boeing 727-100/200 and Boeing 737-100/200 model planes at zero.[18] How did the company justify keeping the rate at 50% in its 767-200 and 767-300 models?

RHEUMATOID ARTHRITIS RETURNS WHEN OXYGEN DROPS BY 50%

A 73-year-old consulted me for rheumatoid arthritis, asthma, and fatigue. She responded well to our program. As is often the case with nondrug therapies in such patients, her initial response was minimal but she improved dramatically after several months. The swelling and pain in her joints decreased and the joint mobility increased. Her severe asthma attacks subsided. The regular use of her arthritis and asthma medications was discontinued.

Three months after I had seen her last, she limped into my office with a full-blown relapse of rheumatoid arthritis. Her hands were diffusely swollen. Her swollen wrists were bent in such a way that she was unable to open her hands and hold anything. Her knees and ankles showed a similar acute inflammatory process. Dismayed, I recalled how bouncy she had looked at the last visit. Here is what she told me:

I was doing very, very well...really the best months I have had in a long time. Then I went down fast.

**I began with what seemed like a common cold.
Next day, I rushed to the emergency room with a
severe asthma attack. They said my oxygen level
was down to 50% and admitted me. They gave me
IV steroids and several other medications. I
stabilized in five days and was sent home on 10 mg
of prednisone for five days. On the third day, my
joints became inflamed. In two more days, I was
just like you see me now.**

WHY IGNORE HYDROGEN?

"Why leave hydrogen out in my theory of aging? Isn't
hydrogen the fuel of life?," some readers might ask. "Doesn't it
provide electrons to oxygen to begin its work in most reactions?,"
they might further argue. It is true that human metabolism uses
hydrogen ions (electron-rich form of hydrogen) as its primary fuel.
Oxygen extracts electrons from hydrogen to initiate most human
metabolic reactions. Most of the hydrogen ions come from hydrogen
atoms contained in fats, proteins, and carbohydrates. During
metabolism of those foods, many toxic organic acids are produced
which the body gets rid of at a substantial energy cost.

**If the fuel could be pure hydrogen, metabolic
mating of oxygen with hydrogen would produce
clean energy and pure water. That, of course,
would be the most desirable energy reaction.**

The problem is while we use so much hydrogen, we

understand very little about it. In recent years, some "hydrogen pills" have been heavily marketed to treat disease and promote health. Alas! Those products have yielded only limited results in my own experience. That did not surprise me, nor should it surprise any serious student of human health. Dysfunctional oxygen metabolism, once established, is far too deep a problem to solve with pills of single remedies, regardless of how effective they might seem in theory. Furthermore, human ecologic systems, once battered, are far too complex to be restored with single therapies. Major ecologic disruptions call for broad-based ecologic-restorative measures.

The theory of "hydrogen economy" seems to make much theoretical sense.[19,20] Indeed, there is much current interest in hydrogen in the energy industry. Consider the following quote from a recent issue of *Nature* (2000;404;233-4):

> **What fuel will drive the coming century? As we look back over the past millennium, the progression of fuel useage has been from wood to coal to oil. Now, at the turn of the millennium, methane gas appears to be the preferred clean fuel of the major electricity generators. But we are moving inexorably towards hydrogen as the ultimate clean power source of the future.**

It seems very likely that hydrogen will become a major, if not the primary, source of energy production. Indeed, in the March 16, 2000, issue of *Nature*, Park and his colleagues described a fuel cell in which hydrogen is directly oxidized to produce energy, thus opening up the possibility of a "flame-free future."

It also seems likely that some effective "hydrogen products" will be developed in the future for medical uses. I look forward to the day when that theoretical possibility turns into a reality, and I can add "hydrogen therapies" to oxy therapies described in this volume.

But, how does the notion of hydrogen economy fit into my oxygen theory of aging and my view of the clinical efficacy of oxy therapies? First, none of the considerations of hydrogen as an antioxidant and as a source of clean energy is in any way inconsistent with my theory or my clinical observations. Second, and more importantly, *oxidation is a spontaneous process of decay and dying, while reduction (where hydrogen comes into play) requires energy. One is a process of breakdown and the other of building up.* Common sense tells us—as does the Second Law of Thermodynamics—that each living being one day must disintegrate and die. Oxygen is the driving force behind that process of decay and death, not hydrogen. Until new information is developed that forces us to consider the roles of oxygen and hydrogen differently, I continue to consider oxygen as *the* organizing influence of human biology.

SUMMARY:
Oxidative-Dysoxygenative States and the
One-Disease/One-Drug Model

The oxidative-dysoxygenative dysfunction (ODD) model of illness has strong explanatory power. It provides answers to many questions not answered by the prevailing classifications of diseases based on microscopic observations *after* the tissues have been injured. However, no medical theory has any validity unless it can be tested with true-to-life situations and real patients. Data obtained with integrated clinical outcome studies and summarized in this chapter provide significant support for the proposed ODD hypothesis. Some may consider most of such evidence indirect. However, it must be noted that the number of biologic variables in any illness is very large. It seems highly unlikely that studies can ever be designed in such a way that direct evidence for one-cause/one-effect relationships between intracellular oxidative-dysoxygenative phenomena and clinical symptomatology can be established. I am confident that the benefits of oxy therapies will be readily attested to by all those who undertake such therapies in earnest.

References
1.   Ali M. Science and angry colleague. In: Intravenous Nutrient Protocols in Molecular Medicine. Mmonograph. 1987. Life Span, Denville, New Jersey.
2.   Ali M, Ali O, Fayemi A, et al: Improved myocardial perfusion in patients with advanced ischemic heart disease with an integrative management program including edta chelation therapy. J Integrative Medicine 1997;1:113-145.
3.   Ali M. Hypothesis: Chronic fatigue is a state of accelerated oxidative molecular injury. J Advancement in Medicine. 1993;6:83-96.
4.   Ali M, Juco J, Fayemi A, et al. Efficacy of ecologic-integrative management protocols for reversal of fibromyalgia, J Integrative Medicine 1999;1:48-63
5.   Ali M: Amenorrhea, oligomenorrhea, and polymenorrhea in CFS and fibromyalgia are caused by oxidative menstrual dysfunction (OMD-I) J Integrative Medicine 1998;2:101-124.
6.   Ali M, Ali O, Alfred et al. Efficacy of an integrative program including intravenous and intramuscular nutrient therapies for arrested growth. J Integrative Medicine 1998;2:56-69.
7.   Ali M, Ali O, Fayemi A, et al: Guidelines for intravenous therapies in integrative medicine. J Integrative Medicine 1998;2:82-95.
8.   Grief R, Akca O, Horn EP, et al. Supplemental Perioperative oxygen to reduce the incidence of of surgical wound infections. N Eng J Med 2000;342:161-7.

9.   Gottrup F. Prevention of surgical-wound infections. N Eng J Med 2000;342:202-3.

10.   Ali M. Oxidative coagulopaty. In: Syllabus of the Capital University of Integrative Medicine, Washington, D.C., 1997.

11.   Ali M. Oxidative plasma membrane injury and magnesium. Environmental Physician. Summer 1992. American Academy of Environmental Medicine, Denver, Colorado.

12.   Ali M, Ali O. AA Oxidopathy: the core pathogenetic mechanism of ischemic heart disease. J Integrative Medicine 1997;1:1-112.

13.   Ali, M. Oxidative menopausal dysfunction (OMD-II); Hormone replacement therapy (HRT) or Receptor restoration theraoy (HRT), J Integrative Medicine 1998;3:125-139

14.   Ali M, Juco J, Ali O, et al. Integrative management of bronchial asthma. Journal of Integrative Medicine. 2000 (in press)

15.   Ali M: Non-pharmacologic management of asthma as a model. Abstract of the annual meeting of the American Academy of Envioronmental Medicine, page 12, 1991.

16.   Ali M, Fayemi AO. The pathology of Maintenance Hemodialysis. Springfield, Illinois,1982.

17.   Ali M. Air travel dysoxygenosis. Journal of Integrative Medicine. (in press).

18.   Foss K. *Globe and mail*, Toronto, April 6, 1999 (as reproduced in *New Scientist* July 1999.

19.   Park S, Vohs JM, Gorte RJ. Direct oxidation of hydrocarbon in a solid-oxide fuel cell. Nature 2000;404:265-7.

20.   Kendall K. Hopes for a flame-free future. Nature 2000;404:233-4.

Appendix

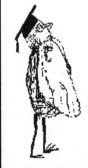

AGING HEALTHFULLY FOOD CHOICES

BEVERAGES		PROTEINS		FATS
1st Choice		**1st Choice**		**1st Choice**
Carbon-filtered water Fresh vegetable juice Ginger water Banch tea Grain coffee Herbal teas Spreing water Deep well water		Protein Peptide Powders Hunted fish Lentils Beans Duck Quail Wild game	Goat Sheep Lamb Guinea hen Muscovy duck Whole grains Spirolina Plankton	Olive oil Ghee Butter Sesame oil Flaxseed oil
2nd Choice		**2nd Choice**		**2nd Choice**
Bottled spring water Bottled deep well water Mineral water Fruit teas Grapefruit juice	Apple juice Soy milk, diluted Rice milk, diluted Sheep's milk Goat's milk Buffalo's milk Green teas	Chicken Turkey Shellfish Cornish hen Egg		Safflower oil Sunflower oil Soybean oil Avocado oil Canola oil
3rd Choice		**3rd Choice**		**3rd Choice**
Skim milk, cow Low fat cow's milk Light Diet Sodas Grape juice Cranberry juice Orange juice Coconut juice Nut milks, diluted Salted vegetable juice		Beef Veal Pork Cultured fish		Corn oil Cottonseed oil
Aging Oxidants		**Aging Oxidants**		**Aging Oxidants**
Coffee Chocolate drinks\shakes Dark sodas Alcohol Tea (common black)		Deli meats Highly-processed meats Highly-spiced meats		Margarine Vegetable shortening Animal fats Cholesterol-free fatty foods

AGING HEALTHFULLY FOOD CHOICES

CARB's	FRUITS	VEGETABLES
1st Choice	**1st Choice**	**1st Choice**
Brown rice Wild rice Amaranth Millet Artichoke Quinoa Tapioca Milo Tofu Tempeh Spelt Kamut Teff Sunflower seeds Sesame seeds Pumpkin seeds	Peach Pear Cherries Berries Avocado Papaya Guava Persimmon Pomegranate Rhubarb Prune Apple Figs	Daikon Burdock Red radish Squash Chinese cabbage Turnips Shiitake Mushrooms Lotus root Ginger Green beans Carrot Collards Kale Spinach Artichoke Asparagus Beets Brussels sprouts Broccoli, Cauliflower Celery, Cucumber Garlic, Okra, Peas Cabbage
2nd Choice	**2nd Choice**	**2nd Choice**
Rye Buckwheat Oats Potato Barley Yam	Lemon Lime Raisins Watermelon Kiwi Grapefruit Cantaloupe Banana	Romaine lettuce Iceberg lettuce Boston lettuce Onion Red peppers Green peppers Eggplant Tomato Mushrooms
3rd Choice	**3rd Choice**	**3rd Choice**
Wheat Corn White rice Cashews Brazil nuts Chestnuts Pecans Peanuts Walnuts Almonds	Orange Pineapple Coconut Strawberries Grapes Honeydew Mangoes Dates Polished fruits Dried fruits	None
Aging Oxidants	**Aging Oxidants**	**Aging Oxidants**
Sugar	None	None

ORGANIC VEGETABLE JUICES

Fresh organic vegetable juice is the very best way to assure an ample supply of nutrients for optimal function of enzymes of human energy, detoxification, digestive/absorptive, and neurotransmitter pathways. Such nutrients include:

1. Minerals 2. Vitamins 3. Enzymes.

For times when fresh juicing is not feasible, bottled organic vegetable juices may be used. Such juices contain all the minerals present in fresh juices (minerals do not degrade with storage). However, bottled juices may not contain many of the vitamins and enzymes present in fresh vegetables.

PEROXIDE-SALT BATH

(Please read this protocol twice before using it.)

First Bath
1. Fill the bath tub with warm water with temperature you prefer.
2. Add one quart of 3% hydrogen peroxide bottle to the bath tub.
3. Add one-half teaspoon of sea salt to the bath water (Baleine is a good brand).
4. Avoid direct contact of the bath tub water with eyes.
5. After five minutes, add a second one quart bottle of 3% hydrogen peroxide to the bath water, if there is no tissue irritation is experienced (see caution note below).
5. After five minutes, add the third quart bottle of 3% hydrogen peroxide to the bath water.
6. Stay in the bath from 20 to 25 minutes.

Second And Later Baths
1. Fill the bath tub with warm water with temperature you prefer.
2. Add three one-quart bottles of 3% hydrogen peroxide to the bath tub.
3. Avoid direct contact of the bath tub water with eyes.
4. Stay in the bath from 20 to 25 minutes.

Caution:
1. Use bath water temperature that is comfortable for you.
2. Some women with symptoms of vaginitis may experience temporary

irritation and may need to use only one-half or one bottle of peroxide until tissue irritation clears up.

3. Some persons experience lightheaded if they stand up suddenly after a warm bath. It is a necessary safety step that this possibility be kept in mind and one should get up slowly, holding the safety bar or the side of the bath tub.

Note:

Brown colored 1 quart bottles of 3% hydrogen peroxide are generally available from drug stores and other stores, such as A&P. It pays to do comparative shopping.

**LIVER CASTOR OIL PACK
AND LIVER FLUSH PROTOCOL**

Two natural therapies that have stood the test of time for liver detoxification are liver castor oil pack and liver flush protocols. As for other specific therapies I include in this volume, I recommend that both liver pack and flush should be undertaken under professional supervision first. I myself prescribe castor oil liver packs to facilitate liver detox and reduce liver congestion as a part of our basic bowel-blood-liver detox program in most patients with chronic ailments.

Steps for the Castor Oil Liver Pack

1. Gently massage the *entire* liver area (upper abdomen and lower chest on the right side) along with the front of the lower abdomen with your left hand for two to four minutes.
2. Prepare a piece of flannel or cotton cloth large enough to cover the liver and abdomen areas when folded twice.
3. Fold flannel or cotton piece and soak it with castor oil (available from most pharmacies).
4. Cover the liver and abdominal areas with the soaked flannel or cotton piece and cover the cloth with a plastic sheet (an opened plastic bag is adequate). Use tape to anchor the plastic sheet.
5. Put a heating pad over as much of the area as possible covered by the pack, favoring the area of the liver. *The heating pad must not be hot.*
6. Leave the castor oil soak for two hours, unless otherwise specified by your physician.
7. Gently wash off the castor oil with a mild soap after finishing the protocol.

Steps for One-Day Liver Flush
1. Drink 5 to 8 (or more if tolerated) glasses of organic apple cider or juice throughout the day. Persons with hypoglycemia or glucose intolerance may substitute organic vegetable juice for apple juice.
2. Drink additional water to maintain a state of overhydration from morning till 6 PM.
3. Take a vegetarian lunch at noon.
4   Continue with your prescribed nutrient and herbal supplements.
5. Three hours after lunch, take two teaspoons of disodium phosphate (or Epsom salt, if disodium phosphate is not available) dissolved in two ounces of hot water. Drink one cup of hot water with a few drops of lemon juice and a pinch of salt to eliminate bad taste from mouth.
6. Two hours later, repeat the above step (# 5).
7. Take an evening meal of grapefruit. (Grapefruit juice may be substituted if the whole fruit is not available. Fresh juice is preferred to canned juice.)
8. At bedtime, drink one cup of an equal-parts mixture of extra-virgin olive oil and lemon juice (1/2 cup of each). Again, fresh juice is preferred.
9. Lie in bed on your right side with knees pulled up for about 30 minutes.
10. Additional vegetarian meals may be taken if needed.
11. Be prepared to experience nausea, some abdominal cramps, and diarrhea during or after taking lemon juice and olive oil. You may need a Tigan suppository if nausea persists (prescription required from your physician).

Steps for Two-Day Liver Flush
1. Drink 5 to 8 (or more if tolerated) glasses of organic apple cider/juice or vegetable juice daily for two days.
2. Three hours after a vegetarian lunch on the second day, take 2 teaspoons of disodium phosphate dissolved in two ounces of hot water. Drink one cup of hot water with a few drops of lemon juice and a pinch of salt to eliminate bad taste from the mouth.
3. Continue with additional steps as for the one-day protocol (steps # 6 to 9).

BOWEL ECOLOGY PROTOCOLS

BOWEL ECOLOGY PROTOCOL #1®
One billion spores of Lactobacillus acidophilus, Lactobacillus bulgaricus, Bifidobacterium in a base of-complex vegetable fiber, Magnesium sulfate, Vitamin B Complex, L-Histidine, L-Arginine, Pantethine, Aloe vera.

BOWEL ECOLOGY PROTOCOL #2®
Alfalfa 500 mg, Pau D' Arco 100 mg, Allium 100 mg, Licorice root extract 200 mg.
BOWEL ECOLOGY PROTOCOL #3®
Calcium 50 mg, Magnesium 50 mg, Grapefruit seed extract 25 mg, Aloe vera 1 mg, Spirulina 10 mg.
BOWEL ECOLOGY PROTOCOL #4®
Grapefruit seed extract 50 mg, Allium 50 mg, Pau D'Arco 500 mg.
BOWEL ECOLOGY PROTOCOL #5®
Par-Quing 150 mg, Pau D'Arco 150 mg, Beet root fiber 200 mg, Guar Gum 100 mg.
BOWEL ECOLOGY PROTOCOL #6®
Echinacea 200 mg, Goldenseal root 150 mg, Astragalus root 150 mg, Burdock root 150 mg.
BOWEL ECOLOGY PROTOCOL #7®
Cascara sagrada 250 mg, Alfalfa 50 mg, Beet root fiber 50 mg, Goldenseal root 50 mg.
BOWEL ECOLOGY PROTOCOL #8®
Beet root fiber 700 mg.
BOWEL ECOLOGY PROTOCOL #9®
Milk thistle extract 200 mg, Goldenseal root 150 mg, Turmeric 150 mg, Jerusalem artichoke 150 mg.
BOWEL ECOLOGY PROTOCOL #10®
Vitamin B-5 165 mg, Folic acid 50 mcg, Pantethine 100 mg, PABA 5 mg, Potassium 2 mg, L-Arginine HCI 25 mg, L-Histidine 25 mg, L-Ornithine 5 mg, Aloe vera 5 mg, Licorice Root 50 mg, Spirulina 10 mg.
BOWEL ECOLOGY PROTOCOL #11®
Senna 50 mg, Psyllium 400 mg, Beet root 100 mg, Glycerin 50 mg.
BOWEL ECOLOGY #12®
Magnesium 150 mg, Potassium 50 mg, Taurine 250 mg.
BOWEL ECOLOGY PROTOCOL #13®
Fenugreek, Fennel Seeds, Pau D'Arco, Licorice Powder
BOWEL ECOLOGY PROTOCOL #14®
Psyllium Hush Powder 4000 mg, Apple Pectin 100 mg

BLOOD ECOLOGY PROTOCOLS

BLOOD ECOLOGY PROTOCOL #1®
Cayenne 150 mg, Turmeric 150 mg, Garlic 150 mg, Dandelion root 150 mg, Ginger 150 mg.
BLOOD ECOLOGY PROTOCOL #2®
Butcher's Broom 150 mg, Hawthorne 150 mg, Mother's Wort 150 mg, St. John's Wort 150 mg, Bilberry 150 mg.
BLOOD ECOLOGY PROTOCOL #3®
Siberian ginseng 150 mg, Mistletoe 150 mg, Linden flowers 150 mg, Schisandra 150 mg, Cranberry 150 mg.

LIVER ECOLOGY PROTOCOLS

LIVER ECOLOGY PROTOCOL #1®
Dandelion root 100 mg; Beet root fiber 50 mg; Black radish 50 mg; Goldenseal 50 mg; Catnip 50 mg; Methionine 400 mg; Choline bitartrate 200 mg; Inositol 20 mg.
LIVER ECOLOGY PROTOCOL #2®
Turmeric 100 mg; Milk Thistle 100 mg; Red clover 100 mg; Ginger root 100 mg; Goldenseal 100 mg; Jerusalem artichoke 100 mg; Fennel seed 100 mg.

ABSTRACT # 1

Improved Myocardial Perfusion in Patients with Advanced Ischemic Heart Disease with An Integrative Management Program Including EDTA Chelation Therapy

Majid Ali, M.D., Omar Ali, M.D., Alfred Fayemi, M.D., Judy Juco, M.D., Carol Grieder-Brandenburger, R.N.

Journal of Integrative Medicine 1997;1:113-142

Objective
    To assess the clinical efficacy of an integrated management program including nutritional and herbal therapies, nongoal-oriented exercise, self-regulation, and EDTA chelation therapy for patients with advanced ischemic heart disease (IHD).

Patients
    Twenty-six consecutive patients who presented with advanced ischemic heart disease and who had fared poorly after one or more coronary bypass operations (5), one or more angioplasty procedures (6), or who failed to respond adequately to multiple drug therapies (15), and who had received a minimum number of 20 EDTA infusions. Duration of follow-up ranged from 15 months to 9 years.

Methods
    1. Clinical evaluation of patients before, during and after the integrated program used in this study. 2. Assessment of myocardial perfusion by comparative study of thallium perfusion scans performed before and after the IHD reversal program.

Clinical Outcome Measures
    The following clinical outcome criteria were semiquantitatively defined: Excellent

outcome, absence of significant symptoms and discontinuance of previously prescribed drug therapies; good, 75%+ relief of symptoms and reduction of drug dose; moderate, 50%+ relief of symptoms and reduction of drug dose; and poor, 25% or less relief of symptoms and reduction of drug dosage. Elements for follow-up included in the clinical outcome sheet were as follows: angina, chest tightness and related discomfort, arrhythmia, other chest symptoms, dyspnea, severity of stress, mood changes, anger, energy level, quality of sleep, appetite, digestion and frequency of bowel movements (all clinical parameters that determine the degree of AA oxidopathy—a state of chronic and insidious accelerated oxidative molecular injury to all elements of the circulating blood which we consider to be the core pathogenetic mechanism of IHD.[1])

Results
      Clinical outcome data are as follows: excellent 61%, good 17%, moderate 13%, and poor 9%. Comparative study of pre- and post-chelation myocardial perfusion scans showed clear, objective evidence of significant improvement in myocardial perfusion in five of six patients in whom such studies were performed. No patients during the study period suffered an acute myocardial infarction or underwent angioplasty or coronary bypass operation.

Conclusion
      Preliminary and limited outcome data in this study indicate significant potential for reversing IHD in patients with advanced ischemic heart disease by an integrated management plan with global emphasis on reducing oxidative stress on the circulating blood, cardiac myocytes and the conducting system of the heart. The program included nutritional and herbal therapies, self-regulation, nongoal-oriented exercise and EDTA chelation therapy. Additional and larger studies are warranted to fully explore the clinical potential of such an integrated management plan.

ABSTRACT # 2

EFFICACY OF ECOLOGIC-INTEGRATIVE MANAGEMENT PROTOCOLS FOR REVERSAL OF FIBROMYALGIA:
An Open Prospective Study of 150 Patients

Majid Ali, M.D., Judy Juco, M.D., Alfred O. Fayemi, M.D., Omar Ali, M.D., Mahboob Baig, M.B.,B.S.; Marta Babol, M.D., Karimullah Zirvi, Ph.D., Carol Grieder-Bradenberger, R.N., Mary Ann Carroll, R.N.

Journal of Integrative Medicine 1999;3:48-64

Objective
      To report the results of an open, prospective trial of broad-based, ecologic-integrative management protocols for the reversal of fibromyalgia in 150 patients.

Patients

One hundred fifty patients who presented at the Institute of Integrative Medicine with fibromyalgia and for whom clinical outcome data were available for at least six months prior were included in this study. There were 116 females (range of age, 13-81 yrs) and 34 males (range of age, 14-68 yrs). The average duration of illness was 6.6 years and the average duration of clinical management was 11.5 months. Patients were divided into three groups: Group 1, when the duration of illness was less than three years; Group 2, when the duration of illness was between three and six years; and Group 3, when the duration of illness was longer than six years.

Ecologic-Integrative Management Protocols

The comprehensive, ecologic-integrative management protocols employed were based on clinical, biochemical, and high-resolution microscopic assessment of the microecologic cellular and macroecologic tissue-organ systems of the body. Such protocols included the following: choices in the kitchen designed to provide for optimal hydration, elimination of foods causing incompatibility reactions and rapid glucose-insulin-adrenaline shifts; supplementation with vitamins, minerals, and some "redox-restorative substances" (RRSs) such as glutathione, taurine, methylsulfonylmethane (MSM), coenzyme Q10, and lipoic acid; ample herbal support for the bowel, blood, and liver ecosystems (including colon hydrotherapy and liver flushes); endocrine support, especially for the thyroid, adrenals, and sex hormones; intramuscular and intravenous nutrient protocols; oxygenative therapies, including nasal oxygen, intravenous infusions of hydrogen peroxide and ozone, and EDTA chelation; gentle stretching and noncompetitive (limbic) exercise; and training in effective methods for self-regulation, stress reduction, and guidance for spiritual surrender.

Assessment of Compliance

Assessment of compliance was based on entries made on a specifically designed clinical outcome sheet during follow-up visits. The following scale of scores was used for assessment of compliance according to predetermined criteria: Class A, a compliance value greater than 75%; Class B, a value between 75% and 50 %; Class C, a value between 50% and 25%; and Class D, a value lower than 25%.

Assessment of Clinical Outcome

Assessment of clinical outcome was based on concurrent evaluation of the progress made, or lack thereof, employing the clinical outcome sheet. The scale of scores for clinical improvement comprised the following: excellent outcome (Category I) when more than 90% relief of symptoms was obtained and all drug therapies were discontinued; good outcome (Category II) when the relief of symptoms was between 90% and 75%, with a similar reduction in use of drugs; fair outcome (Category III) when the relief of symptoms was between 75% and 50% with a similar reduction in symptoms; and poor outcome (Category IV) when the relief of symptoms was less than 50% with a similar reduction in the use of drugs.

Results

The overall final outcome scores for all 150 patients were as follows: excellent outcome, 65.4%; good, 19.3%; fair, 5.3%; and poor, 10%. The final outcome scores for

Group 1 (56) patients were as follows: excellent outcome, 75%; good, 10.7%; fair, 7.2%; and poor, 7.1%. The final outcome scores for Group 2 patients (26) were as follows: excellent outcome, 69.2%; good, 19.2%; fair, 7.7%; and poor, 3.9%. The final outcome scores for Group 3 patients (68) were as follows: excellent outcome, 55.9%; good, 26.5%; fair, 2.9 %; and poor, 14.7%.

Conclusion

The data in this clinical outcome study document the efficacy of the ecologic-integrative management protocols used in reversing fibromyalgia (excellent or good outcome in 84.7%). The results provide empirical support for the view that fibromyalgia is an oxidative-dysoxygenative disorder (ODD) and that disruptions of the bowel, blood, and liver ecosystems play critical roles in its pathogenesis. The data also warrant further and larger clinical outcome studies of the efficacy of the ecologic-integrative protocols such as those employed in this study for reversing fibromyalgia, a disorder for which no pharmacologic regimens have yielded satisfactory results so far.

ABSTRACT # 3

EFFICACY OF AN INTEGRATIVE PROGRAM INCLUDING INTRAVENOUS AND INTRAMUSCULAR NUTRIENT THERAPIES FOR ARRESTED GROWTH

Majid Ali, M.D.; Omar Ali, M.D.; Alfred Fayemi, M.D.; Judy Juco, M.D.; Carol Greider-Brandenburger, R.N.; Mary Ann Carroll, R.N.

Journal of Integrative Medicine 1998;2:56-69

Objective

To report the clinical outcome of an integrated management plan, including the use of intravenous and intramuscular nutrient protocols, for restoring growth in six children and adolescents with arrested growth.

Patients

All six patients who presented at the Institute with arrested growth (no gain in height and weight for a period of nine or more months) were included in this study. Two children had stopped growing after chemotherapy (one for rhabdomyosarcoma and the second for Wilms' tumor). Two girls were severely malnourished due to Crohn's disease treated with long-term immunosuppressant therapies. An 11-year-old boy stopped growing after steroid therapy and multiple hospitalizations for Glanzmann's thrombasthenia. The cause of growth arrest in the sixth patient was obscure.

Methods

The integrated management plan included the following: choices in the kitchen designed to provide for optimal hydration, elimination of foods causing incompatibility reactions and rapid glucose-insulin-adrenaline shifts; supplementation with vitamins, minerals, and some redox-restorative substances (RRS) such as glutathione, taurine, selenium; ample herbal support for the bowel, blood, and liver ecosystems; endocrine support when indicated; intramuscular and intravenous nutrient protocols; gentle stretching and noncompetitive (limbic) exercise; and training in effective methods for self-regulation and stress reduction.

Clinical Outcome Measures
Clinical evaluation using general health parameters and measurements of growth parameters. Weight and height measurements before and after institution of the integerated program lasting for a minimum of nine months.

Results
All six children and adolescents showed satisfactory improvement in general health parameters and resumed growth in height and weight (as well as secondary sexual development in two girls) within six to fourteen months of beginning the program.

Conclusion
Preliminary data of this clinical outcome study show efficacy of an integrated plan for restoring growth in children and adolescents with arrested growth and failure to develop secondary sexual characteristics. If validated by larger clinical trials, such a management plan should be of considerable value for growth failure caused by: (1) chemotherapy; (2) steroid and other immunosuppressive therapies for autoimmune disorders; (3) digestive/absorptive disorders; (4) inflammatory disorders of the bowel; (5) certain constitutional disorders; and (6) some cases of arrested growth of obscure origin.

ABSTRACT # 4

AMENORRHEA, OLIGOMENORRHEA, AND POLYMENORRHEA IN CFS AND FIBROMYALGIA ARE CAUSED BY OXIDATIVE MENSTRUAL DYSFUNCTION (OMD-I)

Majid Ali, M.D.

Journal of Integrative Medicine 1998;2:56-69

It is proposed that amenorrhea, oligomenorrhea, and polymenorrhea in chronic fatigue syndrome (CFS) and fibromyalgia are aspects of an "oxidative menstrual dysfunction" (OMD-I) that occurs as a consequence of global oxidative damage to microecologic cellular and macroecologic tissue-organ ecosystems of the body. Thus, OMD-I is considered as one facet of the broad spectrum of accelerated oxidative injury to: (1) matrix, plasma membranes, and mitochondria (3M ecologies); (2) coagulation cascade, complement system, and capsases (3C pathways); (3) enzyme pathways involved with oxygen transport and utilization; (4) enzyme pathways involved with detoxification pathways; (5) enzyme pathways involved with synthesis of sex and non-sex hormones; (6) enzyme pathways involved in hormone receptor synthesis; and (7) regulatory hormone-receptor- gene dynamics. In support of the OMD-I model, clinical outcome data for 35 women is presented. Menstrual cycles were normalized completely in 12 of 14 amenorrheic women (and improved in the remaining two) and in 19 of 21 women with oligomenorrhea or polymenorrhea with therapies that addressed issues of redox homeostasis and damaged bowel, blood, and liver ecosystems, but did not employ synthetic estrogens or other hormones.

Menstrual irregularities in CFS and fibromyalgia are common and are generally assumed to be due to gonadal insufficiency. The standard therapies for such disorders employ a variety of regimens of synthetic hormones to correct the putative estrogen deficiency. The OMD-I model challenges that view and proposes oxidative pathogenetic mechanisms for hormone-receptor-gene dysregulations in fibromyalgia and CFS. Furthermore, normalization of menstruation in such disorders with therapies that restore oxidatively damaged bowel, blood, and liver ecosystems provides a new insight into the relationship between pathophysiology of those organs and menstrual dysfunction. Some essential aspects of redox and hormonal homeostasis are reviewed to underscore the enormous complexities of the menstrual function, and to show that the prevailing use of synthetic hormones for menstrual dysregulation in fibromyalgia and CFS is neither rational on theoretical basis nor acceptable on empirical grounds.

ABSTRACT # 5

HYPOTHESIS: CHRONIC FATIGUE SYNDROME IS A STATE OF ACCELERATED OXIDATIVE INJURY

Majid Ali, M.D.

Journal of Advancement in Medicine, Volume 6, Number 2, Summer 1993

A hypothesis is proposed that chronic fatigue is a state of accelerated oxidative molecular injury. Evidence supporting the hypothesis includes the following: 1. Spontaneity of oxidation in nature is the basic cause of the aging process for organisms capable of aerobic respiration. Redox dysfunction represent the initial events that lead to clinical disease processes. 2. Incidence of chronic fatigue is increasing, as is the oxidant stress in the Earth's atmosphere. 3. Evidence for oxidative cell membrane injury in chronic fatigue is furnished by changes in intracellular and extracellular ions. 4. Immunologic abnormalities that occur in chronic fatigue are consistent with initial oxidative injury. 5. Commonality of association of antigens of HLA-DR3 region with chronic fatigue syndrome and with other autoimmune disorders such as rheumatoid arthritis, pemphigus vulgaris, systemic lupus erythematosus, and IgA and gold nephropathies. 6. Direct, morphologic evidence of increased oxidative stress on the cell membrane is shown by the fact that we have found deformities in up to 80% of erythrocytes in blood from chronic fatigue syndrome patients. These deformities are quickly reversed by administering ascorbic acid intravenously. 7. Changes in electromyopotentials observed in chronic fatigue patients are consistent with intracellular ionic and membrane changes. 8. Clinical entities commonly associated with chronic fatigue are know to increase oxidative molecular stress. 9. Clinical evidence obtained with relief of fatigue and related muscle symptoms with the use of oral and intravenous anti-oxidant nutrient therapy. From a clinical standpoint, this model for the molecular basis of chronic fatigue is useful for making therapeutic decisions for successful management of chronic fatigue without drug regimens.

Also reprinted in The Canary and Chronic Fatigue, Life Span Press, 1994, 2nd Edition.

Glossary

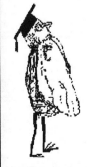

Abscess:

An inflammatory lesion which accumulates a pocket of pus.

Acid:

A substance that can react with alkalis to form salts and can ionize to give hydrogen ions. It turns litmus paper red.

Acidosis:

Acidosis (acid-o-sis) is excess acidity. Acidosis slows or blocks the enzyme systems of the body, including those involved with energy, digestion and absorption, detoxification, muscle function, and neurotransmitters. Enzymes are catalysts that facilitate life processes. Acidosis fans the flames of both oxidosis and dysoxygenosis which, in turn, cause more acidosis.

Adaptation response (general):

A set of biochemical changes that is believed to prepare an organism to cope with stress or a demand for change.

ADD:

Attention deficit disorder.

Adrenal glands:

A pair of glands weighing about one-half ounce and situated above the kidneys. These glands produce adrenaline and steroid hormones. It is commonly—and, in my view, inaccurately—believed to be the primary body organ involved in the stress response.

Adrenaline:

A hormone produced by the adrenal glands, which plays many roles in human biology and is believed to cause the stress response.

Adrenaline roller coasters:

Repeated adrenaline rushes that follow each other, creating sharp peaks and deep troughs of adrenaline levels in the blood and tissues.

Adrenaline rushes:

Blasts of adrenaline produced in sudden shock states that quicken the heart rate, tighten the muscles, and cause anxiety.

Adrenergic hypervigilence:

A state of overproduction of adrenaline hormone and related hormones that keeps various energy pathways revved up and causes molecular burnout.

Aging-oxidant molecules:

A family of oxidant molecules that causes death and decay in cells and tissues. See oxidation.

AIDS:
> Acquired immune deficiency syndrome, generally believed to be caused by HIV.

Alkali:
> A substance that can react awith acids to form salts and can ionise to produce hydroxyl radicals. It turns litmus paper blue.

All-in-the-head syndrome:
> A derisive term used by many doctors to dismiss patients with chronic complaints as malingerers—such symptoms are believed to be false and imaginary. See shirker's syndrome.

Alzheimer's disease:
> A progressive degenerative disorder of the brain in which loss of nerve cells and formation of tangles leads to loss of memory and disintegration of the personality.

Amino acids:
> Building blocks for proteins, amino acids are simple nitrogen-containing molecules.

Angina:
> A painful condition of the heart which causes chest pain that often radiates to the left arm, left side of the face and/or neck. It is caused by inadequate blood supply to the heart due to spasm of coronary arteries or blockage caused by plaque.

Angioplasty:
> A procedure by which an attempt is made to increase the blood supply to the heart by squeezing plaque in coronary arteries resulting in widening. Not recommended. Though theoretically a valid approach, it rarely works in real life because it does not address the underlying problems that cause heart disease.

Antibodies:
> Protein molecules produced in the body by the immune system to fight off microbial infections or deal with foreign materials. Antibodies are quite specific for the molecules against which they are directed.

Antihistamines:
> A class of drugs that controls the symptoms of allergic reactions by blocking the action of histamine, a substance that is released from mast cells and, in turn, causes the release of many inflammation mediators.

Antioxidant:
> Molecule that prevents oxidation (loss of electrons) of other substances.

Antioxidants of interest in human metabolism include vitamins such as vitamins A, C and E as well as minerals such as selenium.

Antioxidant defenses:
Host defenses against oxidative molecular injury. See oxidation.

Anxiety state:
An abnormal state of undue anxiety about real or imagined adverse events. In severe forms, anxiety causes loss of appetite, difficulty with sleep, jitters, indigestion, heart palpitations and missed heartbeats.

Arrhythmia:
Irregular heartbeat. Sometimes the individual can sense the irregular rhythm of the heart as skipped beats.

Arteriosclerosis:
Commonly called hardening of the arteries, arteriosclerosis is a disease process characterized by plaque formation on the inside walls of arteries. It leads to heart attacks, strokes and leg cramps while walking due to insufficient blood supply.

Ativan:
A commonly prescribed antianxiety drug. Generic name: lorazepam.

Attention deficit disorder:
A disorder of children as well as adults characterized by inattentiveness, impulsivity and inability to perform ordinary chores at home and at work. See hyperactivity syndrome.

Autism:
A disorder characterized by severe inability of the subject to react to ordinary stimulations and to communicate with family members and friends. The resulting isolation, unless averted, causes serious developmental problems.

Autoimmune disorders:
An individual's immunity turned against himself. A class of disorders in which an injured immune system produces antibodies directed against the body's own molecules, cells and organs. These autoantibodies may cause widespread tissue damage. See lupus, multiple sclerosis and hyperthyroidism.

Autonomic nervous system:
A part of the nervous system that is believed to be outside voluntary control, for example, nerve cells and nerve fibers that regulate normal heart rhythm and rate.

Autoregulation:
A process by which a person enters a healing energy state.

Azulfidine:
A drug used to suppress symptoms caused by various types of colitis such as ulcerative colitis, Crohn's colitis and others.

Biology:
A branch of science that deals with the structures and functions of living plants and animals.

Blood ecosystem:
A diverse, dynamic and delicate biochemical ecosystem of blood components circulating in blood vessels that actively interfaces with the bowel, liver, brain and other ecosystems. This concept contrasts with the traditional view that sterile blood circulates in a closed system of arteries and veins. The circulating blood is an open ecosystem in the sense that there is an ongoing free entry into it of bacteria, viruses and parasites from the bowel and other ecosystems of the body.

Bowel ecosystem:
A delicate, diverse and dynamic ecosystem composed of chemical (food elements and digestive-absorptive enzymes) and biologic elements (bacteria, viruses and parasites).

Cancer:
A malignant tumor that spreads and invades distant body organs. A growth produced by uncontrolled multiplication of cells.

Candida:
A single-celled fungus (yeast) normally found in the colon of almost all individuals. Furthermore, it is found in the bloodstream of most persons with suppressed immune systems.

Capillary:
A minute blood vessel that represents the narrowest part of the vascular tree.

Cellular ecosystems:
The internal environment of cells and intracellular organelles that sense—and respond to—changes in the tissue fluid that bathes cells.

Cellulitis:
A type of inflammation which spreads rapidly within soft tissues, causing pain, swelling and redness—at times extending into the surrounding tissues as red streaks.

Cell wall deficient organims:
Microbial organims with different structural and functional characteristics than the native species. (Sometimes also called pleomorphic forms).

Chelation:

> A process by which metals are eliminated from the body by binding them to substances with a special affinity for such metals. When used to reverse coronary artery disease, chelation employs EDTA as the chelating agent for calcium deposits in the plaque lining the arteries.

Chemotherapy:

> Treatment with drugs used to control cancer. In general, these drugs are highly toxic and seriously injure the immune system while incompletely killing cancer cells.

Cholesterol:

> A waxy, fatty substance in the blood that is incorrectly considered to be the cause of heart disease, stroke and instances of common heart attacks.

Cholinergic:

> A part of the autonomic nervous system that provides a counterbalance to adrenergic nerve receptors and messenger molecules such as adrenaline. See adrenaline.

Chronic fatigue syndrome:

> A chronic state of undue tiredness that lasts for more than six months and results in more than a fifty percent reduction in physical activity. It is associated with immune dysfunctions; dysfunctions of the thyroid, adrenal and pancreas glands; and disorders of mood, memory and mentation.

Colitis:

> Inflammation of colon, which causes pain, abdominal bloating and cramps. Sometimes bleeding can occur.

Consciousness:

> Traditionally defined as a state or condition of being critically aware of one's own identity and condition. In the context of autoregulation, it refers to an energetic awareness of one's relationship with the larger presence around him.

Coronary arteries:

> Arteries that supply blood to the heart muscle.

Coronary artery disease:

> A disease state created by inadequate blood supply to the heart caused by blockage of the coronary arteries by plaque formation.

Cortical:

> In autoregulation terminology, cortical indicates a thinking state in which the mind counts, calculates, computes, competes, censors and cautions. The cortical mind creates images of suffering and disease. It is a competitive mode in which one yearns for control, further compounding

the problem. In contrast, limbic in autoregulation terminology cares and comforts. It creates images of relief and health, and so mitigates suffering. In the limbic mode, human energy pathways are in a steady state and facilitate the healing response.

Cortical monkey:
In autoregulation terminology, it refers to a mind fixated on itself—recycling past misery unendingly and, when that is not enough, precycling feared, future misery.

Cortical overdrive:
In autoregulation terminology, it refers to relentless—and futile—worrying about things that do not happen.

Cytomegalovirus:
A common virus that causes fever and may involve any body organ, especially when the immune system of the individual is compromised by antibiotic abuse, chemotherapy, radiotherapy and environmental toxins.

DHEA:
Dehydroepiandrosterone, a "mother" hormone produced in the adrenal glands that orchestrates the production of estrogens, progesterones and testosterone in the body. It is also considered to be an anti-aging hormone.

Diagnostic labels:
The diagnostic terms that are employed in drug medicine to justify the use of symptom-suppressing drugs but reveal nothing about the cause of the illness. For instance, irritable bowel syndrome, chronic headache and restless leg syndrome.

Directed pulses:
A term used in autoregulation to indicate enhancement and perception of ordinary arterial pulses in different parts of the body.

Distress:
A state of harmful stress, contrasted to eustress, which is believed to be a helpful state of stress.

Diuretics:
A class of drugs used to treat excessive accumulation of fluids in tissues. These drugs promote loss of fluids via the urine.

Dynamics:
The study of relationships between motion and the forces affecting the motion of physical systems.

Dysautonomia:
A disorder of the autonomic nervous system that often causes

disturbances in heart rate, blood pressure, sweating and control of urination.

Dysfunction:

Malfunction in the cells, tissues and organs.

Dysfunctional oxygen metalolism:

The author's term for impaired oxygen metabolism. It leads to accumulation of certain organic acids in the urine, including lactic acid, and 2-hydroxybutyric acid. It is not merely lack of oxygen due to heart disease or asthma, nor poor transport of oxygen due to anemia. The scientific term for that is anoxia. In dysfunctional oxygen metabolism, there is a failure of cellular oxygen metabolism due to damage to the enzymes of oxygen metabolism. Thus, metabolism due to damage to the enzymes of oxygen metabolism. Thus, DOM threatens the health of every cell, every tissue, every body organ.

Dysoxygenosis:

Dysoxygenosis (dys-oxy-gen-o-sis) is my term for dysfunctional oxygen metabolism. It is not merely lack of oxygen due to heart disease or asthma, nor poor transport of oxygen due to anemia. The scientific term for that is anoxia. Dysoxygenosis is the failure of *cellular* oxygen metabolism due to damage to the enzymes of oxygen metabolism. Thus, dysoxygenosis threatens the health of every cell, every tissue, every body organ.

Dysregulation:

Abnormalities in the regulation of various molecular functions in the body. For instance, ingestion or assimilation of external synthetic chemicals with estrogen-like activities interferes with normal hormonal functions in women and causes such disorders as endometriosis.

Ecology:

Study of relationships between living beings and their environment. In this volume, it is used to focus on interrelationships between the various molecular, cellular and tissue systems of the human body.

Ecotoxins:

Toxic substances in the environment, including man-made synthetic molecules as well as some naturally produced toxins.

EDTA:

Ethylenediaminetetraacetic acid, a substance used in chelation therapy to eliminate toxic heavy metals in cases of metal poisoning, to remove calcium and reverse coronary heart disease.

Electromagnetism:
The study of electricity and magnetism. Also, magnetism arising from an accelerating charge.

EM medicine (energetic-molecular medicine):
A type of medical practice in which therapies are based on energetic-molecular events that occur before cells and tissues are damaged and disease develops, rather than on how tissues look under a microscope after they have been damaged.

EM traffic:
Energetic-molecular events that take place at the cell and plasma membranes in health and disease and represent the essential energy dynamics of living beings.

Endothelins:
Substances produced in the blood vessel wall and other parts of the body that serve a large number of functions, such as the control of blood flow within arteries and the regulation of many hormonal functions.

Energy responses:
In autoregulation terminology, it refers to subtle energy that is perceived during meditation. In some areas as in simple hand warming, energy responses can be readily documented with suitable electronic equipment. In other areas, technology to measure such responses is not yet available.

Enzyme:
Catalysts that facilitate biochemical reactions in the body. Enzymes are delicate proteins that are highly vulnerable to oxidant stress.

Epstein-Barr virus (EBV):
A common virus that causes infectious mononucleosis (kissing disease) and was at one time thought to be the cause of chronic fatigue syndrome.

Estrogens:
A class of female hormones essential for normal fetal development and for maintenance of menstruation and other female reproductive functions. Opposed by progesterones.

Eustress:
Eustress is considered a type of stress with healthful effects.

Fatigue:
Undue tiredness. Also see chronic fatigue syndrome.

Fourth-of-July chemistry:
A state of chemistry in which electrons are fired excessively and randomly in various tissues, causing widespread damage to cellular enzymes, membrane receptors, membrane channels, enzymes, hormones

and neurotransmitters.

Glucaric acid:

A substance that indicates increased detoxification activity by the liver enzymes. Increased urinary amounts are found in chronic fatigue states, chemical sensitivity and other states.

Glucose:

A simple six-carbon sugar molecule that is utilized in the tissues for energy production. In the brain, glucose is almost exclusively utilized for all neurologic functions.

Glucose roller coasters:

A term I use for rapid changes in the blood sugar level, creating high peaks and deep valleys. Synonymous with rapid hyperglycemic-hypoglycemic shifts.

Glyceric acid:

An organic acid produced during oxidative breakdown of sugars, proteins, and fatty acids. It accumulates in excess in the urine in states characterized by dysfunctional oxygen metabolism.

Growth hormone:

A pituitary hormone that promotes growth during childhood and prevents premature aging.

HDL cholesterol:

High-density lipoprotein, the "good" cholesterol that is supposed to prevent coronary heart disease. The higher the blood level, the lower the presumed risk of heart disease. (I say presumed because this is an overly simplistic view.)

Herpesvirus:

A family of viruses that causes common fever blisters in the mouth as well as genital lesions.

High-energy molecule:

A molecule that contains chemical energy bonds that may be broken to release the energy contained in them. For example, glycogen is a high-energy molecule that contains many energy bonds. When it is broken down into smaller sugar molecules, energy is released for muscular activities or other energy functions in the body.

HIV:

HIV (human immunodeficiency virus) causes AIDS (acquired immunodeficiency syndrome).

HMO:
> Health maintenance organizations, in essence, are insurance companies that specialize in reducing costs by controlling the spending of doctors.

Hormone:
> A substance in the body that is produced by glands called endocrine glands. In the past, deemed as a molecule that is produced in one organ and exerts its effects on another. Now some hormones are recognized as produced primarily for local effects, i.e., nitric oxide produced in endothelial cells lining blood vessels.

Hydroxybutyric acid:
> An organic acid produced during oxidative breakdown of sugars, proteins, and fatty acids. It accumulates in excess in the urine in states characterized by dysfunctional oxygen metabolism.

Hyperactivity syndrome:
> A syndrome usually diagnosed in children whereby a child is restless, impulsive and unable to perform common chores at home or at school.

Hyperadrenergic state:
> A state in which excessive release of adrenaline and related stress molecules causes restlessness, anxiety, insomnia, heart palpitations and stress.

Hyperglycemia:
> Opposite of hypoglycemia. A state of raised blood sugar levels. Persistent hyperglycemia is the essential feature of diabetes.

Hyperthyroidism:
> An autoimmune disorder characterized by overactivity of the thyroid gland that causes undue sensitivity to high temperatures, speeded-up metabolism, sweating, weight loss and heart palpitations. See autoimmune disorders.

Hypochondria:
> Neurotic conviction of the existence of an imaginary illness. Derived from hypochondrium—a region of abdomen located below the cartilage of the breast bone—thought to be the seat of melancholy in the past.

Hypoglycemia:
> Opposite of hyperglycemia. A state of low blood sugar—usually lower than 50 mg/Dl—associated with symptoms of weakness, jitters, anxiety, heart palpitations, nausea and sweating.

Hypothyroidism:
> Opposite of hyperthyroidism. An autoimmune disorder characterized by

underactivity of the thyroid gland that causes undue sensitivity to cold temperatures, fatigue, dry skin, weight gain, hair loss and sluggish metabolism.

Hysteria:
A type of neurosis characterized by vulnerability to suggestion, amnesia, emotional instability and related mental disturbances.

ICU:
Intensive care unit in a hospital.

Immune system:
The Body's system of defense against microbes and foreign substances. Specifically, it involves the body's production of antibodies to destroy microbes or neutralize foreign substances.

Immunology:
A discipline in medicine that deals with health and disease of the defense systems of living beings called the immune system.

Infarction:
Death of tissue due to the sudden interruption of its blood supply. Example: myocardial infarction causes heart attack.

Insulin:
A storage hormone produced in the pancreas that regulates blood sugar levels by promoting storage of glucose in tissues as fat. It also facilitates the entry and utilization of sugar in cells.

Insulin roller coasters:
Sharp peaks in blood insulin levels followed by precipitous drops, which represent the dysregulation of insulin production in the pancreas.

Integrative medicine:
A medical philosophy that integrates empirical knowledge of healing nutrients and herbs as well as energy methods with the science and technology of modern medicine. It prescribes what is safe and effective regardless of what disciplines the particular therapy may come from.

Ischemia:
A condition of diminished blood supply to tissues. Examples: ischemia of the heart muscle, which may cause heart attacks, and of the brain, which may lead to stroke.

Klonopin:
A drug used to improve the function of the brain neurotransmitter, GABA, and to promote sleep and control anxiety.

Kukuyu:
The largest native tribe of Africans in Kenya.
Lactic acid:
An organic acid produced during oxidative breakdown of sugars, proteins, and fatty acids. It accumulates in excess in the urine in states characterized by dysfunctional oxygen metabolism.
Language of silence:
In autoregulation terminology, it is an intuitive-visceral stillness that enlightens without any analytical activity: equivalent to a profound meditative state in other disciplines of meditation.
LDL cholesterol:
Low-density lipoprotein that is often considered "bad" cholesterol. A raised blood level of LDL is considered a risk factor for heart disease.
Leaky cell membrane syndrome:
A term used by the author for health disorders that can be traced to consequences of oxidative damage to cell membranes, which increases cell membrane permeability and leads to hemorrhage out of the cell what belongs inside and flooding of cell innards by elements that do not belong to the cell. For example, functional deficiency of magnesium and potassium and functional excess of calcium exists in chemical sensitivity and mold allergy reactions—clinical situations in which supplemental magnesium and potassium and calcium channel blockers are effective.
Life span:
The length of one's whole life. For humankind, it has been estimated to be between 100 and 110 years.
Life span enzymes:
Enzymes that promote health and allow a living being to achieve his or her expected life span. Also see enzyme.
Limbic:
Limbic indicates a calm, comforting, noncompetitive healing energy state. The term autoregulation refers to a nonthinking, noncompetitive, nongoal-oriented, steady healing energy state. The limbic state "cares and comforts," and "creates" images of health and healing that mitigate suffering. The cortical state, by contrast, indicates a thinking state in which the mind counts, calculates, computes, competes, censors and cautions. It creates images of suffering and disease. It is a competitive mode in which one yearns for control, further compounding the problem.

Limbic breathing:

> In autoregulation terminology, a type of breathing that profoundly affects the energy state of an individual. Limbic breathing is an enhanced energy state in which the breathing-out phase of respiration is prolonged in a slow, sustained fashion following a brief, effortless breathing-in period. Very effective for reducing stress, slowing quickened heart rates, normalizing high blood pressure, and managing other chronic disorders.

Limbic calmness:

> In autoregulation terminology, it refers to peace and tranquillity that come with meditative surrendering to the presence that permeates and surrounds each of us at all times.

Limbic exercise:

> A type of non-goal oriented, noncompetitive exercise in which slow, sustained physical exercise is combined with meditation.

Limbic language of silence:

> In autoregulation terminology, this expression refers to reaching higher energy states with periods of silence and meditation.

Limbic silence:

> In autoregulation terminology, it refers to a deep state of visceral tranquillity in which there is no awareness of ordinary stress-inducing perceptions.

Limbic-spiritual

> In autoregulation language, a term for a non-thinking, non-analytical energy healing state in which one surrenders in silence to the larger presence that surrounds and permeates one's being.

Limbic-visceral:

> In autoregulation terminology, a non-thinking energy state—but not quite as spiritual as the limbic-spiritual.

Low-energy molecule:

> A molecule with few energy bonds or electrons available for transfer to other molecules. See high-energy molecule for further explanation.

Lupus:

> An autoimmune disorder in which a confused immune system turns on the body's own tissues and produces destructive antibodies that damage various body organs. Full medical name: systemic lupus erythematosus.

Malignant:

> A term used for cancer, such as a malignant tumor.

Melatonin:
A hormone produced in the pineal gland that promotes natural sleep during night hours. It also helps people and animals adjust to various seasons.

Mercapturic acid:
A substance that indicates increased demand for detoxification in the liver. Increased levels in the urine are seen in chronic fatigue syndrome, chemical sensitivity and many other conditions.

Metabolic roller coasters:
This term is used in this volume for abrupt changes in the blood and tissue levels of sugar, insulin, adrenaline, cholinergic hormones and neurotransmitters. Sharp rises and sudden drops in the levels of such molecules cause a host of symptoms such as anxiety, the jitters, nausea, weakness, sweating and heart palpitations.

Metabolism:
The complex of biochemical and physical processes involved in the maintenance of life. Metabolism comprises reactions necessary for breakdown of food substances for release of chemical bond energy (catabolism) as well as those for synthesis of structural and functional molecules for cellular and tissue buildup (anabolism).

Metaphysical:
Based on abstract or speculative situations. Sometimes considered supernatural.

Microclot:
A microscopic clot composed of coagulated (curdled) blood plasma with or without blood cells entrapped within it.

Microplaque:
A microscopic plaque circulating in the bloodstream composed of clotted blood plasma with entrapped blood platelets, dead and dying blood cells and microbes, including yeast. Microplaques clog blood capillaries in various body organs and cause all patterns of tissue injury and symptomatology.

Mind-body-spirit:
A spurious concept of using the thinking mind to force healing on injured tissues.

Miracle:
A happening that is considered beyond the laws of nature. An act of God. In common language, an exceptionally fortunate event.

Mitral valve prolapse:

A condition in which a chronically overdriven heart muscle stresses the mitral valve. The mitral valve leaflets bulge (prolapse), become floppy, and fail to prevent the backflow of blood from the left lower chamber of the heart to the left upper chamber. Except when it is associated with a mitral valve damaged by rheumatic fever or other conditions, it is not a specific heart defect. The proper holistic approach is to address all the elements that overdrive the heart of each individual patient.

Molecules:

A group of atoms with defined atomic arrangement within its structure.

Morphology:

A scientific discipline that deals with the structure and appearance of living beings as well as nonliving entities.

MRI:

A type of exquisitely sensitive scan that utilizes magnetic energy for creating diagnostic images.

Multiple sclerosis:

An autoimmune disorder that damages the insulation material in nerve fibers called myelin sheaths.

Murmur:

An abnormal heart sound produced by turbulence in the flow of blood within the heart. It may be caused when the heart is overdriven, when one of the heart valves does not open fully (stenosis), or when it does not close fully (regurgitation).

Myocardial infarction:

Death of the heart muscle; heart attack, in common terminology.

Natural selection:

According to Darwin's theory, natural selection is a phenomenon that results in the survival of the fittest individuals and species. Seen in light of modern genetics, natural selection refers to gene mutations that favor survival of the species and so preserve and prolong the survival of the new (genetically altered) species. Mutations that adversely affect the survival result in extinction (being selected out) of that species.

N^2D^2 medicine:

A type of medicine in which a practitioner's work begins with a search for the name of a disease and ends with the selection of a name of a drug. In N^2D^2 medicine, no consideration is given to the ecologic and nutritional factors in the cause of disease. This type of medicine is expressed as follows:

N^2D^2 medicine= Name of a disease x Name of a drug

In N^2D^2 medicine, a doctor begins care of a patient with a disease name and ends with a drug name.

Neuron:

A nerve cell present in the brain and nerve ganglia of many body organs.

Neurotransmitters:

Molecules that facilitate communications between nerve cells.

Nitric oxide:

1) A simple but essential molecule composed of one atom each of nitrogen and oxygen. In human tissues, it regulates the caliber of small blood vessels and so regulates blood pressure within normal limits. It also functions as a hormone in many different organs of the body.

2) A colorless gas composed of one molecule of oxygen and one of nitrogen. It is an important messenger molecule that is produced in the cells lining the blood vessels, brain, immune cells and many other organs. Among its many metabolic roles is regulation of blood circulation.

Organ ecosystems:

An ecologic community of biochemical and biologic elements together with its physical environment situated within a specific body organ. For instance, liver ecosystem, brain ecosystem, etc.

OSHA:

Occupational Safety and Health Administration.

Ovary:

An organ in the female pelvis that produces ova (eggs) for conception and various female hormones.

Oxidation:

Loss of electrons (tiny packets of energy) from an atom or a molecule. In common language, it may be seen as decay of high-energy molecules into low-energy molecules. Oxidation in nature is a spontaneous process—it requires no outside programming. Examples of oxidation in nature include spoiled fruit, rotten fish, rancid butter, decomposed grass, and denatured energy enzymes that cause chronic fatigue.

Oxidative coagulopathy (co-ag-u-lop-athy)**:**

A term used by the author and his collegue, Omar Ali, for a state of accelerated oxidative coagulation of plasma proteins, resulting in formation of protein coagulum, microclots and microplaques in the circulating blood. It is the true cause of coronary heart disease, stroke, and many other chronic degenerative disorders. Oxidative coagulopathy is the process by which clean blood turns into "dirty" blood.

Oxidative-dysoxygenative dysfunction (ODD):

ODD is a state in which: (1) oxidosis is caused by oxidants of *all* three types (metabolic, microbial, and man-made) that threaten health; (2) oxidosis leads to dysoxygenosis (abnormal oxygen metabolism), which slows or blocks *all* life processes; (3) oxidosis and dysoxygenosis together cause acidosis; (4) all three elements (oxidosis, dysoxygenosis, and acidosis) feed upon each other and together fan the flames of oxidative injury. In fibromyalgia, an oxidative-dysoxygenative (OD) state leads to injury to *every microecologic cellular and macroecologic tissue-organ ecosystem of the body.*

Oxidative fires:

A term I use for accelerated oxidative molecular injury that literally cooks enzymes, hormones and other essential molecules in the blood and tissues.

Oxidative injury:

Injury to molecules and tissues in which the mechanism of the injury involves the oxidation or decay of high-energy molecules into low-energy molecules.

Oxidative lymphopathy:

Oxidative lymphopathy (lym-phop-athy) is my term for a process by which lymph becomes oxidized, rancid, thick and *gluey*. Lymph is the pale fluid that drains toxins from tissues. Such fluid stagnates in muscles and other tissues, preventing the free flow of oxygen-rich blood, causing soreness in tissues, and producing trigger points in muscles. I introduced this term in 1998 to focus on issues of stagnant lymph in tissues.

Oxidosis:

Oxidosis (oxi-do-sis) is *excessive* loss of energy through rapid loss of electrons. In the context of aging, oxidosis causes disease and premature aging. Oxidation is loss of electrons. In chemical reactions, electrons are transferred from one atom or molecule to the other. The donor substance loses electrons and is so oxidized. The recipient gains electrons and so is reduced. The gainer becoming reduced seems strange, but that is the awkwardness of the scientific terminology.

Oxyology:

Oxyology (oxy-olo-gy) is the study of oxygen, just as pathology is the study of diseases

Oxygen:
> A colorless, tasteless gas comprising about 80 percent of the air and 85 percent of water, that is necessary for oxidation in nature.

Palpitations:
> A rapid heart rate that causes an uncomfortable perception of heartbeats in the chest.

Pancreas:
> A gland situated behind the stomach in the upper abdomen that produces insulin, glucagon and other hormones for regulation of carbohydrate metabolism, as wellas digestive enzymes in the small intestines.

Panic attacks:
> Attacks of extreme anxiety caused by fear of things that do not happen; for example, a sudden sense of doom and fear of heart attack when such an attack has been ruled out repeatedly.

Pantothenic acid:
> Vitamin B_5. It is a precursor of co-enzyme A, and thus is an essential component of the detoxification system.

Pathology:
> The study of disease processes and their clinical and laboratory manifestations.

pH:
> Measure of acidity or alkalinity of a solution. Neutral solutions have a ph value of 7. Its value is calculated as the common logarithm of the reciprocal of the hydrogen ion concentration in moles per cubic decimeter of solution.

Phlebitis:
> Inflammation of the vein wall accompanied by clotting of blood within the vein. Clinically, it is recognized as painful, tender linear thickening extending along the vein wall.

Phobia:
> An irrational, often morbid, fear of things that may or may not take place.

Photosynthesis:
> A process by which sunlight strikes and agitates chlorophyll molecules, thus producing minute electric currents which, in turn, split water in plants into oxygen and hydrogen. Oxygen escapes into the atmosphere, while hydrogen is combined with carbon dioxide to form sugar molecules. Thus is created the chemical bond energy of plants, which begins the food chain on planet Earth.

Physiology:
> The branch of biology concerning the function of organisms.

Plaque:
> An area of swelling involving the inner lining of an artery caused by tissue injury and accumulation of oxidized and denatured fats, with or without surface ulceration or blood clot formation.

Platelets:
> Irregularly shaped particles in circulating blood that contain essential blood clotting factors.

PMS:
> Premenstrual syndrome consisting of irritability, cramps, headache, mood swings and water retention that often precedes the menstrual flow. PMS is caused by hormonal imbalance.

Precycling feared future misery:
> In autoregulation terminology, it is a neurotic compulsion to indulge in disturbing thoughts about the future.

Primordial life forms:
> The author's term for life forms with a "primordial metabolism." Specifically, such life forms hate oxygen, love acidity, and thrive on decaying organic matter. PLFs include the bowel anaerobic flora, yeasts, yeast-like organims, mycoplasma, nanobacteria, and others.

Progesterone cream:
> A progesterone cream derived from wild yam.

Progesterones:
> A class of female hormones that provides a counterbalance to another class of female hormones called estrogens.

Prostate:
> A gland in male mammals that secretes a fluid which becomes a part of semen. In men, it is the size of a walnut and is located at the neck of the urinary bladder. Both benign prostate enlargement and prostate cancer are quite common. In the author's view, the current pandemic of prostate cancer in men is due to an excess of synthetic estrogens and xenoestrogens in the environment.

Protoplasm:
> Thick fluid that is the soup of life in all living beings. It performs most of the basic life functions.

Psychoneuroimmunology:
> A branch of medical science that deals with links among aspects of the psyche, the brain and the immune system.

Psychosomatic:

A disease process that is assumed to be caused by disorders of the mind.

Pyridoxine:

Vitamin B_6

Pyruvic acid:

An organic acid produced during oxidative breakdown of sugars, proteins, and fatty acids. It accumulates in excess in the urine in states characterized by dysfunctional oxygen metabolism.

Quran:

The holy book of Islam. It is the sacred text of revelations made by Allah to Prophet Muhammad. The holy book is often referred to as the Koran by non-Muslims.

RDA:

An abbreviation for the recommended dietary allowance, RDA refers to amounts of nutrients considered sufficient to prevent a handful of nutrient deficiency diseases. RDA is the prevailing —and a pernicious—notion that holds that nutrients play no roles in the healing phenomena in injured tissues, and thus are of no value in the clinical management of ecologic, immune and nutritional disorders.

Reactive hypoglycemia:

Abnormally low level of blood sugar thought to be caused by anxiety and emotional disorders. True hypoglycemia, by contrast, is considered to be caused by a dysfunction of the pancreatic release of insulin. This distinction, in my view, is artificial and clinically irrelevant.

Receptors:

Molecules that provide "docking" sites for attachment to cell membranes for hormones and related substances. For example, receptors for estrogen and progesterone hormones.

Reduction:

In scientific chemistry terminology, the term reduction refers to the gain of electrons by molecules—the opposite of oxidation. When oxidation and reduction occur together, it is called a redox reaction.

Relaxation response:

A set of exercises designed to reduce stress and a set of biochemical changes associated with relaxation described by Harvard professor, Herbert Benson, M.D.

Resonance:

The quality of enhancement of response of a system to a periodic driving force when the driving frequency is equal to the frequency of the system. In autoregulation terminology, it is the energy response of molecules, cells and tissues to energy fields that surround them.

Ritalin:

A drug that stimulates the nervous system and is used for patients with attention deficit disorder.

Selye, Hans:

A noted stress expert credited with popularizing the fight-or-flight stress response.

Silence of stone:

In autoregulation terminology, it is a method of achieving an intuitive-visceral stillness by simply looking at a stone. No attempt is made to banish one's thoughts during this practice.

Somatic nervous system:

A part of the nervous system that is under voluntary control. Examples: use of legs for walking and of hands for holding.

Somatization:

Development of bodily dysfunction in response to emotional triggers.

Somatopsychic:

An adjective for organic medical conditions that secondarily affect the mind.

Spirituality:

Dimensions of human existence that cannot be perceived by physical senses and are beyond the reach of human intellect. I consider spirituality to be the linkage with that larger presence that surrounds and permeates each of us at all times. In my view, it has nothing to do with clever thinking and is quite distinct from intellectual achievement.

Spontaneity of healing:

A natural healing phenomenon that occurs without external aid. In essence, all healing is spontaneous.

Spontaneity of living:

A philosophy of life that fosters heeding natural impulses of essential human goodness. In autoregulation terminology, it is living a life uncensored by the cortical monkey.

Spontaneity of oxidation:

A natural phenomenon in which high-energy molecules spontaneously undergo decay and are turned into low-energy molecules.

Steroids:

These are a family of powerful hormones produced by the adrenal gland (cortisone), ovaries (progesterone), testes (testosterone), and some other body organs that perform a large variety of hormone functions in the body, including maintaining sexual functions.

Stress:

Usually defined as a fight-or-flight response to demand for change. The term was coined by Walter Cannon and popularized by Hans Selye. In this book, stress is regarded as the motivating factor in the process of decay and dying in living beings—the injury-healing-injury cycle of life.

Stress test (of the heart):

A test for adequacy of the blood supply to the heart muscle. In this test, the heart is first stressed by exercise (treadmill or exercise cycle) and then its performance is evaluated with a cardiogram or a thallium scan.

Syndrome of just being sick:

A term first coined and later abandoned by the noted stress expert, Hans Selye.

T_3:

A hormone produced by the thyroid gland to regulate metabolism and body temperature. It is formed by the breakdown of its parent (precursor) hormone called T_4.

T_4:

Thyroxine hormone produced by the thyroid gland to regulate metabolism and body temperature.

Taurine:

A derivative of the amino acid cysteine, 2-aminoethanesulfonic acid. It is an important cell membrane stabilizer which is found in all cells. For this reason it is liberally used in clinical nutritional medicine. Taurine was so named because it was first isolated from ox bile (taurus in Latin means bull).

Thallium scans of the heart:

A type of heart scan that shows patterns of circulation in the heart muscle and is used for diagnosing coronary artery disease.

Thyroid gland:

A gland situated in the front of the neck that produces hormones to regulate metabolism. Underactivity of the gland is called hypothyroidism; overactivity is called hyperthyroidism.

Trigger points:
>Chronically painful and tender areas located in sprained or partially torn ligament, tendons and muscles.

Triglycerides:
>A type of fatty substance in the body which, when present in excessive amounts, is considered to be a risk factor for common heart attacks and strokes. In my view, this risk is grossly exaggerated by physicians who prefer to prescribe drugs rather than take a natural approach to the prevention of heart disease.

Vasodilatation:
>Opening up of blood vessels—a process of relaxation of the muscle in the walls of arteries that results in improved blood circulation and oxygenation of tissues.

Vasospasm:
>Spasm of the blood vessels.

Viruses:
>A family of microbes that cannot be seen with ordinary microscopes and generally can thrive only within the host's cells. Examples: HIV, EBV, CMV and herpesviruses.

Visceral-intuitive:
>In autoregulation terminology, it refers to an energy state in which enlightenment comes though nonanalytical mediums. Also see Limbic-visceral and Limbic-spiritual.

Yeast:
>Any of the single-celled fungi. In the opinion of the author, among the four groups of microbial invaders of the human body (viruses, bacteria, yeast and parasites), yeast pose the most significant threat to human health.

Index

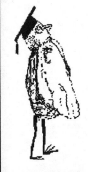

Other works by Majid Ali, M.D.

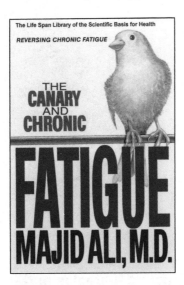

The Life Span Library of the Scientific Basis for Health

REVERSING CHRONIC FATIGUE

THE CANARY AND CHRONIC FATIGUE

MAJID ALI, M.D.

The Canary and Chronic Fatigue
Majid Ali, M.D. ISBN 1-879131-04-8 582 pages $20.00

The classic work on the subject! Hailed by medical organizations, support groups, academic institutions as *THE* definitive book on chronic fatigue. Dr. Ali spells out the three R's of chronic fatigue; it's Real; it's Reversible; and injured energy enzymes cannot be Revived with drugs. Chapters include *What is Chronic Fatigue?; On Reviving Injured Enzymes; Choices in the Kitchen; Oral Nutrient and Herbal Protocols; Intravenous Nutrient Protocols; Battered Bowel Ecology; On Hope, Spirituality and Chronic Fatigue.*

Other works by Majid Ali, M.D.

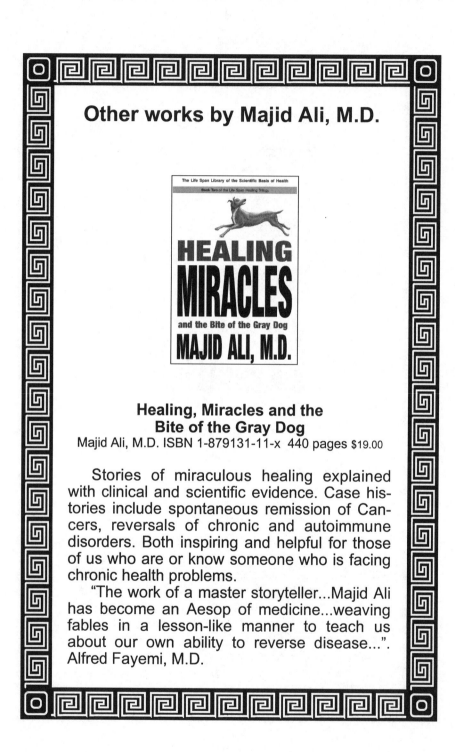

Healing, Miracles and the
Bite of the Gray Dog
Majid Ali, M.D. ISBN 1-879131-11-x 440 pages $19.00

Stories of miraculous healing explained with clinical and scientific evidence. Case histories include spontaneous remission of Cancers, reversals of chronic and autoimmune disorders. Both inspiring and helpful for those of us who are or know someone who is facing chronic health problems.

"The work of a master storyteller...Majid Ali has become an Aesop of medicine...weaving fables in a lesson-like manner to teach us about our own ability to reverse disease...".
Alfred Fayemi, M.D.

Other works by Majid Ali, M.D.

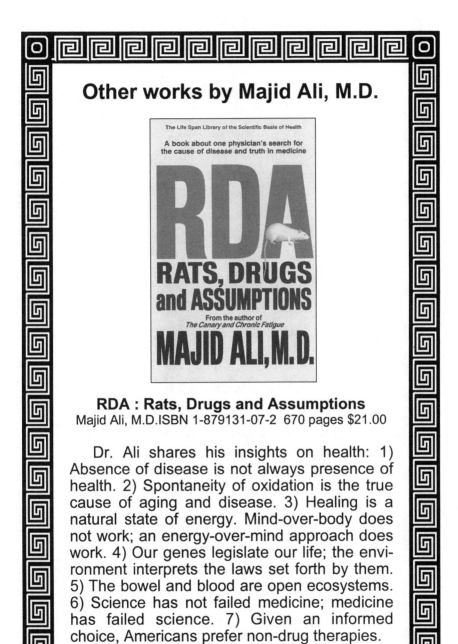

The Life Span Library of the Scientific Basis of Health

A book about one physician's search for
the cause of disease and truth in medicine

RDA

RATS, DRUGS and ASSUMPTIONS

From the author of
The Canary and Chronic Fatigue

MAJID ALI, M.D.

RDA : Rats, Drugs and Assumptions
Majid Ali, M.D.ISBN 1-879131-07-2 670 pages $21.00

Dr. Ali shares his insights on health: 1) Absence of disease is not always presence of health. 2) Spontaneity of oxidation is the true cause of aging and disease. 3) Healing is a natural state of energy. Mind-over-body does not work; an energy-over-mind approach does work. 4) Our genes legislate our life; the environment interprets the laws set forth by them. 5) The bowel and blood are open ecosystems. 6) Science has not failed medicine; medicine has failed science. 7) Given an informed choice, Americans prefer non-drug therapies.

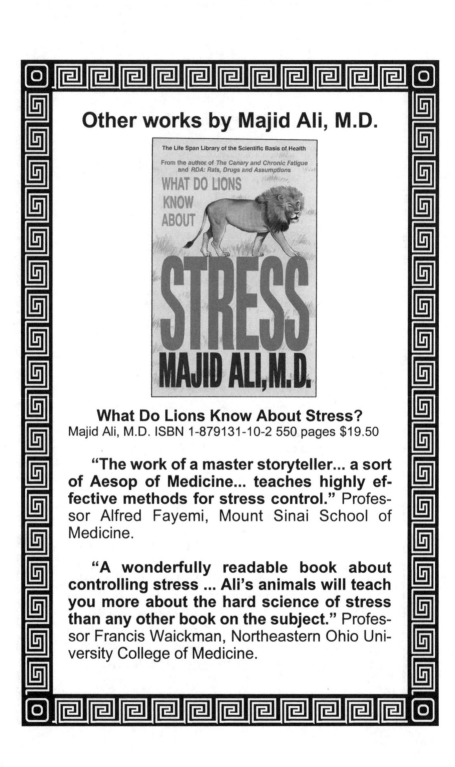

Other works by Majid Ali, M.D.

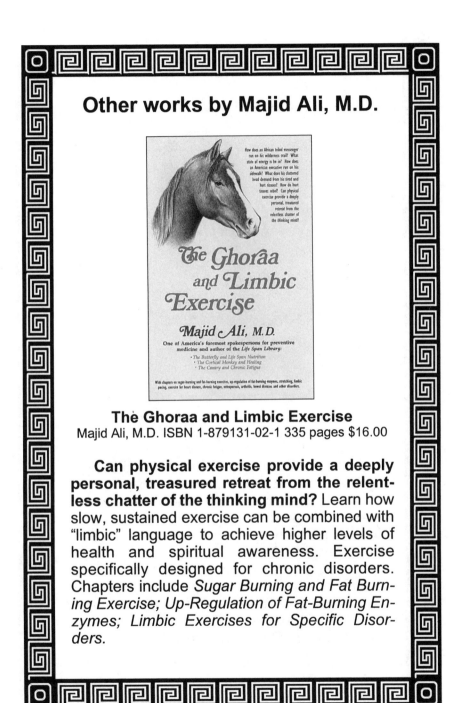

Other works by Majid Ali, M.D.

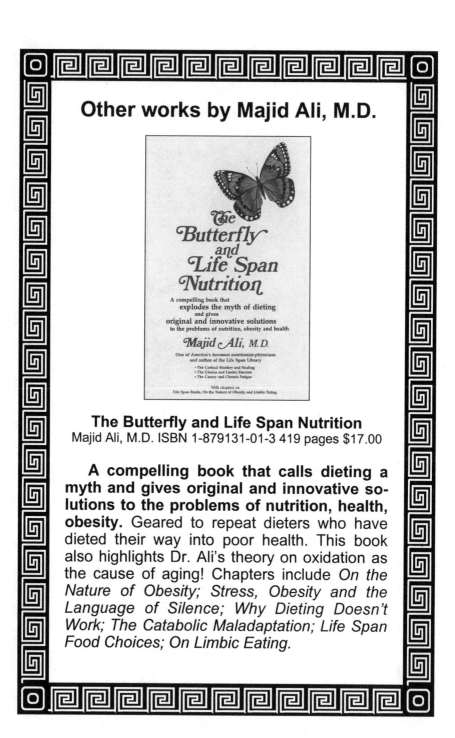

The Butterfly and Life Span Nutrition
Majid Ali, M.D. ISBN 1-879131-01-3 419 pages $17.00

A compelling book that calls dieting a myth and gives original and innovative solutions to the problems of nutrition, health, obesity. Geared to repeat dieters who have dieted their way into poor health. This book also highlights Dr. Ali's theory on oxidation as the cause of aging! Chapters include *On the Nature of Obesity; Stress, Obesity and the Language of Silence; Why Dieting Doesn't Work; The Catabolic Maladaptation; Life Span Food Choices; On Limbic Eating.*

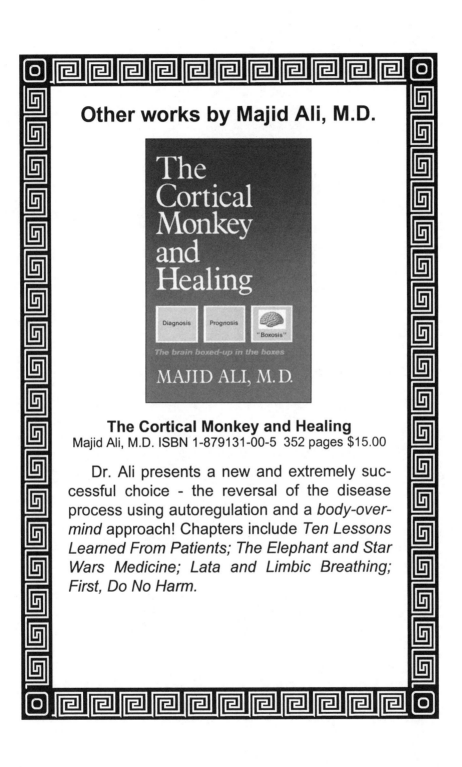

Integrative Medicine Videos Hosted By Majid Ali, M.D.

- Add & Hyperactivity
- Allergy
- Arthritis
- Asthma
- Cancer Part 1
- Cancer Part 2
- Cholesterol
- Chronic Fatigue Part 1
- Chronic Fatigue Part 2
- Chronic Fatigue Part 3
- Depression
- Fibromyalgia

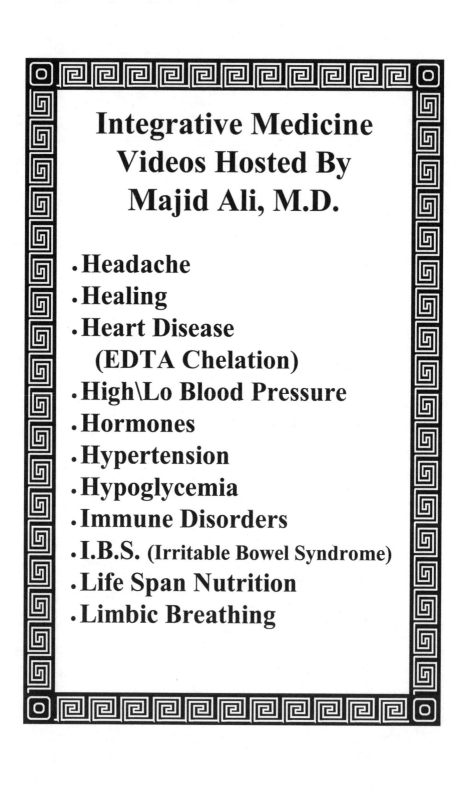

Integrative Medicine Videos Hosted By Majid Ali, M.D.

- Headache
- Healing
- Heart Disease
  (EDTA Chelation)
- High\Lo Blood Pressure
- Hormones
- Hypertension
- Hypoglycemia
- Immune Disorders
- I.B.S. (Irritable Bowel Syndrome)
- Life Span Nutrition
- Limbic Breathing

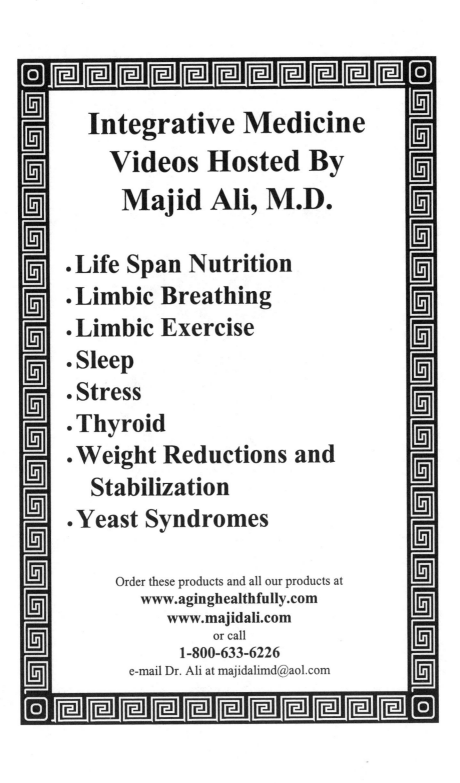

Integrative Medicine Videos Hosted By Majid Ali, M.D.

- Life Span Nutrition
- Limbic Breathing
- Limbic Exercise
- Sleep
- Stress
- Thyroid
- Weight Reductions and Stabilization
- Yeast Syndromes

Order these products and all our products at
www.aginghealthfully.com
www.majidali.com
or call
1-800-633-6226
e-mail Dr. Ali at majidalimd@aol.com

Future works by Majid Ali, M.D.

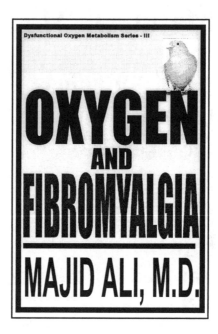

Dysfunctional Oxygen Metabolism Series - III

OXYGEN
AND
FIBROMYALGIA
MAJID ALI, M.D.

Fibromyalgia is a reversible
disorder caused by
cellular dysfunctional oxygen metabolism

Future works by Majid Ali, M.D.

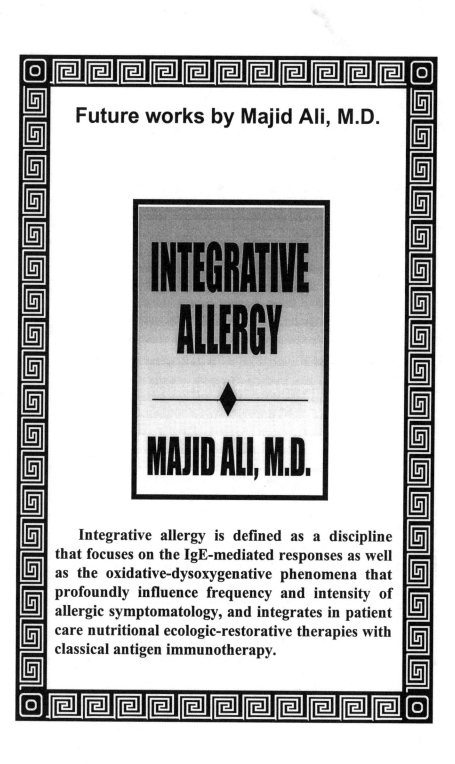

Integrative allergy is defined as a discipline
that focuses on the IgE-mediated responses as well
as the oxidative-dysoxygenative phenomena that
profoundly influence frequency and intensity of
allergic symptomatology, and integrates in patient
care nutritional ecologic-restorative therapies with
classical antigen immunotherapy.

Perfection of means and confusion of goals seem -- in my opinion -- to characterize our age.
Albert Einstein

In acute illness, our perfection of means is astounding. Advances in medical technology are breathtaking. Our surgical prowess is daunting; the potency of our drugs limitless.

In chronic illnesses, our confusion of goals is equally astounding. We seem to think nutritional medicine is a hoax; environmental medicine, a treatment of non-existent disease; and self-healing, a wishful and simple-minded pursuit.

We seem to think that molecular and electromagnetic events which initiate disease, and cell membrane dynamics which perpetuate it, are of little relevance to clinical medicine. We seem to think that to name a disease is to understand it; to classify it is to conquer it; to suppress its symptoms with drugs is to cure it.

Our principal strategy seems to be this: Disease prevention is a patient's responsibility; when a patient is acutely ill, we pull him out of the jaws of death with miracles of modern medicine.

How could we, the healing profession, be so wrong?